Postgraduate Medical Studies in Kuwait

1. 1. 1981 – 30. 6. 1982

**Edited by
Dr. Edward Ruzyllo**

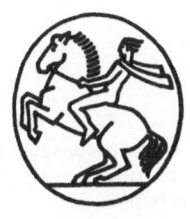

Springer-Verlag Wien GmbH

ISBN 978-3-662-23177-7   ISBN 978-3-662-25167-6 (eBook)

DOI 10.1007/978-3-662-25167-6

© 1983 by Springer-Verlag Wien

Originally published by Springer Vienna in 1983.

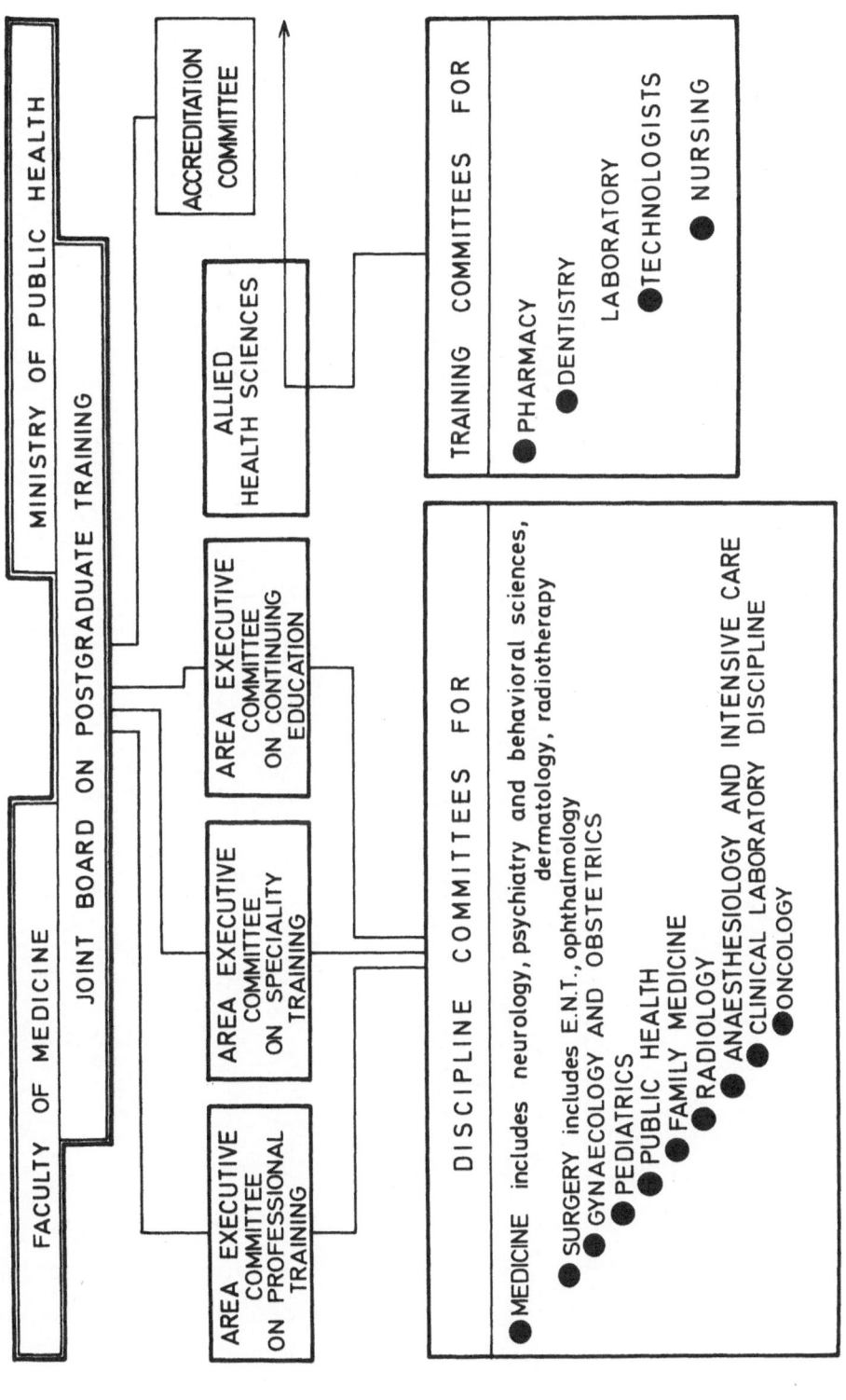

MINISTRY OF PUBLIC HEALTH

FACULTY OF MEDICINE

JOINT BOARD ON POSTGRADUATE TRAINING

ACCREDITATION COMMITTEE

ALLIED HEALTH SCIENCES

AREA EXECUTIVE COMMITTEE ON PROFESSIONAL TRAINING

AREA EXECUTIVE COMMITTEE ON SPECIALITY TRAINING

AREA EXECUTIVE COMMITTEE ON CONTINUING EDUCATION

TRAINING COMMITTEES FOR
● PHARMACY
● DENTISTRY
  LABORATORY
● TECHNOLOGISTS
● NURSING

DISCIPLINE COMMITTEES FOR
● MEDICINE includes neurology, psychiatry and behavioral sciences, dermatology, radiotherapy
● SURGERY includes E.N.T., ophthalmology
● GYNAECOLOGY AND OBSTETRICS
● PEDIATRICS
● PUBLIC HEALTH
● FAMILY MEDICINE
● RADIOLOGY
● ANAESTHESIOLOGY AND INTENSIVE CARE
● CLINICAL LABORATORY DISCIPLINE
● ONCOLOGY

CONTENTS

Part One

Page

I. **Organisation and Function of the System of Postgraduate Medical Education** 3
  1. Joint Board of Postgraduate Medical Education 3
     Summary of Organisation 3
     Detailed Organisation 3
  2. Area Executive Committees 4
     Summary of Organisation 4
     Detailed Organisation 5
  3. Discipline Committees 6
     Summary of Organisation 6
     Detailed Organisation 6
     Preparation of the Yearly Programme 7
     Programme Characteristics and Requirements 8
     Organisational Performance of the Study (Course, Seminar etc.) . . 9
     Educational Assistance to Nurses 9
     Important Course (IC) of our Postgraduate Teaching Program . . . 9
     Evaluation of the Course 11
  4. Committee Secretariat of the Joint Board 11
     Summary of Organisation 11
     Detailed Organisation 12
  5. Basic Requirements for Postgraduate Medical Teaching 14
     Hospital Accreditation 14
     Teaching Staff Accreditation 17
     Director of Education in the Teaching Hospital 19
     Tutor-Coordinator for Given Clinical Discipline in the Hospital for
     Professional and Continuing Medical Training 21
     Programme Director of Specialisation 21
     Programme Director of Each Study (Course, Seminar etc.) of the
     Nation-Wide Postgraduate Continuing Medical Education 21
     Executive Administrator of the Course 23
     Criteria for Selecting for Appointment Doctors for the Residents or
     Assistant Registrars Posts 24
     Principles of Accreditation of Continuing Postgraduate Medical
     Studies 25
     Recognition Awards 25
     Visitors and Their Role in Postgraduate Medical Education 26
     Form for Invitation of Foreign Lecturers (Visitor) Academic Year:
     1982—83 27
     General Rules Applicable to Doctors Working in the Ministry of
     Public Health in Relation to the Postgraduate Training Programme 27
     Leave Arrangements in Relation to the Postgraduate Training Pro-
     gramme 28
  6. Course Identifying Numbers (C.I.N.) 28
     Speciality Identifying Numbers 29
     Speciality Identifying Numbers in Alphabetic Order 31

II. **Terms of the Joint Board of Postgraduate Medical Education in Kuwait** . . 34
     Philosphy of the Activities of the Joint Board for Postgraduate
     Medical Education in Kuwait . . . . : 34

III. **Members of the Organisation** 36
     Decision of the Minister of Public Health on the Actual Term of the Joint
     Board. 27. 5. 1981—26. 5. 1983 36
          Composition of the Joint Board for the Third Term (1981—1983) . 38
          Area Executive Committees 38
     Discipline Committees 40
          Discipline Committee for Medicine 40
          Discipline Committee for Surgery 40
          Discipline Committee for Obstetrics and Gynaecology 41
          Discipline Committee for Paediatrics 42
          Discipline Committee for Family Medicine 42
          Discipline Committee for Public Health 43
          Discipline Committee for Radiology 43
          Discipline Committee for Clinical Laboratory Medicine 44
          Discipline Committee for Anaesthesiology and Intensive Care . . . 44
     Training Committees 45
          The Training Committee for Pharmacy 45
          The Training Committee for Dentistry 45
          The Training Committee for Laboratory Technologists 45
          The Training Committee for Nursing 46
     Accreditation Committee 46
     Decision of the Minister of Public Health on the Membership of the
     Accreditation Committee 46
          Composition of the Accreditation Committee 47

Part Two

I.   **Programmes of the Postgraduate Medical Studies in the Period Between**
     1. 1. 1981—30. 6. 1982 51
     1. Professional Training 51
        a) for E.C.F.M.G. and V.Q.E. Examinations 51
           Kuwait Miami Comprehensive Medical Education Programme.
           First V.Q.E. Course 51
           English Languages Course for Students of the First V.Q.E. Course 53
           Self-Learning Seminars for After the First V.Q.E. Course Period . . 54
           Basic Medical Sciences Repetitorium as Preparation for the Sec-
           ond V.Q.E. Course 56
           English Language Course as a Preparatory Course for the Second
           V.Q.E. Course 58
           Kuwait-Miami Comprehensive Medical Education Program. Sec-
           ond V.Q.E. Course 59
           Instructions for Pleno Titulo Coordinators 65
        b) Rotating Internship 67
           Medicine 67
           Dermatology 69

Surgery 71
Ophthalmology 75
E.N.T. 76
Anaesthesiology and Intensive Care 77
Paediatrics 80
Gynaecology and Obstetrics 82
Community Medicine and Primary Health Care 85
Community Medicine 86
Primary Health Care — Six Months 87
Psychiatry — Two Months 88
Clinical Laboratory Medicine 88
    1. General Idea of the Training 89
    2. Methodology 90
    3. Laboratory Medicine — Twelve Months 91
    4. Public Health — Twelve Months 91

2. Speciality Training 91
    Part I and II of the Course Preparing for the Examination for Membership of the Royal College of Physicians (M.R.C.P.—U.K.) 91
    Part I and II of the Course Preparing for Examination for Membership of the Royal College of Physicians (M.R.C.P.—U.K.) 98
    List of Lecturers 103
    M.R.C.P. Part II Course 104
    M.R.C.P. Part II Course 106
    M.R.C.P. Part II Course 108
    Part I (Basic Sciences) Course Preparing for Examination for Fellowship of the Royal College of Surgeons (F.R.C.S.—Dublin) . . . 109
    Part I (Basic Sciences) Course Preparing for Examination for Fellowship of the Royal College of Surgeons (F.R.C.S.—Dublin) . . . 117
    Part I (Basic Sciences) Course Preparing for Examination for Membership of the Royal College of Obstetrics and Gynaecology (M.R.C.O.G.—London) 124
    Course in Basic Sciences for Anaesthesists. Part I (F.F.A.R.C.S.—England) Programme 132
    Primary F.F.A.R.C.S. Examination in Kuwait, June, 1982. Revised Programme 138
    Primary Dental Fellowship Course 138
    Report on the Course Preparing for Mock Examination for Membership in the Royal College of Physicians 146
    Report on Primary Fellowship (F.R.C.S.—Dublin) Course and Examination 147
        1. Preface 147
        2. Planning 147
        3. Candidate Selection 147
        4. The Primary Fellowship Course 148
        5. The Primary Fellowship Examination 151
        6. Comparative Data of the Past Four Years 153
        7. Observations and Recommendations 153
        8. Vote of Thanks 154
    Report on Primary F.F.A. Course and Examination 154
        1. Preface 154
        2. Planning 155

3. Candidate Selection 155
4. The Primary F.F.A. Course 156
5. The Primary F.F.A. Examination 157
6. Observations and Recommendations 159
7. Vote of Thanks 160
Appendix I. List of Selected Candidates for the Primary
F.F.A.R.C.S. Course in Kuwait 1981—1982 160
Appendix II. List of Candidates Accepted for the Primary
F.F.A.R.C.S. Examination in Kuwait 1981—1982 161
Report on Primary F.F.D. Course and Examination 162
I. Introduction 162
II. Course 162
III. Primary F.F.D. Examination 165

3. Continuing Medical Education 168
a) Local (In-Service) Continuing Medical Education 168
Sabah Hospital, Amiri Hospital, Farwania Hospital, Adan Hospital, In-Service Training in Medicine October 1981—June 1982 Programme 168
Amiri Hospital In-Service Training in Medicine 18. 4. 1981—6. 6. 1981 Programme 168
Amiri Hospital In-Service Training in Medicine 28. 4. 1982—17. 6. 1982 Programme 170
Sabah Hospital In-Service Training in Paediatrics 3. 2. 1982—2. 6. 1982 Programme 172
Mubarak Al-Kabir Hospital In-Service Training in Radiology ... 174
Sabah Hospital In-Service Training in Radiology 1981—1982 Academic Year General Programme 174
Ibn Sina Hospital In-Service Training in Radiology 1981—1982 Academic Year General Programme 175
Farwania Hospital In-Service Training in Radiology 1981—1982 Academic Year General Programme 175
Jahra Hospital In-Service Training in Radiology 1981—1982 Academic Year Programme 176
Sabah Hospital In-Service Training in Anaesthesia and Intensive Care. 3. 9. 1981—8. 4. 1982 Programme 176
Mubarak Hospital In-Service Training in Anaesthesia and Intensive Care. 11. 2. 1982—11. 3. 1982 Programme 178
Farwania Hospital In-Service Training in Anaesthesia and Intensive Care. 10. 9. 1981—18. 2. 1982 179
Sulaibikhat Hospital In-Service Training in Anaesthesia in Intensive Care. November 1981—March 1982 Programme 180
Maternity Hospital In-Service Training in Anaesthesia and Intensive Care. 1. 10. 1981—16. 6. 1982 Programme 181
b) Nation-wide (institutional) Continuing Medical Education 183
Biostatistics for Clinical Use 183
Some Clinical Aspects of Allergy and Immunology 184
Applied Immunology in Medicine 185
First Workshop on how to do Simple Illustrations Yourself 188
Second Workshop on how to do Simple Illustrations Yourself ... 188
Third Workshop on how to do Simple Illustrations Yourself 189
Fourth Workshop on how to do Simple Illustrations Yourself ... 189

Report by Antonia Land and Doig Simmonds, Royal Postgraduate
Medical School, London on 4 Workshops on "How to do Simple
Illustrations Yourself" 190
Cardiology 197
Cardiomyopathies 198
Seminar on Cardiology 198
Seminar on Academic Education 201
Seminar on Gastroenterology 202
The Nephrology Seminars 203
Seminar on Endocrinology 205
Advances in Medicine, Particularly in the Field of Haematology . 206
Haematological Seminar 208
Seminar on Haematology 209
Seminar on Hyperlipidemia 211
Seminar on Rheumatology 212
Transplantation Surgery 213
Seminar on Surgery 216
Seminar, Conference, Lectures, etc. 217
Cardiosurgical Seminar 219
Seminar on Cardiac Surgery 220
Seminar on Vascular Surgery 222
Surgery of the Alimentary System 223
Urinary Calculi 230
Distal Ureteric Structures in Bilharzia 231
Course in Surgery of the Hand 232
Paediatric Surgery 234
Seminar on Paediatric Surgery 236
Seminar on Paediatrics 238
Course in Paediatric Gastro-Enterology 239
Recent Advances and Current Paediatric Gastro-Enterology 241
Intensive Course in Gynaecology and Obstetrics 244
Seminar on Obstetrics and Gynaecology 246
Family Medicine Practice 247
Two Months Refresher Course for Primary Health Centre Doctors 250
Ultra-Sound in Ophthalmology 251
Retinopathy 252
Seminar on Ophthalmology 254
Clinical Seminar on Ophthalmology 254
Seminar on Dermatology 258
Medical Mycology 258
Seminar on Dermatology 259
The Neurology Seminars 261
Neurological Seminar 262
Seminar on Neurology 263
Seminar on Psychiatry 264
Radiological Seminar 265
Seminar on Paediatric Radiology 266
Seminar on Radiology 267
Overview of Nuclear Medicine 268
Nuclear Medicine and its Clinical Application 270
Cancer Education and Control 271
Advances in Anaesthesia and Intensive Care 275

Recent Advances in Open Heart Surgery, Anaesthesia and Intensive Care 278
Initiation of Primary F.F.A.R.C.S. Course in Kuwait 280
Advances in Neurosurgical Anaesthesia and Intensive Care 282
Epidural Analgesia for Labour 284
Seminar in Anaesthesia and Intensive Care 286
Recent Advances in Anaesthesia 289
Haematolgy and Blood Banking 290
The Histopathology Course 292
The Microbiology and Parasitology Course 294
Medical Biochemistry 296
The Integral Course 298
Use and Abuse of Antibiotics 299
Infection Control 300
Seminar of Infectious Diseases 303
Third Epidemiological Seminar 304
Fourth Epidemiological Seminar 307
Course for Potential Head Nurses 309
Course for Head Nurses 311
Refresher Course for Head Nurses 311
Course for School Health Nurses 312
Course for School Health Supervisors 312
Potential Assistant Directors of the Nursing Course 313
Course for Clinical Instructors 314
Course for Assistant Nurses 317
Course for Midwives 319
Refresher Course for Medical Nurses 320
Refresher Course for Paediatric Nurses 321
Refresher Course for Surgical Nurses 323
Refresher Course for Psychiatric Nurses 324
Course for School Health Nurses 324
c) International Meetings 325
1st Kuwait International Medical Sciences Conference 325
Cancer and Immunology 326
Respiratory Diseases 328
Neurotransmitters 328
Liver Diseases 329
Epidemiology 330
Cardiology 331
2nd Kuwait International Medical Conference 332
Bulgarian-Kuwaiti Medicine Week 337

II. List of Medical Sciences (in Alphabetic Order). Subjects for Postgraduate
Studies, Presented by Course Identifying Numbers 340
Allergology 340
Anaesthesiology and Analgesia 340
Bacteriology and Virology 340
Basic Medical Sciences 340
Behavioral Sciences 340
Biostatistics 341
Cardiac Surgery 341
Cardiology 341

Clinical Laboratory Medicine 341
Community Medicine 341
Dentistry 341
Dermatology 341
Dietetics 341
Education and Teaching Facilities 341
Endocrinology 342
Environmental Health 342
E.N.T. 342
Epidemiology 342
Family Medicine 342
Gastroenterology 342
Gynaecology and Obstetrics 342
Health Education 342
Haematology 342
Hygiene 342
Industrial Medicine 342
Immunobiology 342
Infectious Diseases 343
Intensive Care 343
Internal Medicine 343
Metabolic Diseases Including Diabetology 343
Nephrology 343
Neurology 343
Neurosurgery 343
Nuclear Medicine 343
Nursing 343
Nutrition 344
Occupational Therapy 344
Oncology 344
Ophthalmology 344
Orthopaedic Surgery 344
Paediatrics 344
Paediatric Surgery 345
Parasitology 345
Pharmacology 345
Pharmacy 345
Physical Medicine 345
Plastic Surgery 345
Preventive Medicine 345
Primary Health Care 345
Professional Diseases 345
Psychiatry 345
Public Health 345
Pulmonology 345
Radiology 345
Radiotherapy 345
Radiation Protection 345
Rehabilitation 345
Rheumatology 346
Surgery 346
Thoracic Surgery 346

Toxicology 346
Tropical Medicine . . . . : 346
Urology 346
Venerology 346
Virology 346

III. Invited (Foreign) Lecturers 347

IV. Annual Reports of Committees 358
   1. Area Executive Committee for Professional Medical Training 358
   2. The Area Executive Committee for Medical Speciality Training 358
      Structure and Organisation 358
      Activities of the Committee 359
   3. Area Executive Committee for Continuing Medical Education 359
   4. Accreditation Committee 360
      Surgery 362
      Medicine 362
      Paediatrics 362
      Gynaecology and Obstetrics 363
      Medical Records 363
   5. Discipline Committee for Medicine 363
   6. Discipline Committee for Surgery 364
      Introduction 364
      Organisation and Meetings 364
      Activities . . . . : 364
      Postgraduate Programme in Surgery 365
      Postgraduate Courses and Symposia Held in 1981—1982 366
      Visitors 367
      General Visitors . . . . : 367
      Future Plans and Goals 367
      Recommendations 368
      Summary 369
   7. Discipline Committee for Obstetrics and Gynaecology 370
   8. Discipline Committee for Paediatrics 370
      General Paediatric Subjects . . . . : . . 371
      Lectures by Visiting Experts 372
      Neonatal Problems and Procedures 372
   9. Discipline Committee for Public Health 373
   10. Discipline Committee for Family Medicine 373
   11. Discipline Committee for Radiology 373
   12. Discipline Committee for Anaesthesiology and Intensive Care 374
      1. Postgraduate Training in Anaesthesiology and Intensive Care . . 374
      2. Activities Accomplished During the Last Year 374
   13. Discipline Committee for Clinical Medical Laboratory 376
   14. Training Committee for Dentistry 376

V. Preparatory Steps for a New Programme for Postgraduate Medical Education for the Academic Year 1982—1983 378
   CIRCULAR NO. 1, Regarding the Programme of Education for
   1982—1983 378

CIRCULAR NO. 2, Regarding the Programme for Postgraduate Medical Education for 1982—1983 379
CIRCULAR NO. 3, Regarding the Programme of Education for 1982—1983 381
Memorandum. Area Executive Committee for Continuing Medical Education 382

Part Three

A Short History of Postgraduate Medical Education in Kuwait (Dr. Nouri Al Kazemi) 387
Teaching and Learning Processes (Dr. E. Ruzyllo) 395
Methodology of Self-Education of Doctors (Dr. E. Ruzyllo) 399
The Importance of Subjective Examination in the Diagnosis of Disease (Dr. E. Ruzyllo) 404
Organisational Forms of Postgraduate Medical Studies (Dr. E. Ruzyllo) 407
The Library as a Base for Postgraduate Teaching, Learning and Self-Education (Dr. E. Ruzyllo) 411
General Outline of Postgraduate Medical Education in Oncology as an Example of Forming a Teaching Program (Dr. E. Ruzyllo) 413
Community Medicine-Personal (Individual) Medicine (Dr. E. Ruzyllo) 418
Preparatory Steps for Introducing Family Medicine Practice (Dr. E. Ruzyllo)   423
        Report on a Visit by the President and Chairman of Council of the Royal College of General Practitioners of the United Kingdom — February 1981 423
        The Role of the Family Doctor and His Place in the National Health System 430
        Report on a Visit by the President and Chairman of Council of the Royal College of General Practitioners of the United Kingdom — February 1981 433
        The Role of the Family Doctor and His Place in the Kuwait National Health System. An Implementation Report 434
Trend of the Evolution of Medical Postgraduate Education (Dr. E. Ruzyllo) . 439

Part One

I. Organisation and Function of the System of Postgraduate Medical Education

1. Joint Board of Postgraduate Medical Education

Summary of Organisation

1. The Joint Board is the policy making body of postgraduate medical education in the country on behalf of the Ministry of Public Health and the Faculty of Medicine, and has the authority to decide its organisational forms and implementations.
2. The Joint Board is the body that approves all programmes, i.e. it sets the minimum requirements, monitors the implementation, making sure that the programme, the staff, and the teachers of the postgraduate programmes are all properly accredited and evaluated from time to time. The implementation of programmes is the responsibility of coordinators, approved by the Joint Board.
3. Responsibility for the implementation of policies is delegated to the major policy-making bodies, because the way in which a policy is implemented is critical to the achievement of its purpose. By giving both functions to the Area Executive Committees it is hoped that a more effective implementation of policies will be secured.
4. The planning of management policies for the government of all postgraduate training programmes is the responsibility of the Joint Board.
5. The planning of policies for postgraduate training is the responsibility of the Area Executive Committees in their respective areas of responsibility in consultation with the Discipline Committees. These policies are submitted to the Joint Board for approval and returned to the appropriate Area Executive Committee for implementation.
6. Implementation of policies is the responsibility of the chairmen of the Area Executive Committee assisted by the Committee Secretariat.
7. Members of the Joint Board are to be the chairmen of the Area Executive Committees.

Detailed Organisation

In accordance with Ministerial Decree No. 293/79 and Ministerial Decree No. 72/79 the Joint Board shall be responsible for:

Medical Professional Training;
Medical Speciality Training and
Continuing Medical Education.

a) Membership

Ex-officio members:

Undersecretary of the Ministry of Public Health;
Dean of the Faculty of Medicine;
Head of the Training Division. Secretary.

Four members nominated by the Dean of the Faculty of Medicine.
Four members nominated by the Undersecretary of the Ministry of Public Health, one of whom shall be a chairman.
Two doctors—representatives of the doctor-residents and assistant registrars.

b) Functions and Responsibilities

It shall decide the general policies for managing postgraduate professional training.
It shall decide the terms of reference of the Area Executive Committees for Medical Professional Training, Postgraduate Medical Speciality Training, and Continuing Medical Education.
It shall appoint the members of the Area Executive Committees for Medical Professional Training, and Continuing Medical Education.
It shall decide the terms of reference of the Discipline Committees.
It shall appoint the members of the Discipline Committees.
It shall receive and approve Professional, Speciality and Continuing Medical Education programmes.
It shall receive and approve curricula for Professional, Speciality and Continuing Medical Education programmes.
It shall receive and approve the regulations, criteria and procedures for the appointment of course coordinators and tutors.
It shall receive and approve the regulations, criteria and procedures for the accreditation of departments, units and number of tutorial posts.
It shall receive and approve the accreditation of individual departments, units and tutorial posts.
It shall receive and approve the regulations, criteria and procedures for the admission of candidates.
It shall receive the names of those candidates who have satisfactorily completed a course.
It shall approve the annual budget.
It shall review regulations for licensing.
It shall revise and review the annual reports of the Area Executive Committees.
It shall monitor the progress of all programmes and the performance of the personnel responsible for them.

The procedures by which the Joint Board and its subcommittees are to conduct their business is laid down in the executive regulations of the Ministry of Public Health.

2. Area Executive Committees

Summary of Organisation

In accordance with Ministerial Decree No. 293/79 and Ministerial Decree No. 72/79 the Joint Board shall be responsible for: Medical Professional Training; Medical Speciality Training; and Continuing Medical Education.

Detailed Organisation

To satisfy these requirements accordingly three Area Executive Committees have been organised:

Area Executive Committee on Medical Professional Training;
Area Executive Committee on Medical Speciality Training;
Area Executive Committee on Continuing Medical Education.

a) Membership

Membership shall be decided by the Joint Board. A member of the Joint Board shall be Chairman. The Assistant Head of the Training Division shall be an ex-Officio member and act as Secretary.

b) Functions and Responsibilities

The Area Executive Committees are subcommittees of the Joint Board and are responsible for the planning of policies for recommendation to the Joint Board and the implementation of policies approved by the Joint Board.

1. The Area Executive Committee for Medical Professional Training should prepare at the end of the two-year course of report on each candidate and make appropriate recommendations to each candidate and inform the Joint Board.

2. a) The Area Executive Committee for Medical Speciality Training should review the requirements for new speciality training programmes and plan and recommend policies for their implementation and evaluation.

   b) It shall evaluate and submit reports on all speciality examinations held in Kuwait.

Their detailed functions and responsibilities are in the status of the Joint Board. The chief functions and responsibilities of the Area Executive Committees are:

Review, recommend, and monitor the training programmes.
Review and recommend the curricula and content of the training programmes.
Review, recommend and monitor the activities of Tutor-coordinators of hospitals (see page 21).
Plan and recommend the regulations, criteria and procedures for the accreditation of departments, units and number of tutorial posts.
Recommend the accreditation of individual departments, units and tutorial posts.
Review, recommend and execute the policy governing the supply, to hospitals and other appropriate centres, of books, journals and audio-visual software, and identify the means of accommodating and controlling their use.
Plan and recommend the regulations, criteria and procedures for selecting staff to coordinate and conduct the programme of medical education.
Plan and recommend policies with regard to overseas travel with or without scholarships.
Approve recommendations from the Discipline Committee for the award of individual scholarships.
Review the education programmes submitted by the various Discipline Committees and the role of foreign medical staff invited to participate.
Plan and recommend the policy on admission to the training programme.

Execute admission procedures, including the selection of candidates.

Submit biannual reports to the Joint Board once in the first week of December and the next in the first week of June.

Prepare its annual budget for submission to the Joint Board.

3. Discipline Committees

Summary of Organisation

The Discipline Committees are responsible to the appropriate Area Executive Committee for submitting recommendations to them according to the postgraduate area under consideration, and for routine administration.

Detailed Organisation

a) Membership

The members of the Discipline Committees should be:

i) Heads of the divisions of discipline in the hospitals.
ii) Members appointed by the Joint Board.
iii) The number of members of a Discipline Committee as a general rule should be between 5 and 10.
iv) Chairmen of all Discipline Committees will be chosen by the Joint Board.
v) There will also be Deputy Chairmen and Secretaries in each Discipline Committee, who will be elected by the Committee.

The Discipline Committee may have subcommittees for specialities belonging to or depending on a basic speciality. Such a subcommittee is constituted by the Joint Board and its chairman, and members are appointed by the Joint Board.

The subcommittes shall work along with the general policy given by the basic discipline committee.

The secretaries shall be elected by the members of each Discipline Committee from amongst themselves to hold office for two-year, renewable terms.

b) Meetings

The Discipline Committees shall meet at least once a month.

c) Functions and Responsibilities

They plan and recommend to the appropriate Area Executive Committee their respective training programmes and curricula.

They are responsible for organising approved programmes in their respective disciplines. (See "Preparation of the Yearly Programme" and "Basic Requirements of Postgraduate Medical Teaching".) They are responsible for the day-to-day coordination and programming of clinical meetings.

They organise conferences with tutors for clinical discipline committees discussing methods and level of postgraduate studies (see page 21).

They recommend to the appropriate Area Executive Committee all tutors, course coordinators and tutorial posts in accordance with agreed regulations, criteria and procedures.

They evaluate and recommend to the appropriate Area Executive Committee all candidates who complete training programmes.

They recommend to the appropriate Area Executive Committee individual candidates for the award of scholarships, according to policies agreed upon.

They are responsible for planning and recommending to the appropriate Area Executive Committee visits by "experts" in their respective disciplines and for preparing programmes for such visits (objectives, topics, coordinators, participants, duration, time place, budget).

They are obliged to teach doctors sensitivity towards moral and ethical aspects of their professional activities.

The Chairman, after a consultation with the majority of the members of the committee, may invite one more local or foreign specialist of the appropriate discipline to attend the meeting of the committee.

They must submit biannual reports to the Area Executive Committee once in the first week of November and the next in the first week of May.

Preparation of the Yearly Programme

According to the decision of the Joint Board for Postgraduate Medical Education, Kuwait, the postgraduate medical education programmes should be formed for the fiscal year which begins on the 1st of July and ends on the 30th of June the following year.

Experience shows that a delay in the proper management of organisational preparations delays a programme of teaching, and in many instances forces a change of projected activities. When discussing the next year's training programme, the whole field of Postgraduate Medical Education should be taken into consideration, and accordingly, suggestions, remarks or changes should be proposed for:

professional training
speciality training
topics and forms of continuing medical education activities.

So far as continuing medical education is concerned, it is the wish of the Joint Board that training programmes should take into consideration proportionately the requirements of the whole system of National Health Care. That means, it should be prepared

for doctors with primary health care duties (general Practitioners, Family Medicine doctors)
for doctors working in hospitals on Registrar and Sr. Registrar level positions and finally for Consultants.

These 3 levels of postgraduate medical programmes may be performed in the best way if one main topic for such training is chosen. The programme for teaching of this main topic should be prepared for GPs, after a short time the same topic should be accordingly discussed for the requirements of Registrars and Sr. Registrars, and finally again after a short time, these topics should be discussed during the postgraduate medical teaching programme on the level of Consultants (conference or seminar).

The programme of the conference prepared for Consultants should have aspects of the previous 2 programmes (for GPs and for Registrars) just to give them possibilities for discussions, and to clarify some problems initiated during the respective courses.

In elaborating the yearly teaching programme the following periods should be performed:

1. A Preparatory Period

Between *September and February* the educational programme for the teaching year should be thoroughly discussed by the Discipline Committees. The outline of different requirements on medical studies should be taken under consideration and accordingly the names of programme Directors of studies and the names of foreign lecturers should be considered (see pages 26, 27). In this preparatory period necessary letters should be sent to proposed foreign lecturers.

2. Area Executive Committees Approval

In March the outline of the programme of studies (courses, seminars, workshops, lectures, conferences, other clinical activities, etc.) should be sent by Discipline Committees to Area Executive Committees for final discussion and decisions. This programme should consist also of code identifying numbers (C. I. N.) according to the instructions of the Joint Board for Postgraduate Medical Education (see page 28).

3. Joint Board Approval

In April the programmes accepted by the Area Executive Committees should be sent to the Joint Board for final approval for the next teaching year.

Programme Characteristics and Requirements

a) The programme should be *very exact in its objectives,* should be sent to all concerned in advance, and should be in detail covering lectures, days, hours, place, etc.
b) The programme is aimed not only at specialists but at all doctors attending lectures or any other form of medical studies. These doctors require *early and detailed information* (seminars, lectures, etc.)
c) The programme should be aimed also at doctors from different specialities, because one of the purposes of postgraduate medical education is to give a *general outlook* on all medical problems of different specialities.
d) The Joint Board of Postgraduate Medical Education decided that all kinds of medical studies should be presented in the same *organisational form* which is as follows:

Course Identifying Number (C.I.N.)
Title of the Course (seminar, conference, lecture, etc.)
Objectives
Place
Duration (dates) from—till
Organiser
Programme Director (person responsible)
Participants (for whom the course is organised in detail)
Programme in detail.

Organisational Performance of the Study (Course, Seminar, etc.)

The Discipline Committee which organises its teaching programme and the *Secretary of this Discipline Committee* should deal with all necessary arrangements.

The Discipline Committee should also *give the authority to one of the doctors* who may or may not be a member of the Discipline Committee (to engage anyone from outside this Committees e.g. a head of the department or other hospital unit) giving him the responsibility for organisational arrangements as the *Programme Director* of the study.

The Programme Director along with the Secretary of the Discipline Committee should cooperate with the Secretary of the relevant Area Executive Committee (see pages 21, 22).

Educational Assistance to Nurses

Having in mind the importance of cooperation with doctors and nursing staff each Discipline Committee may forsee the possibility of initiating and assisting in the continuing medical education of nurses. A doctor's course or seminar may be utilised for that purpose.

It could be organised along the following principles:

The Training Committee for Nursing (see page 46) should delegate 2 to 3 *observers* to doctors' courses or seminars and later on to organise on the same topic the seminar for nurses. The organisation of such a seminar for nurses should have the following points:

1. General introduction to the subject given by *the tutor doctor* delegated by the programme director of the course or seminar for doctors on the same subject.
2. Nurse observers should act as *rapporteurs* of the doctors' courses or seminars emphasizing the medical problems of importance for nurses.
3. *General discussions*, film (video) presentations with the comments of the tutor doctors attending the seminar and nurse rapporteurs.

Important Course (IC) of our Postgraduate Teaching Program

Definition of an Important Course

The postgraduate medical education programme should be thoroughly thought over and properly prepared and the form should represent an important part of the whole programme of postgraduate medical education.

Some of the subjects of teaching may have exceptional character either because of the subject itself, which may have a basic meaning for many fields of theoretical and practical medicine, or because of the special organisational form of the course.

When we invite many outstanding lecturers for a broad and comprehensive programme, and when the number of participants foreseen is big; the course is usually held in bigger accommodations, and is given the character of a traditional doctors' meeting, in the form in which up-to-date medical societies and other social and professional meetings are organised.

Differentiation between a Traditional Meeting Organised by the Medical Society and a Course which is a Part of the Postgraduate Medical Education Programme

We all have a tradition of organising *conferences* and meetings as members *of medical societies*. If a decision is taken to organise a conference the society calls an organising committee which deals with every matter connected with scientific and organisational problems. A programme for such a conference is proposed to members of the society and they declare whether they would like to participate by sending a proper declaration. Then they share the cost of the conference by paying the appropriate fees.

The course organised *by institutions of postgraduate* medical *education* applies a different form of organisation and budgeting. First, the programme of the conference, a part of the general programme of postgraduate medical education, is discussed and accepted by the appropriate body. This body also decides who should participate in the course, and the programme of the course must be agreeable to the doctors. Second, the budget which covers the cost comes out of the budget of the postgraduate medical education institution.

In the organisation of postgraduate medical education, the Discipline Committee and the Area Executive Committee for Continuing Medical Education should decide who is obliged to attend the course. In some cases they may even name the doctors who should attend the courses. In such a case, these doctors automatically get permission from the respective authorities and are released from their work. They do not pay a fee and if catering is provided they may pay for that. In many instances the catering could be included in the budget of the course or it could be outside the jurisdiction of the institution of postgraduate medical education. All organisational activities and procedures should be arranged by the Secretary of the Area Executive Committee for Continuing Medical Education. It is up to this committee to decide what kind of help and assistance should be given to the Secretary to fulfil his duties.

How the Course is Marked as an Important Course (IC)

The Discipline Committee may suggest that some of the postgraduate medical education courses may be considered as bigger and more important for the programme of postgraduate medical education. It would mean that a bigger number invited for a lecture could be engaged, and also a bigger number of local doctors could participate in it. Also it would mean that such a course could take from 3 to 6 days. It obliges the Discipline Committees who organise such a course to make a different organisation. In such a situation the Discipline Committee which proposes organising this important course (IC) should produce for the Area Executive Committee for Continuing Medical Education the following information and details:

1. List of foreign visitors which should, as a principle, include at least one lecturer from an Arab country.
2. Place in which the course should be conducted.
3. Number of doctors participating and their required professional characteristics.
4. List of the Organising Committee who will look after the proper organising of the course.
5. Budget required for such a course.
6. Comments and recommendations at the end of the course.

Foreign Participants of the Important Course (IC)

Some of the important courses (IC) organised by the Area Executive Committee for Continuing Medical Education may also serve foreign doctors as a gesture of hospitality and goodwill from the Kuwait side.

If a Discipline Committee proposes to make a course with international participation it should suggest the doctors from each country whom they wish to invite and also the number of doctors to be invited. This invitation will be sent by the Secretary of the Area Executive Committee for Continuing Medical Education through the Ministry of Public Health, having previously been approved by the Chairman of the Joint Board. Such information and invitation should be sent at least 3 months before the course begins, explaining objectives of the course, methods used and giving some names of the lecturers. Hotel arrangements for such a doctor should be discussed by the Secretary of the Area Executive Committee with the proper unit of the Ministry of Public Health.

Foreign participants of the course should send to the Secretary of the Area Executive Committee their declaration and fee for participation.

Evaluation of the Course

Evaluation is a systematic way of learning from experience and using the lessons learned to improve current activities and promote better planning by careful selection of alternatives for future action.

Evaluation is a difficult task. It requires from relevant people abilities for proper measurement, quantified objectives, qualitative judgement, quantified information and finally, sensitive indicators.

The purpose of evaluating postgraduate medical education is to improve health programmes and the health infrastructure for delivering them, and to guide the allocation of resources and future programmes.

After each postgraduate medical study (conference, seminar, etc.), the *programme director* should present a short evaluation of the course. The evaluation should be prepared according to the following scheme:

a) That the course fulfilled its objectives.
b) General remarks on the organisation of the course.
c) General remarks on the level of teaching.
d) General remarks on the attendance of doctors (numbers and the active participation).
e) Final evaluation which should suggest that the course be repeated, changed or not repeated, etc.

4. Committee Secretariat of the Joint Board

Summary of Organisation

In the committee organisation governing postgraduate training programmes, the Committee Secretariat has a crucial role to play in coordinating the work of the committees, in ensuring that policy planning follows stipulated channels, and in making certain that policies are implemented according to approved procedures. It also has to coordinate the collection of feedback on agreed policies by monitoring their effectiveness.

Detailed Organisation

, To facilitate the Secretariat's functions, the Head of the Training Division is the Secretary to the Joint Board and the Area Executive Committees. This is done on the principle that it is most effective for the administrative officer concerned with a particular area of administration to service the committees with responsibility for that particular area.

Secretary to the Joint Board—Head of the Training Division

Field of activities and responsibilities:

a) Implementation of the policies being formed by the Joint Board.
b) Continuation of the development of the objectives and forms of postgraduate medical studies.
c) General policy of the library and its utilisation for postgraduate medical education and in the field of pedagogy, didactics, and teaching facilities.
d) Cooperation with the Medical Faculty with regard to postgraduate medical studies.
e) General management of the Committee Secretariat.
f) Planning and organising of the policies and procedures by which it carries out its tasks.
g) Annual performance evaluation of the individual secretariat staff members.
h) Planning of staff resources, and preparation of an annual report and budget. As the Head of the Committee Secretariat of the Joint Board of Postgraduate Education he is expected to:

coordinate the work of the three Area Executive Committees;
convene, when necessary, ad-hoc meetings of the three Area Executive Committee Chairmen;
function as a management information system;
evaluate the results of postgraduate studies.

Deputy Head of the Training Division for Professional and Specialisation Training

Field of activities and responsibilities:

a) Forming programmes and steadily developing them in the field of professional and specialised training in the country.
b) As secretary of the Area Executive Committees on Professional Training or an Speciality Training he will co-ordinate the work of the Committees in ensuring that policy-planning follows stipulated channels and in making certain that policies are implemented according to approved procedures. This is especially important with Area Executive Committees on Speciality Training in close cooperation with the Postgraduate Committee of the Faculty of Medicine.

He will also have to co-ordinate the collection of feedback on agreed policies by monitoring their effectiveness.

He will cooperate administratively with Secretaries of the following Discipline Committees, by advising procedures and showing principles:

Discipline Committee for Medicine
Discipline Committee for Surgery
Discipline Committee for Gynaecology and Obstetrics
Discipline Committee for Paediatrics

Discipline Committee for Public Health
Discipline Committee for Family Medicine
Discipline Committee for Radiology.

c) To cooperate with the Kuwait representatives to the Arab Board of Specialisation within the framework of the Joint Board on Postgraduate Medical Education.

In brief his formal duties are as follows:

— To study advances in postgraduate training with the aim to discuss them with
proper people or proper units. Good solutions should be implemented in the
Kuwaiti system of postgraduate education.
— To cooperate with the chairmen of the Executive Committees in setting up the
educational programme for a proper fiscal year. The final programme elaborat-
ed by the Executive Committees should be presented to the Joint Board (see
page 8 during the first week of April.
— To ensure the effective feedback of information between the above mentioned
Area Executive Committees and all Discipline Committees.
— To arrange systematic meetings with Tutor-coordinators of the hospitals (page
21).
— To see to it that invited visitors fulfil the requirements given by the Joint Board.
— To prepare the agendas in consultation with committee chairmen. The secretary
should keep a record of all business and all activities in his administrative area
so that he can keep his committee chairman informed of the status of all activities under a committee's jurisdiction. If there are papers to be prepared to support items on the agenda, he must ensure that these are ready to be circulated
with the agenda. Often, he may write such papers himself.
— To make certain that the Area Executive Committee Chairman is thoroughly
briefed before a meeting.
— To follow up all Area Executive Committees' decisions and to ensure that they
are communicated to the appropriate bodies for execution (see page 5, 6).
— To record all programmes of postgraduate medical studies and present them
with the annual report of the activities of the Area Executive Committees.
— To prepare an annual report for the first week of June each year.

Deputy Head of the Training Division for Continuing Medical Education, Allied
Health Sciences and Nursing

Field of activities and responsibilities:

a) Forming programmes and their steady developments in the field of:

Continuing Medical Education
Allied Health Services
Nursing Training

b) To cooperate administratively with secretaries of the following Discipline Committees and Training Committees by advising procedures and showing principles:

Discipline Committee for Anaesthesiology and Intensive Care
Discipline Committee for Clinical Laboratory Medicine
Discipline Committee for Oncology

Training Committee for Pharmacy, Dentistry, Laboratory Technologists and Nursing.

c) Remaining duties as for Deputy Head for Professional and Speciality Training.

Deputy Head of the Training Division for Administrative Affairs

Field of activities and responsibilities:

a) General management of the Training Division in all aspects of economic, material organisation, manpower utilisation and administration to fulfil the requirements of the postgraduate medical education in the country.

b) To cooperate on behalf of the Head of the Division with all units in the Ministry of Public Health and the Medical Faculty.

c) He will look after proper elaboration of the budget for the fiscal year. The budget should be based on the programme given by the 3 Executive Committees of the Joint Board. The programme should include also the names of the visitors and their place in the respective courses or symposia. The budget should be finished and presented to the Ministry of Public Health in the first week of April each year.

d) He is responsible for the preparation of an annual report for the first week of June each year.

e) He is responsible for the administration and supervision of didactic areas of the Training Division at Al Adan and Farwania Hospitals. According to his instructions and regulations and his consultation with the Head of the Training Division, the proper equipment of these areas should be made and kept in good order. Apparatus required for a given course may be sent by the Pedagogy, Didactic and Teaching Facilities Units and after the course, returned to the units.

f) The Deputy Head for Administrative Affairs has general charge of the material state of the Training Division and its accommodation surveys, yearly cleaning and repairs. He looks after proper equipment and repairs of the apparatus used in the Training Division.

g) He should see to the implementation of new and important apparatus, furniture and especially, pay attention to the utilisation of typewriters, photocopy machines, stationery, etc.

h) He controls and advises the utilisation of the communication services.

i) He is directly responsible for the computerised information unit, looking after proper input and output information. The quality of information should be continually developed and apparatus continually improved.

j) He will give special attention to the Pan Arab Board for Specialisation.

5. Basic Requirements for Postgraduate Medical Teaching

Hospital Accreditation

Criteria for Recognition of Eligible Hospitals for Training in Kuwait

General Terms

1. All clinical departments (and units) in the existing as well as in the new hospitals should be utilised in the training of graduates entering the professional Training Program. Consequently, all departments and units should qualify or be made to qualify for this purpose.

2a. A training unit of 60 beds in Medicine, Surgery, Gynaecology and Obstetrics, Paediatrics and Psychiatry should comprise:

Two Consultants   — One Head of unit, one Assistant Head of unit
One Senior Registrar
Two Registrars
Two Assistant Registrars
Two Residents

---

9 Total Number

2b. In other subspecialities, the training unit should comprise:

Two Consultants   — One Head of unit, one Assistant Head of unit
One—two Senior Registrars
Two—three Registrars
One—two Assistant Registrars

with a maximum total number of seven staff members in each unit.

It was noted that although the training programme is the responsibility of the consultants and Senior Registrars, the Registrars have a role in the day to day activities and practices.

3. The hospital must be a general hospital with the following departments:

a) Internal Medicine
b) General Surgery
c) Paediatrics
d) Gynaecology and Obstetrics

4. The capacity of the General Hospital is normally around 500 beds.

a) The hospital should have a laboratory to satisfy the modern requirements of laboratory diagnostics with access to tissue examination.
b) The hospital must have a proper X-ray department.
c) The hospital must have out-patient clinics.
d) Proper hospital accident-emergency clinics.
e) Intensive care unit.
f) Vital Statistics and Medical Records.
g) A library of medical books and medical periodicals must be in every hospital.
h) A proper conference and lecture hall must be available.
i) The hospital must have proper nursing staff and administration.

Medicine

Size and Structure: The Unit (60 beds) should comprise at least 2 wards each comprising not less than 30 beds for males and 30 beds for females.

The *Department* should have an Intensive Care Area including coronary care.

Facilities:

1. A departmental library supplied with basic books and manuals.
2. A room for departmental group meetings for teaching purposes for residents.
3. Facility in the hospital for clinical meetings (including lectures, demonstrations, clinical presentation of cases) for residents as well as for the regular all-departmental staff clinical meetings.

Activities:

1. *Teaching round:* conducted by the consultant once per week at least, in addition to those carried by Senior Staff.
2. *Clinical meetings:* held once weekly. The meetings at the Unit/Departmental level should actively involve the residents in the presentation of cases and in subsequent discussions. Lectures should include topics on common practical problems.
3. *Clinical-Pathological meetings.*
4. *Out-patient Sessions:* at least once weekly; should be managed by senior medical staff.
5. *Casualty Reception Service:* should be run by the Unit/Department.

Surgery

Size and Structure: The Unit (60 beds) should comprise at least 2 wards, each comprising not less than 30 beds for males and 30 beds for females.

120 beds in surgery for teaching purposes must be found as a minimum. The surgical admittance for hospitals must be on an average of 35 patients yearly for each bed. The total amount of surgical operations must not be less than 3,000 operations each year. The operation theatres must not be less than three theatres for every 100 beds.

Facilities: Same as in General Medicine.
Activities: Same as in General Medicine.

Paediatrics

Size and Structure: The *Unit* should comprise at least 2 wards, each comprising not less than 30 beds.

The *Department* should include a Neonatology Section.
Facilities: Same as in General Medicine.
Activities: Same as in General Medicine.

Obstetrics and Gynaecology

1. *Size and Structure:* The Unit should be responsible for not less than 60 beds and the department should have at least 10—15 beds allocated for labour and delivery.

   The postnatal beds should comprise no more than 50% of the total number of beds.

   The beds allocated for gynaecological cases should not be less than 8 beds per unit.

   The rest of the beds should be allocated for antenatal and abortion cases.

2. *Facilities:*

   Facilities as stated in the section on General Medicine.

   The Department should have facilities for modern Obstetric care including fetal heart rate monitoring and Ultrasonography and facilities for radiological investigation, i.e. Hysterosalpingography and Pelvimetry.

   Facilities for minor and major operative procedures.

3. *Activities:* The following activities should be run by the unit at least once weekly:
   Teaching round conducted by the consultant/senior registrar.
   Operative session attended by consultant/senior registrar.

Labour ward and obstetric/gynaecologic emergency service.
Scientific meeting with active involvement of the residents at least twice during the training period.
Out-patient session supervised by consultant/senior registrar. This includes minor operative procedures on out-patients.

Teaching

1. Each resident should be responsible for a minimum of 15 beds during his training.
2. The sub-specialities must be taken into consideration in case of recognition.
3. There must be in each department of each hospital scientific meetings (three times every week) as follows:

   a) Bedside wards meetings.
   b) Journals meetings (clubs).
   c) Seminars.
   d) Big bedside wards rounds.
   e) Laboratory clinical seminars.
   f) Specialised lectures in addition to daily rounds in different wards.

4. Two full time Consultants or Senior Registrars must be appointed for each department of 30 beds to each unit.
5. The above mentioned specialists must have a scientific degree. One of them should have previous experience in academic teaching and scientific research.
6. It is not permissible to have more than three fellow doctors for the three years of medical training and that means one fellow doctor yearly for every 20 beds.

Teaching Staff Accreditation

Criteria for Accreditation of Clinical Staff for Purposes of Postgraduate Speciality Training

The following shall be the minimum criteria for accreditation of clinical staff:

1. The consultant should have postgraduate professional qualifications which are required for a consultant's post in the English-speaking world, or its equivalent as determined by an Accreditation Committee, e.g. (see page 46).

Surgery	— F.R.C.S. (Ireland or U.K.), the American Board of Surgery, or F.R.C.S. (C)
Medicine	— M.R.C.P. (Ireland or U.K.), the American Board of Internal Medicine
Gynaecology and Obstetrics	— M.R.C.O.G. (Gyn, Ireland), the American Board of Obstetrics/Gynaecology or F.R.C.S. (C) (GYN).
Paediatrics	— M.R.C.P. (Paed) (Ireland or U.K.), the American Board of Paediatrics, or F.R.C.P. (C).
Anaesthesiology	— F.F.A.R.C.S. (Ireland or U.K.)
Public Health (Community Medicine)	— MFCM: Member of the Faculty of Community Medicine.

Family Medicine (General
Practice, Primary Health
Care)

MFOM: Member of the Faculty of
Occupational Medicine.
— MRCGP: Member of Royal College of
General Practitioners.

2. The individual clinician must have 5 years of professional and teaching experience after postgraduate speciality qualifications. In Public Health (Community Medicine) and in Family Medicine (Primary Health Care) the individual physician must have 4 years of professional and teaching experience after postgraduate speciality training. But due to the fact that the above mentioned qualifications are limited to those with full registration in the U.K. The Master in Community Medicine, the Master in Occupational Medicine or MRCGP should be considered as the common academic core and the basic postgraduate degree but accreditation should be given after 6 years.

3. It is desirable that a Consultant should have academic accomplishments, e.g. research and publications in his field.

4. The Consultant should be of sufficiently high moral and ethical standing as judged by acceptable referees.

5. The Consultant and his department *(medicine, surgery etc.)* should have adequate and acceptable facilities and staff for postgraduate training, and should be actively involved in clinical and other postgraduate meetings and conferences (see Hospital Accreditation).

6. The consultant and his department: Medicine, Surgery, Public Health (Community Medicine, Epidemiology and Occupational Medicine) and Family Medicine (General Practice) should have adequate and acceptable facilities and staff for postgraduate training and should be actively involved in field and community work as well as in postgraduate meetings and conferences.

   a) There should be at least 2 senior Registrars (higher specialist training), 1 registrar and 2 residents attached to the consultant concerned.

   b) There should be at least one unit of activity under the consultant concerned whether in Public Health (Community Medicine, Epidemiology, Occupational Health) or Family Medicine (General Practice). The functions of such units are specified (see Hospital Administration).

7. In addition to the usual working day, the consultant concerned must be willing to organise and participate in clinical meetings and conferences in the afternoons.

8. There should be evidence of a sufficiently high standard of professional practice in the unit in which the doctor concerned works. There should also be evidence that bedside or ambulatory teaching is a regular activity of the Unit. In Family Medicine (General Practice) as well as in Public Health (Community Medicine, Epidemiology and Occupational Health) there should be evidence of a sufficiently high standard of practice in the unit supervised by the consultant. There should be evidence through proper evaluation that the functions of the unit are fully carried out.

9. An Accreditation Committee is appointed (see page 46).

   a) to implement the above mentioned recommendations, and

   b) to review accreditation procedures and consultants' posts at 3-yearly intervals.

Director of Education in the Teaching Hospital

The Director of Medical Education in the teaching hospital is proposed by the Director of the hospital and approved by the Joint Board of Postgraduate Medical Education.

The appointment of the Director of Medical Education in the hospital should be reviewed at 1 year intervals by the Joint Board.

The chief purpose of the Director of Medical Education in the hospital is:

1. To coordinate the programme of medical education in the hospital in all three areas of training.

   Professional training
   Speciality training
   Continuing Medical Education

   by having continuous contact with the tutor-coordinator for clinical discipline in the hospital and with the program director of specialisation (see p. 21).
2. To create the best conditions for teaching and learning. It is recommended that the clinical side be stressed and theoretical knowledge acquired through more active participation and effort by the trainee himself rather than by spoon-feeding him knowledge by classical lectures, which he may or may not attend (and he may be inattentive if he does). Hence the suggestion of having discussion sessions about cases he is personally looking after with the senior registrar and the consultant.

   The suggestion that the trainee should prepare papers (of course under the guidance of his seniors) about a topic related to one of his cases is an important addition to the old scheme of training. Apart from the knowledge gained, it will teach the trainee how to research a subject, how to look up the literature, etc.

   The director of medical education in the teaching hospital should consider incentives and disciplinary measures, which may improve interest in the training program.

   As regards incentives, the Discipline Committee should think of ways to reward the deserving resident, e.g. giving him priority for registrarship appointments, study leaves abroad etc.

   As for disciplinary measures, the resident may be kept for another training period. This should be in addition to the complete rotation programme and not at the expense of any part of it (or it will lose its significance). Any other disciplinary measure can be suggested in addition, but these measures should be made very clear to the residents from the start and should be enforced very strictly.
3. To organise and conduct in-service postgraduate education programmes in the hospital.
4. To evaluate the results of training in all three areas of training.
5. To supervise the training of the residents (professional training) according to the following instructions:

Interviewing the Residents

At the beginning of training, the director of medical education in the hospital should meet with the residents and dedicate a special session to introduce them to the programme. The director of education with the cooperation of tutor-coordinators for clinical discipline in the hospital will instruct them fully about training. He will give them a detailed outline evolving:

a) The objectives of training.
b) The programme for training.
c) Methods and procedures adopted to implement such a programme.
d) Schedule and curriculum of lectures, outpatient and inpatient sessions, clinical rounds, clinical meetings, other teaching activities (seminars, general duties, etc.).

Orienting the Trainee to His New Work and Activities

The resident must be well acquainted with his duties and role during his training period. This calls for his active participation in his training process. He should be well informed with the expected procedures which should follow in the patient's care as far as he is responsible (history taking, thorough physical examination, writing sheets, study files, etc.).

The trainee must be directed towards his duties and responsibilities both in outpatient and inpatient care.

Procedures Adopted for Direction and Supervision

The machinery of work in the wards must be explained to the trainee. The link between candidate and staff to whom he may resort or report and who the senior staff member responsible for his training in the ward is. Who supervises his activities, and how he shall be evaluated must be explained to him.

Relationships

The placement of the resident amongst other serving staff should be clear. An important fact that should be borne in mind is that residents are medical graduates on their postgraduate training. They should always be treated on that basis. Staff doctors, nurses and technicians must realise this fact. Such a consideration will have a positive effect on the attitude and inclination of residents, helping them to benefit from their training.

Distribution of Trainees on Various Training Units

Effective training goes hand in hand with:

1. Readiness to train. How ready the Unit is to train him.
2. The satisfactory criteria for training (place, facilities, personnel).
3. Interest of staff to train.
4. Acceptable trainee/bed ratio.
5. Proper evaluation of training process and trainee.

The director of medical education in the teaching hospital must consider such factors in distributing residents among various units.

Written notes or booklets containing most or some of these points would help the trainee to realise what he is up to. In principle the approved programmes for training should be given to the trainee's trainer to follow with a certain flexibility.

The director of medical education may help to produce such handbooks and gives them to each resident when he joins the training department. Other functions and responsibilities are well illustrated in the decisions made and distributed by the Joint Board.

Tutor-Coordinator for Given Clinical Discipline in the Hospital for Professional and Continuing Medical Training

The Tutor-Coordinator for a given clinical discipline in the hospital for professional and continuing medical training responsible for the education of the doctor trainees in a given medical discipline. He is appointed by the Departmental Council of each speciality in each teaching hospital and approved by the Joint Board of Postgraduate Medical Education.

A Tutor-Coordinator for clinical discipline in the hospital will act in the name of the chairman of the department who is ultimately responsible for the training programme.

The appointment of the Tutor-Coordinator for clinical discipline should be reviewed at 1 year intervals by the Joint Board.

The Tutor-Coordinator should be in a position to dedicate most if not all of his time to carrying out the following responsibilities:

1. Interviewing the trainees directed to his clinical discipline unit.
2. Orienting them to their new work and duties.
3. Placement and rotation of trainees within the different units of the same discipline.
4. Executing the teaching and training programme.
5. Periodic follow up of each trainee for the achievement of the programme.
6. Counselling with the trainee or his registrar or consultant regarding the performance, the complaints (of either side) or the hardships.
7. Supervision of attendance of the trainees at all activities assigned to them.
8. To check continuously if criteria for recognition of eligible hospitals for training are actually carried out. In the case of any discrepancies arising the Joint Board should be notified.
9. To cooperate with the director of medical education in the hospital.
10. Final evaluation of the performance of trainees.

Programme Director of Specialisation

1. The Chairman of the accredited department of any hospital shall be responsible for the implementation of the programme as *Programme Director of Specialisation* in his hospital.
2. The Programme Director of Specialisation shall report in a regular manner to the corresponding Discipline Committee.
3. *The Selection Committee* for a given speciality programme shall be composed of:

   the Postgraduate Dean of the Medical Faculty, as Chairman,
   the Programme Director of Specialisation in a given hospital,
   representative of the concerned Discipline Committee,
   the Director of the given hospital, and
   Chairman of any other department.

Programme Director of Each Study (Course, Seminar etc.) of the Nation-Wide Postgraduate Continuing Medical Education

The Programme Director of each course is nominated by the Discipline Committee and accepted by the relevant Area Executive Committee. As Programme Director, he realises both teaching programme and all methodological and organisational aspects of the course according to the instructions laid down by the Discipline Committee.

In some instances the Discipline Committee may form an Organisation Committee for a given postgraduate medical course. In such a situation, the Organisation Committee'takes on its own shoulders the responsibility and duties of the Discipline Committee regarding a given postgraduate medical course.

The Programme Director should pay attention both to the scientific and didactic level of teaching during the course, as well as its proper organisation. Lectures and bedside practical activities have to find the proper proportion during each course.

The chief purpose of the Programme Director (coordinator) is:

1. To form organisational conditions so as to satisfy requirements of lecturers, allowing them in the most optimal way to realise the task given them by the programme director of the course.

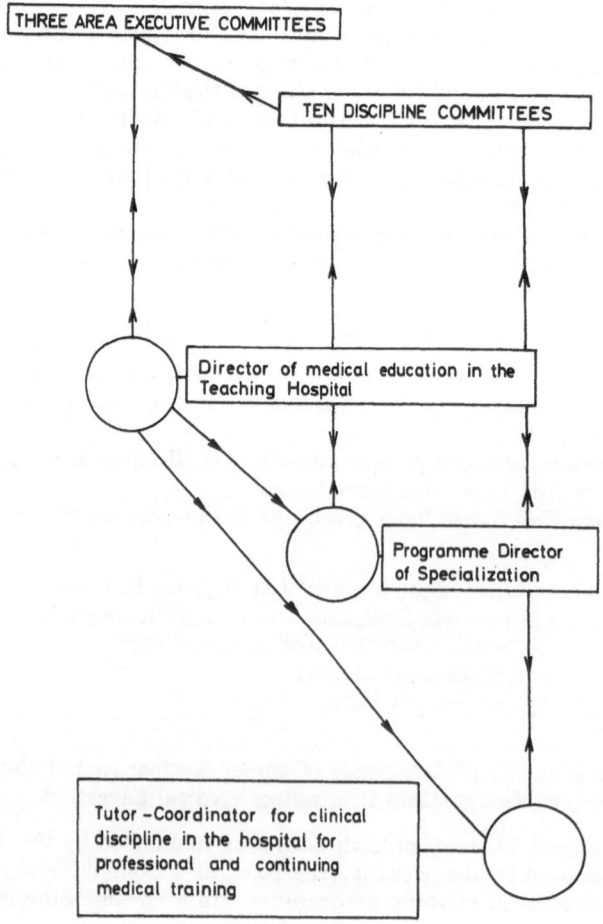

2. To create conditions which can fully utilise the wisdom of the lecturers.
3. To create the best didactic programme.
4. One of the final aims of the activities is to achieve the best results of training by doctors in the course.
5. To best execute his duties, the Programme Director should be well informed about the needs and requirements of the lecturers.
6. Before the beginning of the course, the Programme Director (coordinator) should make sure that all the needs and requirements, technical and didactic, of the lecturers are fulfilled.
7. He should also confirm the information about the course for doctor students and see to their proper preparation for the course.
8. Strict attention should be given to proper organisation of the lecture room. This should also be done by the Organising Committee of the given course and supervised by the Programme Director, but in this respect the Training Division could also assist in the field of teaching facilities.
9. It is advisable that the Organising Committee of the course should nominate the host of the lecture room. He should look to such details like proper utilisation of the microphones by lecturers, discussing participants, proper settlement of teaching facilities and their proper utilisation and so on.

Executive Administrator of the Course

Between many forms of postgraduate medical studies there may be courses of complex organisation for a long period, requiring constant administration and organisation direction. Independent of the Programme Director, it is required to have an Executive Administrator of the Course.

The task of the Executive Administrator is to prepare and conduct a smooth running course and to satisfy its organisational and material needs.

The Executive Administrator of the course begins his duties two weeks before the opening of the course and finishes one week after the course is completed.

Responsibilities of the Executive Administrator of the Course are:

In the Organisation Period of the Course (two weeks before the course begins). The responsibilities are to get a thorough understanding of the programme of the course and the conditions in which the course will be conducted; to learn about the accommodation and transportation requirements, teaching facilities and food or any kind of refreshments which are planned; to prepare a proper documentation of the course, a list of attendants of the student-doctors, service of attendants and all other requirements which are usually required of such a course and which a programme direction may demand.

For the good procedure of the course, the Executive Administrator should, generally speaking, remember during the preparatory period what needs are required for the sake of the programme director, lecturers, and student-doctors.

During the session of the course his responsibilities are: permanent supervision of the order and settling organisational and administrational requirements, particularly the organisational discipline of the course (time-table for lectures and the attending student-doctors); a list of attendance should be kept by the Executive Administrator to whose responsibilities also belong the permanent supervision of the teaching facilities, their technical efficiency, discipline, efficiency of the technical personnel connected with electrical services for the needs of the lecturers and the lecture room, everyday attention to the punctuality and quantity of refreshments given to the student-doctors, and also attention to the transportation arrangements for lecturers and student-doctors.

In the period after the course (one week after the course). He is responsible to give instructions connected with the accommodations used for the course, the furniture and all kinds of instruments and materials used, to look after the proper conservation of the apparatus particularly used for teaching facilities, and transfer them to the institution from which they were borrowed for the course.

He will write a short report on the course with evaluating remarks.

Criteria for Selecting for Appointment Doctors for the Residents or Assistant Registrars Posts

The following criteria or preference is to be given when selecting/appointing doctors for the Residents or Asst. Registrars posts:

1. The number of Resident jobs and Asst. Registrars jobs in the Ministry of Public Health should be known to both the Department of Hospital/Administration and the Training Division.
2. These jobs should be filled by Kuwaiti doctors.
3. If the number of Kuwaiti doctors is not sufficient to fill the vacancies, priority for appointing non-Kuwaiti doctors should be as given below:

   a) Doctors born in Kuwait, studied in Kuwaiti schools up to Secondary School and were living in Kuwait with their families;
   b) One of their parents worked as a doctor for the Government of Kuwait, in Kuwait, for 12 years at least;
   c) Doctors who have obtained their Hons. Degree at least with a very good grade.

4. Doctors appointed as Residents after April 1977 will have to do the basic rotation of:

   6 months in surgery, 6 months in medicine,
   3 months in Gynae. and Obst., 3 months in Paediatrics,
   2 months in Psychiatry and 3 months in Community medicine and Primary Health Care,

   and Imtiaz, Internship or any other training done elsewhere will not be taken into consideration.
5. *Procedure:* According to the above criteria, the Ministry should send the Residents to the Training Division once they are appointed. The Training Division will give them details about the whole training programme and decide where to post them. They will then be sent to the Director of Hospital Administration, who will take from them various details required in his office, and will then send them on to the Hospital Director of the hospital where he/she is being posted by the Training Division.

Continuing Medical Education

Continuing education based on self-education is a moral obligation of doctors. This obligation should be succoured by professionally and institutionally motivated educational activities.

Local or in-service continuing medical education is organised by each unit of the national health care system. The organisational structure of the national health care system should have an influence on the level and methodology of the local (in-service) training. The Joint Board of Postgraduate Education controls, advises and supports heads of the units (centre, hospital) in their duties of running in-service medical education.

Nation-wide (institutional) continuing medical education is organised by the Area Executive Committee for Continuing Medical Education. The nation-wide programme of education should supplement the programmes of the in-service continuing medical education.

Principles of Accreditation of Continuing Postgraduate Medical Studies

1. The effectiveness of postgraduate medical education depends on the systematic continuity of learning and of the logical problem of its performance. These two principles have a basic influence on the effectiveness of the postgraduate medical studies process. Its proper organisation should ensure economy of effort during this process, both of the learning doctors and the organisational efforts of the teachers.
2. Assuming that each practising doctor contribute at least three hours a week for his own medical study, it can be expected that during approximately 10 months of *each year* this doctor should contribute *at least 120 hours* for studying his professional problems and looking into the advances of medicine.

    Half of this time (60 hours) should be accepted as a minimum time for self-learning and the second half (60 hours) as a minimum time for taking active part in the organised postgraduate medical educational programme.

    Then we may accept that 60 hours should be accredited during a one year period and accordingly recorded.
3. The above mentioned criteria present the minimum requirements. They should be augmented by the proper Area Executive Committee on the motion given by the different Discipline Committees.
4. The number of accredited hours obligatory for post-graduate medical education should be limited by the given Discipline Committees, with the statements on which hours, and how many hours of each course should then be accredited.
5. For accreditation hours the doctor-student will be given certificates.

Recognition Awards

1. Those student-doctors on postgraduate medical education programmes who have demonstrated their commitment to the studies by attending many lectures of the programme, shall receive *Recognition Awards of the Kuwait Postgraduate Continuing Medical Education.*
2. There are 3 grades of yearly recognition awards depending on the number of credit hours achieved by a doctor, during one academic year (fiscal year), and a Certificate of Acknowledgement.

    A. Grade award
    When achieving 90—100% of all accredited hours.

    B. Grade award
    When achieving 80—89% of all accredited hours.

    C. Grade award
    When achieving 70—79% all accredited hours.

    Certificate of Acknowledgement for fulfiling the minimum requirements for accreditation of postgraduate medical studies.
3. A ceremony for presenting yearly recognition awards shall be arranged by the Joint Board of Postgraduate Medical Education.

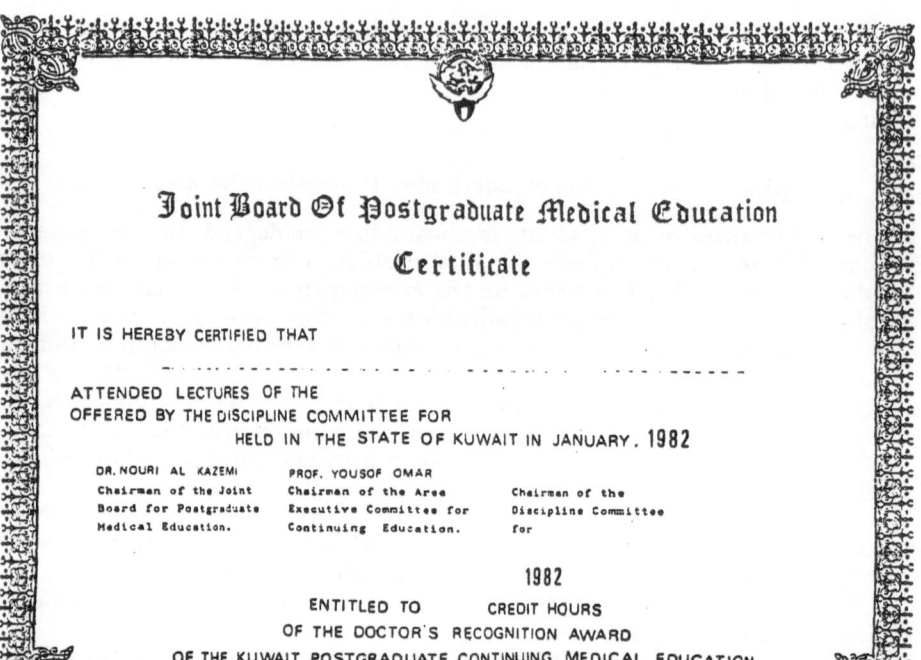

Visitors and Their Role in Postgraduate Medical Education

There will always be the need to improve skills and performance or to implement new programmes or develop new techniques. Visitors from foreign countries are to be invited to satisfy various needs in the many fields of activity of the Divisions of the Ministry of Public Health and of the Medical Faculty of Kuwait University.

Most of these purposes of inviting visitors may and should usually be linked together. This would mean that foreign visitors would be fully utilised to all purposes for which they might serve.

The Joint Board recommends the following guidelines to invite experts from abroad:

a) Doctors or units who are inviting foreign visitors should have clear and identified objectives.
b) They should have in mind all directives for the utilisation of the consultants.
c) In order to limit the total number of visitors per year, the more general lecture component of postgraduate education should be given by local staff.
d) A general education programme should be organised on one symposium per discipline per year.
e) Clinical expertise of visitors should be made available to Kuwaiti citizens who seek medical advice from overseas physicians, thus precluding the necessity of sending so many patients abroad.

Invited Visitors shall cooperate, advise and assist in various areas of activities such as:

1. Postgraduate Medical Education (lectures and clinical work)
2. Organisation methods
3. Diagnostic procedures
4. Professional consultation for particular patients
5. Administration and general management, etc.

According to the decision of the Ministry of Public Health, names of invited visitors should be submitted by the Training Division to the Undersecretary's Office in April of each year, so that appropriate administrative and financial arrangements can be made for them accordingly.

A form for each invited visitor was outlined as follows:

Form for Invitation of Foreign Lecturers (Visitor)
Academic Year: 1982—83

C.I.N.... (see page 28)

Visitor:
1. Full *name* with titles:

2. Professional *position*, address of the institution in which invited visitor works:

Programme:
1. Forms of utilisation for postgraduate education (course, seminar, conference, lecture, etc.):

2. Titles of *lectures* to be given:

3. Course Identifying Number (C.I.N.) in which the visitor will be engaged:
Reason or justification for invitation

This invitation is proposed by the Discipline Committee of: ...

General Rules Applicable to Doctors Working in the Ministry of Public Health in Relation to the Postgraduate Training Programme

— The newly qualified medical graduates who apply to work in the Ministry of Health must undergo three years compulsory professional training.
— The newly qualified graduates are advised not to do the Imtiaz, as this will not be recognized in most circumstances.
— The Kuwaiti graduates will have first preference for the training posts.
— Non-Kuwaiti doctors will be considered if vacancies are available in the training programme.
— The resident, after his appointment in the Ministry of Health, should consult the Head of the Training Division, who will allocate to him the training rota.
— New doctors will be given provisional registration. Full registration can be granted after satisfactory completion of three years of training.
— No doctor will be allowed to go abroad for clinical training on scholarship either from the Ministry of Health or from the Faculty of Medicine unless he is fully registered.
— After satisfactory completion of two years general professional training the candidate is eligible for promotion to Assistant Registrar status.

— On achieving full registration, the candidate is eligible for a Junior Registrar post.
— A candidate who satisfactorily completes the three year professional training programme will be eligible for Part I, Doctor of Medicine (D.M.) examination conducted by the Faculty of Medicine.

Leave Arrangements in Relation to the Postgraduate Training Programme

During the first year there is an allowance of three weeks leave (you can simply arrange this directly with the Head of your Department, who should agree on the dates with you). If not taken then, it cannot be taken until during the third year.

In the second year there is an allowance of 30 days leave. This leave can only be taken during the one-month linked with the two-month training programme in Psychiatry. If part or all of that one month is not taken at that time, you may spend the remainder or the whole of that month working in any hospital department of your choice. For this, you should personally arrange the matter with the head of Psychiatry and the department of choice. Please contact them early, so that they can arrange a programme for you. The difference between leave actually taken and the 30 days, can be taken during the third year or later.

In the third year there is an allowance of 30 days leave. You may also take the number of days (if any) remaining from the first and second year entitlements.

6. Course Identifying Numbers (C.I.N.)

For organisational and practical purposes all forms of postgraduate medical training shall be recorded. This will allow us to have the possibility of proper planning of postgraduate medical education, to make possible an evaluation of the whole programme of training in the country, as well as a judgement of the training activities in a given field of medical science.

C. I. N. will be composed of four particulars:
— *Teaching year* (see "Note" page 33) in which a given form of postgraduate medical education (course, seminar, conference, etc.) is performed.
— *Area* of postgraduate training
— *Speciality number*
— *Consecutive numerals* of any form of postgraduate medical education *in a given field of medical* (paramedical, nursing) *sciense.*
Symbols accepted for above mentioned particulars:
— The year in which a given form of postgraduate medical education is performed will be shown by the two last numerals of the year (teaching year = fiscal year, starts 1.7. and ends 30.6. of the next year). So the course performed in the teaching year which starts in 1980 will have the first particular of its C.I.N.—"80" even though the second half of the teaching year will be in 1981.
— The *Area* of postgraduate training will be shown by a capital letter (character) as follows:
  A — Professional training
  B — Specialisation
  C — Continuing medical education
  D — Allied health sciences personnel (paramedical) education
  E — Continuing nursing education

Speciality Identifying Numbers

Would be as follows:

in numeral order . . . Page 29
in alphabetic order . . . Page 31

01 — Basic Medical Sciences
02 — Biostatistics
03 —
04 —
05 —
06 —
07 — Immunobiology and Allergology
08 — Bacteriology and Virusology
09 — Education and Teaching Facilities
10 —
11 —
12 — Medicine (General, Internal Medicine)
13 — Cardiology
14 — Gastroenterology
15 — Pulmonology
16 — Nephrology
17 — Endocrinology
18 — Haematology
19 — Metabolic Diseases including Diabetology
20 — Rheumatology and Arthritis
21 —
22 —
23 — Surgery (General)
24 — Cardiac Surgery
25 — Thoracic Surgery
26 — Urology
27 — Orthopaedic Surgery
28 — Plastic Surgery
29 — Paediatric Surgery
30 — Neurosurgery
31 —
32 —
33 — Paediatrics
34 —
35 —
36 —
37 — Gynaecology and Obstetrics
38 —
39 — Infertility
40 — Perinatology
41 —
42 —
43 — Family Medicine
44 — Primary Health Care
45 — Intensive Care
46 —
47 — E.N.T. General
48 — Otology

49 — Rhinology
50 — Laryngology
51 — Audiology
52 —
53 —
54 — Ophthalmology
55 —
56 — Dermatology (General)
57 — Venereology
58 —
59 — Neurology,
      Neurosurgery – see 30
60 —
61 — Psychiatry and Behavioral Sciences
62 —
63 — Radiology
64 —
65 — Oncology
66 — Radiotherapy
67 — Nuclear Medicine
68 —
69 — Anaesthesiology and Analgesis
70 —
71 — Clinical Laboratory Medicine
72 —
73 — Pharmacology
74 — Toxicology
75 — Pharmacy
76 — Dentistry
77 —
78 — Infectious Diseases
79 — Parasitology
80 — Tropical Medicine
81 —
82 — Public Health
83 — Hygiene
84 — Nutrition
85 — Preventive Medicine
86 — Environmental Health
87 — Radiation Protection
88 — Epidemiology
89 — Community Medicine
90 — Industrial Medicine
91 — Professional Diseases
92 —
93 — Dietetics
94 —
95 — Occupational Therapy
96 — Physical Medicine and Rehabilitation
97 —
98 — Health Education
99 — Nursing

Speciality Identifying Numbers
In Alphabetic Order

Allergology — 07
Analgesis — 69
Anaesthesiology — 69
Anatomy — 01
Andrology — 17
Arthritis — 20
Audiology — 51

Bacteriology and Virusology — 08
Basic Medical Sciences — 01
Behavioral Sciences — 61
Biology — 01
Biochemistry — 02
Biostatistics — 02

Cardiac Surgery — 24
Cardiology — 13
Clinical Laboratory Medicine — 71
Community Medicine — 89

Dentistry — 76
Dermatology — 56
Diabetology — 19
Dietetics — 93

Education — 09
Endocrinology — 17
Environmental Health — 86
E.N.T. — 47
Epidemiology — 88

Family Medicine — 43

Gastroenterology — 14
Gynaecology and Obstetrics — 37

Health Education — 98
Haematology — 18
Hygiene — 83

Industrial Medicine — 90
Immunobiology — 07
Infectious Diseases — 78
Infertility — 39
Intensive Care — 45
Internal Medicine — 12

Laboratory Medicine — 71
Laryngology — 50

Medical Biochemistry — 01
Medicine (General) — 12
Metabolic Diseases — 19

Nephrology — 16
Neurology — 59
Neurosurgery — 30
Nuclear Medicine — 67
Nursing — 99
Nutrition — 84

Obstetrics — 37
Occupational Therapy — 95
Oncology — 65
Ophthalmology — 54
Orthopaedic Surgery — 27
Otology — 48

Paediatrics — 33
Paediatric Surgery — 29
Parasitology — 79
Pathology — 01
Perinatology — 40
Pharmacology — 73
Pharmacy — 75
Physical Medicine — 96
Physiology — 01
Plastic Surgery — 28
Preventive Medicine — 85
Primary Health Care — 44
Professional Diseases — 91
Psychiatry — 61
Public Health — 82
Pulmonology — 15

Radiology — 63
Radiotherapy — 66
Radiation Protection — 87
Rehabilitation — 96
Rheumatology — 20
Rhinology — 49

Serology — 05
Surgery — 23

Teaching facilities — 09
Thoracic Surgery — 25
Toxicology — 74
Tropical Medicine — 80

Urology — 26

Venereology — 57
Virusology — 08

The consecutive number of the course (seminar, conference, etc.) in a given field of medical science will have its normal mathematical consecutive figures.

Example of how C.I.N. is formed:

Teaching Year	Area of Training	Speciality	Consecutive number in a given field of medicine
80	A	23	12

80A—2312 this C.I.N. explains that it is the 12th course in General Surgery performed in the 1980 teaching year in the area of professional training.

Second Example

80C—1805

This C.I.N. explains that it is the 5th Course in the 1980 teaching year in haematology in the area of continuing medical education.

Third Example

80D—0803

This C.I.N. explains that it is the 3rd course in the 1980 teaching year in bacteriology and virusology in the area of education for allied health sciences (paramedical) personnel.

Fourth Example

80E—2318

This C.I.N. explains that it is the 18th course in the 1980 teaching year in continuing nursing education for nurses to work (in surgery theatre).

Note: Teaching year = fiscal year starts on the 1st of July and ends on the 30th of June the next year.
The course performed in the teaching year, which starts on the 1st July 1980 will have the first particular of its C.I.N.—"80".
The course performed in the teaching year, which starts on the 1st February 1981 will have the first particular of its C.I.N.—"80".

II. Terms of the Joint Board of Postgraduate Medical Education in Kuwait

First Term: Was established by Ministerial Decree No. 293/76 dated *2. 8. 1976.* It has functioned for 2½ years.

Second Term: Was established by Ministerial Decree No. 72/79 dated *19. 4. 1979.* It has functioned for 2 years.

Third Term: Was established by Ministerial Decree No. 168/81 dated *27. 5. 1981.* It shall function for 2 years.

Philosophy of the Activities of the Joint Board for Postgraduate Medical Education in Kuwait

The Joint Board for Postgraduate Medical Education was formed in 1976 to serve the Ministry of Public Health and the Medical Faculty of Kuwait University in organising and conducting postgraduate medical education.

This very wise decision was based on the conviction that the Faculty should cooperate by sharing its wisdom and experience of theoretical and practical approaches in teaching and general understanding of the development of science with the Ministry of Public Health, which is responsible for the level of National Health Care and should lay down initiatives and policies which would assure the best level of National Health Care.

In these circumstances the Joint Board forms a very important and most modern organisation to fulfil the expectation of the development of the high standard of the National Health Care System in Kuwait.

The members of the Joint Board are represented in equal parts from the Faculty of Medicine and the Ministry of Public Health. Three Area Committees have been formed as Executive Bodies of the Joint Board.

The *Area Executive Committee for Professional Training* was comprised of the representatives of the Faculty and of the Ministry of Public Health and should be lead, as in fact it is, by the very experienced and esteemed Chairman both in academic and professional activities.

In that period of education the young doctor would like to be still linked with University teachers. But at the same time he naturally is very keen to meet and to listen to the doctor teachers who are experienced in the work of the national health care system.

Professional training is a very important period in the formation of the doctor's attitudes. This period means that a graduated doctor has to be confronted with practical conditions of life, and execute his newly acquired knowledge in practice. This period means a more educational approach than professional teaching. Moral and ethical problems are taken into consideration during this training as well as a good understanding of the general policy of the national health care organisation.

The Area Executive Committee for Speciality Training

This Area Executive Committee is comprised of the members of the Faculty because its responsibility is traditionally linked with University activities, not only by giving recognised Diplomas and Certificates, but also by training doctors in different fields of medical specialities.

Methodological teaching for specialisation and for medical degrees is best done by the Faculty. That is why, from a scientific point of view the process of specialisation is an academic subject. But this kind of teaching should be primarily conducted in specialised departments of hospitals.

The Area Executive Committee for Continuing Medical Education

This area of medical education has to deal with a number of doctors who not only belong to different specialities and sub-specialities, but also whose professional activities and experience may be different according to their length of professional work. Postgraduate Medical Education in this field should serve directly the needs of the National Health Care system.

The advances of the medical sciences, basic and clinical, should be first checked up on and introduced into practise if conditions suit us or allow us to do it. Members of the Continuing Medical Education Area Executive Committee serve the Ministry of Public Health and should be closely linked with the organisational system of National Health Care, fulfiling the trends of the policy of the Ministry of Public Health.

Principles of Cooperation

The above laid down description persuades everyone of the importance of cooperation between the Ministry of Public Health and the Medical Faculty of Postgraduate Medical Education. There is no other way than close cooperation. It is impossible to achieve good results if this cooperation is not a full one. It is easy to understand the cooperation in ideas, but when we come to do organisational activities, we may have a lot of inconvenience which we should understand and overcome, having in mind the above mentioned principles. To escape the difficulties we should have in mind that the Joint Board is a common body which serves the Ministry of Public Health and the Faculty of Medicine, and it should be utilised by both parties as a serving body for each of them and simultaneously for both of them.

One principle should be accepted which may eliminate all normal difficulties. Namely, that instructions, information and requests will be addressed to the Joint Board Secretariat (Training Division) which should amalgamate all information and decisions to serve the general purpose of the Joint Board and to satisfy the requirements of the Ministry of Public Health and the Faculty of Medicine.

If we would use no other way of arranging postgraduate medical activities, then we would escape from a lot of problems and inconveniences. All instruction and information coming from top to bottom and from bottom to top should come through the Secretariat of the Joint Board which should specialise in the amalgamation of every disposition and assure a proper order and proper information for all concerned bodies.

If we do not keep this basic principle of cooperation, we are, in fact, hindering the formation of a good system of postgraduate medical education in the country.

III. Members of the Organisation

Decision of the Minister of Public Health on the Actual Term of
The Joint Board
27. 5. 1981—26. 5. 1983

Translation from Arabic Text (see page 37)

Ministry of Public Health
State of Kuwait

Public Health & Planning Department
Training Divison
No. 4/2/1—1036
Date: 2/6/1981

Ref: S 43/1—4526
Dated: 27. 5. 1981

Ministerial Decision No. 168/81 regarding establishment of the Joint Board on Postgraduate Medical Education.

The Minister — After going through the first item of the Ministerial Decision No. 293/76 regarding establishment of the Joint Board on Postgraduate Medical Education,
— and according to the recommendations of the above mentioned Committee, that its membership shall be rotated after a 2 year term,
— and as the Faculty of Medicine's nominated representatives are to be in the above mentioned Board,

has decided as under: —

First Item

The Joint Board on Postgraduate Medical Education is to be reconstituted as follows:

1. Dr. Nouri Z. Al-Kazemi—Chairman
2. Dr. Abdullah Al Rashied
3. Dr. Basil Al Naqeeb
4. Dr. Yousof T. Omar
} MINISTRY OF PUBLIC HEALTH

5. Dr. Abdul Razzak Al Yousof
6. Dr. Naser El Din A. Mahmoud
7. Dr. F. F. Fenech
8. Dr. Merghani Y. Ali
} FACULTY OF MEDICINE

9. Dr. E. Ruzyllo—Secretary
   Head of Training Division

Second Item

Dr. Na'il A. Al Naqeeb (Undersecretary/MPH) and Dr. Abdul Mohsen Al Yousof (Dean, Faculty of Medicine) are to be appointed as EX OFFICIO members.

Third Item

The period of membership is for two years effective from the date of this decision.

Fourth Item

This decision is to be conveyed to all those responsible to act, considering it effective from 27. 5. 1981

Sd/–
Dr. Abdul Rehman Al Awadi
H. E. THE MINISTER OF PUBLIC
HEALTH

Translation from Arabic Text

Ministerial Decree No. 413/81

Ref: S. 43/1—10701
Dated: 1st December, 1981

Minister of Public Health:

— After going through the Ministerial Decree No. 25/81 regarding two members joining the Joint Board on Postgraduate Medical Education,
— and according to the Ministerial Decree No. 186/1981 to re-form the Joint Board on Postgraduate Medical Education,
— and according to the recommendation of the above mentioned Committee, two doctors should be elected to represent (Residents/Registrars).

It was decided as under: —

First Item

1. Dr. Mohammed Ahmed Al Jarallah
2. Dr. Abdel Nabi Mohamed Hassan Al Altar
   will join the membership of this Committee.

Second Item

The Decree No. 25/80 should be cancelled.

Third Item

This decision should be informed to whom it may concern to take action from this date.

Sd/–
Dr. Abdul Rehman Al Awadi
H. E. THE MINISTER OF PUBLIC
HEALTH

Composition of the Joint Board for the Third Term
(1981—1983)

1. Dr. Nouri Z. Al Kazemi—Chairman
2. Dr. Abdullah Al Rashied   } MINISTRY OF PUBLIC
3. Dr. Basil Al Naqeeb   HEALTH
4. Dr. Yousof T. Omar

5. Dr. Abdul Razzal Al Yousof
6. Dr. Naser El Din A. Mahmoud   } FACULTY OF MEDICINE
7. Dr. F. F. Fenech
8. Dr. Merghani Y. Ali

9. Dr. E. Ruzyllo—Secretary

10. Dr. Mohammed Ahmed Al Jarallah
11. Dr. Abdel Nabi Mohamed Hassan Al   } REPRESENTATIVES OF
    Altar   RESIDENTS/REGISTRARS

Dr. Na'il Al Naqeeb
Prof. Abdul M. Abdel Razzak Al   } EX-OFFICIO
Yousof

Area Executive Committees

Area Executive Committee on Medical Professional Training

1. Professor Abdul Razzak Al Yousof—CHAIRMAN
   Head of Internal Medicine Department
   Sabah Hospital.
2. Dr. Promoda Mullick
   Consultant Paediatrician
   Paediatrics Department
   Sabah Hospital.
3. Dr. Ahmed Abu Gabal
   Head of Surgery Department
   Farwania Hospital.
4. Dr. Samir Kamel
   Head of Gynaecology and Obstetrics Dept.
   Al Adan Hospital.
5. Dr. Saleh Al Kanderi
   Deputy Head
   Infectious Diseases Hospital.

Area Executive Committee on Medical Speciality Training

1. Prof. F. Fenech—CHAIRMAN
   Chairman Dept. of Medicine
   Sabah Hospital.
2. Prof. G. M. Abouna
   Professor of Surgery
   Mubarak Al Kabir Hospital.

3. Prof. Hassan Hathout
   Head of Dept. of Gynaecology and Obstetrics
   Maternity Hospital.
4. Dr. Abdulla Rashied
   Chairman
   Dept. of Paediatrics
   Sabah Hospital.
5. Prof. P. Vassalo Agius
   Head of Dept. of Paediatrics
   Faculty of Medicine.
6. Prof. M. Khojali
   Associate Professor
   Community Medicine and Behavioural Sciences Dept.
   Faculty of Medicine.
7. Prof. S. Roy Choudhury
   Dept. of Anatomy
   Faculty of Medicine.

Area Executive Committee on Continuing Medical Education

1. Dr. Y. T. Omar—CHAIRMAN
   Head of Radiotherapy Dept.
   Sabah Hospital.
2. Dr. Naser El Din Mahmoud
   Vice Dean
   Faculty of Medicine.
3. Dr. J. B. Katheimer
   Manager, Laboratory Superintendence
   Ministry of Public Health.
4. Dr. Amin Maarafi
   Dept. of Medicine
   Al Adan Hospital.
5. Dr. Basil Al Naqeeb
   Head of Internal Medicine Dept.
   Amiri Hospital.
6. Dr. Ma'Moon Haj Ali
   Asst. Head of Unit, Maternity Hospital.
7. Dr. Nelly Fernando
   Head of Paediatric Division
   Al Adan Hospital.
8. Dr. Ja'far Ezzat
   Head of Preventive Medicine Unit
9. Dr. Joseph Cheriyan
   Dept. of Surgery
   Al Adan Hospital.

Discipline Committees

Discipline Committee for Medicine
(including Psychiatry, Dermatology)

1. Prof. F. Fenech—CHAIRMAN
   Chairman of Medicine
   Mubarak Hospital.
2. Prof. Abdul Razzak Al Yousof—VICE-CHAIRMAN
   Head of Internal Medicine Division
   Sabah Hospital.
3. Dr. Basil Al Naqeeb—SECRETARY
   Head of Gastroenterology
   Unit, Amiri Hospital.
4. Dr. Ahmed Ghamrawy, Head of
   the Internal Medicine Division
   Amiri Hospital.
5. Dr. Mohamed Kamel Amara, Head of
   the Internal Medicine Division
   Adan Hospital.
6. Dr. Ashmawi Abdul Wahab, Acting
   Head of the Internal Medicine Division
   Farwania Hospital.
7. Raid Al Nafesi, Head of Internal
   Medicine Dept., Farwania Hospital.
8. Dr. Hussein Darwish, Head of
   Psychiatric Unit, Psychiatric Hospital.
9. Dr. Mohy Al Din Salem, Head of Skin
   Diseases Division, Khaldiya Clinic.
10. Dr. Samir Mutawah, Deputy Head
    Radiotherapy Division, Sabah Hospital.
11. Dr. Abdel Raaof Lulu, Chairman, Dept.
    of Medicine, Jahra Hospital.

Discipline Committee for Surgery
(including ENT, Ophthalmology)

1. Prof. G. M. Abouna—CHAIRMAN
   Professor of Surgery
   Mubarak Al Kabir Hospital.
2. Dr. John R. McCallum—VICE-CHAIRMAN
   Head of ENT Division
   Sabah Hospital.
3. Dr. Abdulla Behbehani—SECRETARY
   Registrar "A" Surgery
   Mubarak Al Kabir Hospital.
4. Prof. Bo Eklof
   Head of Surgery Dept.
   Mubarak Al Kabir Hospital.

5. Dr. Sodad Sabri
   Head of Surgery Dept.
   Sabah Hospital.
6. Dr. Joseph Cheriyan
   Head of Surgery Dept.
   Al Adan Hospital.
7. Dr. Ahmed Abu Jabal
   Head of Surgery Dept.
   Farwania Hospital.
8. Dr. Hani Shuhibar
   Asst. Head of Heart Surgery Unit
   Chest Diseases Hospital.
9. Dr. Mohamed Al Sharief
   Head of Ophthalmology Division
   Sulaibikhat Hospital.
10. Dr. J. James
    Orthopaedic Consultant
    Sulaibikhat Hospital.
11. Dr. Moktar Al Mehdi
    Neurosurgeon
    Iben Sina Hospital.
12. Dr. Mohamed Essa
    Paediatric Surgeon
    Iben Sina Hospital.
13. Dr. Mohamed Sa'ed Al Manee
    Surgery Department
    Al Adan Hospital.
14. Dr. Mohamed Sami Khalifa
    Asst. Head of Surgery Unit
    Sabah Hospital.

Discipline Committee for Obstetrics and Gynaecology

1. Prof. Hassan Hathout—CHAIRMAN
2. Dr. Samir Mustapha Kamel—VICE-CHAIRMAN
   Head of Gynaecology and Obstetrics
   Adan Hospital.
3. Dr. Ma'meon Haj Ali, Asst.—SECRETARY
   Head of Unit, Maternity Hospital.
4. Salim Yassin, Head of Dept.
   of Gynaecology and Obstetrics
   Jahra Hospital.
5. Dr. Hani Mahmoud Auda, Acting
   Head of Gynaecology and Obstetrics Dept.,
   Farwania Hospital.
6. Dr. Saed Abdullah Al Othman, Deputy
   Director of Maternity Hospital.
7. Dr. Ali Taneer, Director of
   Maternity Hospital.
8. Dr. Talat Al Kassabi, Head of
   Gynaecology and Obstetrics Unit
   Maternity Hospital.

Discipline Committee for Paediatrics

1. Dr. Abdulla Al Rasheed—CHAIRMAN
   Head of Paediatrics Dept.
   Sabah Hospital.
2.   — VICE-CHAIRMAN
3. Dr. Promoda Mullick—SECRETARY
   Paediatric Consultant
   Sabah Hospital.
4. Dr. Yousef Nuwaiyhed, Head of
   Paediatrics Division, Amiri Hospital.
5. Dr. Nellie Fernando, Head of
   Paediatric Division, Adan Hospital.
6. Dr. Hassan Wasfi Abdul Majed
   Acting Head of Paediatrics Division
   Mubarak Hospital.
7. Dr. Aza Shaltout, Senior Registrar
   Sabah Hospital.
8. Prof. Paul Vassalle Agius
   Faculty of Medicine.
9. Dr. Mellery C. G. Hunt, Head of
   Paediatric Dept., Jahra Hospital.
10. Dr. Ahmed Fuad Khalil
    Chairman of Department
    Farwania Hospital.
11. Dr. Mohamed Abu Al Maged
    Paediatrics Orthopaedics Surgery.
12. Dr. Ghaleb Khmash
    Infectious Diseases Hospital.
13. Dr. Mohamed Essa
    Paediatric Surgeon
    Iben Sina Hospital.

Discipline Committee for Family Medicine

1. Professor of Family Medicine   — CHAIRMAN (Vacant)
2. Prof. Mustafa Khogali   — ACTING CHAIRMAN
   Associate Professor
   Community Medicine and Behavioural
   Sciences Dept.
   Faculty of Medicine
   (Dr. Khogali to withdraw when the
   new professor is appointed)
3. Dr. Ibrahim Majdi   — SECRETARY
   Bayan Health Centre.
4. Dr. Leila Dousary   — VICE CHAIRMAN
   Deputy Head
   External Medical Services Dept.
5. Dr. Saad Zaghloul   — MEMBER
   Director
   Farwania Hospital

6. Dr. Ashmawi Abdel Wahab
   Consultant, Medicine Dept.
   Farwania Hospital.
7. Dr. Mohamed Abdul-Kader Elhabali
   Maidan Hawalli Clinic.
8. Dr. Mohd Sami Matar   — EX-OFFICIO
   Head
   External Medical Services Dept.

Discipline Committee for Public Health

1. Dr. M. Sami Mattar—CHAIRMAN
   Head of External Services
   Dept., Ministry of Public Health.
2. Prof. Mustapha Khojali—VICE-CHAIRMAN
   Faculty of Medicine.
3. Dr. Ali Al Seif—SECRETARY
   Preventive Medicine Division.
4. Dr. Jaffar Ezzat, Head of
   Preventive Medicine Division.
5. Dr. Saleh Al Kandarai, Deputy
   Head of Infectious Diseases Hospital.
6. Dr. Ahmed Bayoumi, Community Medicine
   & Behavioral Sciences, Faculty of
   Medicine.
7. Dr. Mohamed Abdulhai Suliman
   Head of Dispensaries.
8. Dr. Laila Al-Dousri
   Head of M.C.H. Centre.

Discipline Committee for Radiology

1. Dr. Leo Steinhart—CHAIRMAN
   Radiology
2. Prof. Hussein M. Abdel Dayem—CO-CHAIRMAN
3. Dr. Fatemah Al Gharbawi—SECRETARY
   Mubarak Hospital.
4. Dr. Mohamed Ahmed Radwan
   Sabah Hospital.
5. Dr. Hussam Basyuni
   Sabah Hospital.
6. Dr. Mohi Din Al Tamami
   Al Adan Hospital.
7. Dr. Mohammed Shafeeq
   Farwania Hospital.
8. Dr. Mohammed Zahran
   Jahra Hospital.

Discipline Committee for Clinical Laboratory Medicine

1. Prof. Ladislav Chrobak—CHAIRMAN
   Professor of Haematology
   Faculty of Medicine.
2. Dr. Sayed Mukram Ali—VICE-CHAIRMAN
   Head of Histopathology
   Sabah Hospital.
3. Dr. Phylip Colin Reavey—SECRETARY
   Asst. Director
   Amiri Hospital.
4. Dr. Kamal Mustafa El-Hag
   Bacteriology Division
   Mubarak Al Kabeer Hospital.
5. Dr. Y. Watanabe
   Manager, Laboratory Superintendence
   Ministry of Public Health.
6. Dr. St. Lopaciuk
   Haematological Laboratory
   Ibn Sina Hospital.
7. Dr. M. S. Adnani
   Faculty of Medicine
   University of Kuwait.
8. Dr. Aida Sherbini
   Dept. of Clinical Biochemistry
   Mubarak Hospital.
9. Dr. Thomas Lipzic
   Haematological Laboratory
   Ibn Sina Hospital.

Discipline Committee for Anaesthesiology and Intensive Care

1. Dr. Mohamed Mutaweh—CHAIRMAN
   Sabah Hospital.
2. Dr. Omran Quader—VICE-CHAIRMAN
   Suliebekhat Hospital.
3. Dr. Ahmed Saed Okasha—SECRETARY
   Maternity Hospital.
4. Dr. Hussien Abdul Fatah
   Sabah Hospital.
5. Dr. M. M. Yacoub
   Mubarak Hospital.
6. Dr. Ahmed Jalal El-Gohary
   Al Adan Hospital.
7. Dr. Khairy Naguib
   Farwania Hospital.
8. Dr. A. El-Mohsen Hassanaine
   Jahra Hospital.

Training Committees

The Training Committee for Pharmacy

1. Dr. Abdulla Ali Al Khars, B.Sc., M.Sc., Ph.D.—CHAIRMAN
   Asst. Prof. Pharmacy
   Faculty of Medicine.
2. Dr. Ali Qassem Hasien—SECRETARY
3. Pharmacist Sameha Al Flage
   Pharmacy Division.
4. Pharmacist Murtada Magdass
   Pharmacy Division, Mubarak Hospital.
5. Dr. Riad Al Alami
   Head of Pharmacy Division.

The Training Committee for Dentistry

1. Dr. Mahmoud Rajaii Al Mustahi—CHAIRMAN
   Dental Centre—Kuwait.
2. Dr. Jawad Behbehani—SECRETARY
   Dental Centre—Kuwait.
3. Dr. Fatmah Al-Za'abi
   School Health—M.P.H.
4. Dr. Nahoud Al Zahain
   Dental Centre—Kuwait.

The Training Committee for Laboratory Technologists

1. Dr. J. B. Kotheimer—CHAIRMAN
   Manager, Laboratory Superintendence.
2. Dr. Thomas Lipzic—VICE-CHAIRMAN
   Consultant Haematologist,
   Al Adan Hospital.
3. Mr. Suliman Marzook—SECRETARY
   Deputy Manager, Laboratory
   Superintendence.
4. Dr. Barbara Malkiewicz-Wasowicz
   Head of Laboratory,
   Al Adan Hospital.
5. Dr. Kamal Mustafa El-Hag
   Bacteriology Division
   Mubarak Al Kabeer Hospital.
6. Dr. S. M. Ali
   Consultant Histopathologist
   Al Sabah Hospital.
7. Dr. P. R. Hira
   Consultant Parasitologist
   Infectious Diseases Hospital.

The Training Committee for Nursing

1. Miss Awatef Al Qattan—CHAIRMAN
   Head of Nurses Training and Planning Unit.
2. Miss Shoaa Said Al Essa
   Deputy Assistant Head of Nursing Dept.
   for Hospital Affairs.
3. Miss Sameera Abdulla Al Razzak Al Motaweh—SECRETARY
   Teacher in Nursing Institute.

Note: Educational assistances to Nurses see pages 309—324.

Accreditation Committee

The Joint Board at its third meeting dated 5. 7. 1981 decided to form an Accreditation Committee to accredit the conditions of the teaching hospitals and to cooperate with the Pan Arab Medical Board.

It also agreed that this Committee shall be composed of 3 Chairmen of the Area Executive Committees, a member chosen by the Chairmen from their respective Committees, and the Secretary of the Joint Board.

Decision of the Minister of Public Health on the Membership of the Accreditation Committee

Ministry of Public Health
State of Kuwait

Translation from Arabic Text

Ministerial Decree No. 445—81

Public Health and Planning Dept.   Ref: 43/1—11538
Training Division   Dated: 26. 12. 1981
No. 4/2/1/—9362

Date: 30. 12. 1981

Minister of Public Health: — After looking at the Ministerial Decree No. 168/81
                                regarding forming the Joint Board on Postgradu-
                                ate Medical Education,
                             — and according to the recommendation of the
                                above mentioned Committee to name the members
                                of the Accreditation Committee,
                             — and according to the Chairman, Joint Board opin-
                                ion,

it was decided as under:

First Item:

To form Accreditation Committee for Hospitals and Units as follows:

1. Dr. Basil Al Naqeeb   — CHAIRMAN
2. Dr. Abdel Razzak Al Yousof — MEMBER
3. Dr. F. Fenech   — MEMBER
4. Dr. Yousof T. Omar   — MEMBER

5. Dr. G. Abouna	— Member
6. Dr. Samir Kamel	— Member
7. Dr. Edward Ruzyllo	— SECRETARY

Second Item:

This Committee should work according to the rules and regulations of the Joint Board on Postgraduate Medical Education. The Committee may also seek professional assistance as and when necessary for fulfiling its function.

Third Item:

This decision should be informed to whom it may concern to take action from this date.

Sd/—
Dr. Abdul Rehman Al Awadi
H. E. THE MINISTER OF PUBLIC
HEALTH

Translation from Arabic Text

Ministry of Public Health
State of Kuwait

Ministerial Decree No. 13/82

Public Health and Planning Dept.   Ref: C 43—1—512
Training Division   Dated: 19. 1. 1982

Minister of Public Health: —   After looking at the Ministerial Decree No. 445/81 regarding forming an Accreditation Committee for hospitals and units,
—   and according to the Undersecretary's opinion,

it was decided as under: —

First Item:

1. Dr. Mahmoud Al Bader will join the membership of this Committee.
   This decision should be directed to whom it may concern to take action from this date.

Sd/—
Dr. Abdul Rehman Al Awadi
H. E. THE MINISTER OF PUBLIC
HEALTH

Composition of the Accreditation Committee

1. Dr. Basil Al Naqeeb	— CHAIRMAN
2. Dr. Abdul Razzak Al Yousof	— MEMBER
3. Dr. F. Fenech	— MEMBER
4. Dr. Yousof T. Omar	— MEMBER
5. Dr. G. M. Abouna	— MEMBER
6. Dr. Samir Mustafa Kamel	— MEMBER
7. Dr. Mahmoud Al Bader	— MEMBER
8. Dr. Edward Ruzyllo	— MEMBER AND SECRETARY

Part Two

I. Programmes of the Postgraduate Medical Studies in the Period between 1. 1. 1981—30. 6. 1982

1. Professional Training

a) for E.C.F.M.G. and V.Q.E. Examinations

81A—01/12/23/33/3701
Kuwait Miami Comprehensive Medical Education Programme. First V.Q.E. Course

Objectives:	To prepare doctors for Visa Qualifying Examination.
Place:	Al Adan Hospital.
Duration:	January 12th—May 29th, 1981.
Methods of Instruction:	Lectures: 4 hours daily (24 hours weekly), during twenty consecutive weeks. Other educational activities to be conducted at hospitals, out-patient clinics, public health departments, and industries, with active participation of faculty (guest and local) and registrants. Before the opening session registrants will receive educational material that the faculty will recommend.
Organiser:	a) The University of Miami School of Medicine. b) The Joint Board on Postgraduate Training which represents common plans, activities and responsibilities both of the Ministry of Public Health of the State of Kuwait and the Faculty of Medicine, Kuwait University.
Programme Director:	Dr. Rafael Penalver (Miami University).
Participation:	36 doctors — 32 doctors from Kuwait and 4 doctors from Bahrain.

Name	Present post and place of work
1. Dr. Abdulaziz Hamad Mohammad	Asst. Registrar Infectious Diseases Hospital

2. Dr. Khyaria M. Al Mazeedi   Asst. Registrar
                                          Mansorya Dermatology Clinic

3. Dr. Zaidan Mansoor Al Mazidi   Registrar
                                          Paediatrics, Sabah Hospital

4. Dr. Fawziyha Abdullah A. Mandani   Asst. Registrar
                                          Paediatrics, Sabah Hospital

5. Dr. Khalid Jassim Al Othman   Asst. Registrar
    Al-Khudhairi   Surgery, Amiri Hospital

6. Dr. Abdul Rahman Saleh Al Naseem   Asst. Head
                                          E.N.T., Military Hospital

7. Dr. Abdullatif A. Aziz Khalifa   Asst. Registrar
                                          Surgery, Sabah Hospital

8. Dr. Kismat Abdullah Al Matrouk   Asst. Registrar
                                          Medical Microbiology/Virology
                                          Kuwait University

9. Dr. Ghuffran Ahmad Akasha   Asst. Registrar
                                          Medicine, Sabah Hospital

10. Dr. Fahed Mohamed Al Abdulhadi   Registrar
                                          Maternity Hospital

11. Dr. Dalal Abdulaziz Al Salem   Asst. Registrar
                                          Maternity Hospital

12. Dr. Abdul Khuder Nasser Al Najdi   Registrar B.
                                          Paediatrics, Adan Hospital

13. Dr. Mohammed Mansour   Asst. Registrar
    Al-Ghanem   Paediatrics, Sabah Hospital

14. Dr. Jawad Abdulkarim H. Al   Asst. Registrar
    Momen   Paediatrics, Sabah Hospital

15. Dr. Aiad Askar B. Al Anazy   Asst. Registrar
                                          Medicine, Sabah Hospital

16. Dr. Tarik Abdul Mohsen   Asst. Registrar
    Al-Mukhaizeem   Medicine, Sabah Hospital

17. Dr. Ahmad Awad Maatooq   Registrar,
                                          Surgery, Amiri Hospital

18. Dr. Abdulla Saad Al Khattaf   Asst. Registrar
                                          Psych. Hospital

19. Dr. Abdul Razzaq Abdul Aziz Al   Asst. Registrar
    Adwani   Maternity Hospital

20. Dr. Ahmed Abdul Rahman A. Al   Registrar B.
    Rowaih   Orthopaedics, Adan Hospital

21. Dr. Hussein Mohammed Merza   Registrar
    Dashti   Surgery, Farwania Hospital

22. Dr. Nima Gholoum Nima Zaid Al   Asst. Registrar
    Awadhi   Surgery, Farwania Hospital

23. Dr. Yousef Ahmad Al Nessef   Asst. Registrar
                                          Medicine, Sabah Hospital

24. Dr. Mohammad Abbass Ridha Ali   Asst. Registrar
    Morad   Central Laboratory, Sabah Hospital

25. Dr. Adnan Ahmed Al Gharabally   Asst. Registrar
                                             Laboratory, Sabah Hospital

26. Dr. Kamel Abdul Mohsin   Asst. Registrar
     Mohammad El Reshaid El Bader   Medicine, Amiri Hospital

27. Dr. Iqbal Mohammad Al Rasheed   Asst. Registrar
                                             Paediatrics, Sabah Hospital

28. Dr. Moneira Mutlak Al Arouge   Registrar,
                                             Medicine, Amiri Hospital

29. Dr. Naima Al Ali   Asst. Registrar
                                             Surgery, Amiri Hospital

30. Dr. Farida Yassin Ali Al Ali   E.N.T. Sabah Hospital

31. Dr. Yaqoub Abdullah Saad Rashid   Registrar B.
                                             E.N.T. Sabah Hospital

32. Dr. Ali Mohammed Ahmed Hassan   Asst. Registrar
                                             Surgery, Farwania Hospital

The candidates from Bahrain

33. Dr. Abdul Jabbar Al Abbasy   M.P.H. Bahrain
34. Dr. Abdul Hadi Ebrahim   M.P.H. Bahrain
35. Dr. Layla Ameen   M.P.H. Bahrain
36. Dr. Masoud Zeerah   M.P.H. Bahrain

Programme:
Curriculum: Classification scheme for items in the curriculum: Biological structure, biochemistry, cardiology, dermatology, endocrinology, gastroenterology,
haematology, microbiology, obstetrics and gynaecology, pathology, paediatrics,
pharmacology, physiology, preventive medicine and public health, psychiatry, radiology, surgery.
Preliminary and Final Tests: Each test will consist of 180 multiple-choice type
questions. To be conducted during the first and last weeks of the course by the Programme Director.
Certificate of Attendance: A certificate stating the number of credit hours will be
presented to registrants with an attendance at lectures of 80% or higher.

81A—0902
English Language Course for Students of the First V.Q.E. Course

Objectives:	The course is to meet the needs of postgraduate doctors presently preparing for study abroad in the United States. The *immediate needs* of these postgraduate doctors is to raise their level of English to a standard which will enable them to pass the required examinations for admission to study abroad.
Place:	Training Division, Ministry of Public Health.
Duration:	The English language course is divided into 3 parts and will be given on Saturdays, Sundays, Mondays and Wednesdays between 4 p.m. and 6 p.m. *Course "A"* begins on 25. 4. 81 and ends on 4. 6. 81.

Course "B" begins on 9. 5. 81 and ends on 4. 6. 81.
Course "C" begins on 5. 6. 81 and ends on 18. 6. 81.
Course "C" is conducted for all members attending the V.Q.E. Course.
Smaller groups of doctor-students will be formed according to teaching requirements.

Organiser: Training Division, Department of Public Health and Planning, Ministry of Public Health.

Programme Director: Dr. Abdul Qatum Safi, Center for Evaluation and Measurement, Kuwait University.

Participation: Doctors who are present in V.Q.E. Course (81A—01/12/23/33/3701).

Programme: An intensive course stressing basic grammar review, and exercises in the improvement of reading and listening skills, emphasizing listening and reading comprehension skills, and the grammar for test-taking.

81A—01/12/23/33/3703
Self-Learning Seminars for After the First V.Q.E. Course Period

Objectives: The course is organised for didactic activities (self-learning, group discussions, different forms of assessment and evaluation) of student-doctors preparing for V.Q.E. examination. The self-learning course will give the student-doctors full possibilities for self-learning, and obliges them to assume moral responsibility for the full and proper use of their time for study. During this time there will also be assessment and evaluation performed.

Place: Conference Room, Training Division, Department of Public Health and Planning, and Centre of Measurement and Evaluation, Kuwait University.

Duration: 102 days, from 30th May 1981 till 8th Sept. 1981.

Organiser: Training Division, Department of Public Health and Planning, Ministry of Public Health.

Programme Director: Head of Training Division.

Participants: Student-doctors on the V.Q.E. course who applied for ECFMG and V.Q.E. examinations. (Total: 34.)

Names of doctors attending
Abdulaziz Hamad Mohammad Juwair
Zaidan Mansoor Al Mazidi
Ibrahim Abdulaziz Al Muzairi
Khalid Jassim Al Othman Al Khudhairi
Abdullatif A. Aziz Khalifa
Kismat Abdullah Al Matrouk
Ghuffran Ahmad Akasha
Fahed Mohamed Al Abdulhadi
Dalal Abdulaziz Al Salem

Abdul Khuder Nasser Al Najdi
Mohammed Mansour Al-Ghanem
Jawad Abdulkarim H. Al Momen
Aiad Askar B. Al Anazy
Tarik Abdul Mohsen Al-Mukhaizeem
Abdulla Saad Al Kataf
Abdul Razzaq Abdul Aziz Al Adwani
Ahmed Abdul Rahman A. Rowaih
Hussein Mohammed Merza Dashti
Adil Mubarak Abdullatif Al Asfour
Yousof Ahmad Al Nessef
Mohammad Abbas Ridha Ali Morad
Adnan Ahmed Al Gharabally
Kamel Abdul Mohsin Mohd El Reshaid El Bader
Iqbal Mohammad Al Rasheed
Moneira Mutlak Al Arough
Naima Yassin Mula Al Ali
Farida Yassin Ali Al Ali
Yaqoub Abdullah Saad Rhashid
Ali Mohammed Ahmed Hassan
Abdul Jabbar Al Abbasy
Abdul Hadi Ebrahim
Layla Ameen
Masoud Zeerah

Programme:

25th April, 1981 — 18th June, 1981

English Language Course
   The English Language Course is divided into 3 parts and will be given on Saturdays, Sundays, Mondays and Wednesdays, between 4 p.m. and 6 p.m.

Course "A" begins on 25. 4. 81 and ends on 4. 6. 81
Course "B" begins on 9. 5. 81 and ends on 4. 6. 81
Course "C" begins on 5. 6. 81 and ends on 18. 6. 81

Course "C" is conducted for all members attending the V.Q.E. Course.
Smaller groups of doctor-students will be formed according to teaching requirements. See 81A—0132 Course Programme.

18th June, 1981

English Language Test
   This test will be performed in the conference room of the Training Division, Department of Public Health and Planning, Dasmah.

19th June, 1981 — 26th June, 1981
   Self-learning, group discussions.

27th June, 1981

ECFMG Mock Examination
   This examination will be performed in the Kuwait University Centre for Measurement and Evaluation, in the exact conditions in which real ECFMG examinations will be performed.

28th June, 1981—3rd July, 1981

Self-learning, group discussions.

4th July, 1981

English Language Test
The English Language Test will be performed in the Centre of Measurement and Evaluation, Kuwait University, in the exact conditions in which real examinations of the English Language Test will be performed.

5th July, 1981—26th July, 1981

Self-learning, group discussion.

22nd July 1981—Official E.C.F.M.G. examination
15th August 1981—V.Q.E. mock examination
9th and 10th Sept. 1981—Official V.Q.E. examination.

To   23rd April, 1981

Dr. Nouri Al Kazemi

English Language course from 25th April till 18th June 1981
After discussions with representatives of doctor-students on the V.Q.E. course, evaluation of the English language efficiency has been done and the decision taken that doctor-students should have additional courses in the English language.
With the agreement with the Centre for Measurement and Evaluation, Kuwait University, such a course has been organised.
Please find enclosed a programme of "English Language Course" for doctor-students V.Q.E. Course (81A—0132 Course).

Self-learning post V.Q.E. course from 30th May till 8th Sept. 1981
To give the doctors full possibility of concentrating on self-learning, a special course has been organised for them. Please find enclosed programme for the course "Self-learning Post V.Q.E. Course" (81A—0107).
By organising this course, the Department of Public Health and Planning, Training Division, had in mind to keep the group of doctors together in a disciplined group obliging them to self-learning and group discussions and also performing a few evaluations during the course.
The evaluation will concern both English language efficiency and medical preparedness for final examinations. During the course the following evaluation will be performed:
The programme has been discussed with representatives of doctor-students and they agree upon it.

Dr. E. Ruzyllo
Head of Training Division

Encl: As above

81A—0104
Basic Medical Sciences Repetitorium as Preparation for the Second V.Q.E. Course

Objectives: The Repetitorium is organised for didactic activities (self-learning, group discussions) for doctors who will start their V.Q.E. Course on January 9th, 1982.

The objective of the Repetitorium is to enable doctors to refresh their knowledge of the science learned during their medical university study.

Place: Al-Adan Hospital—Didactic Area of the Training Division.

Duration: Every Thursday from 19th November, 1981 till 7th January, 1982.

Organiser: Joint Board of Postgraduate Education.

Programme Director: Head of the Training Division.

Teachers (Local Faculty):
Anatomy   Dr. Nabil Azzam
Physiology   Prof. J. S. Juggy
Pathology   Dr. M. S. Al-Adnani
Biochemistry   Dr. Farida Mohamed Ahmed Al Awadi
Microbiology   Dr. T. D. Chugh

Participation: Doctors who begin their Course for V.Q.E. in January 1982.

Programme:

Thursday, 19th November, 1981

9.00 a.m.   The Repetitorium begins at 9 o'clock on 19th November 1981. All lecturers (local Faculty) representing Anatomy, Physiology, Biochemistry, Microbiology, and Pathology will be present.
                            The chairman of the first meeting will be Prof. Nabil Azzam.
                            The aim of the first meeting is to discuss the requirements of doctor-students, and to settle the organisation of self-learning and probably group discussions. During this meeting decisions will be taken in the form of didactic activities during the period of the whole course, i.e. up to 7th January, 1982. For future meetings all Thursdays are reserved, but it should also be studied and discussed by the lecturers and doctor-students themselves.

Thursday, 26th November, 1981
The Gastrointestinal Tract and Liver

8.00 a.m.—9.50 a.m.   Anatomy: Developmental—Gross and Microscopic
10.00 a.m.—11.50 a.m.   Biochemistry and Physiology
11.50 a.m.—12.10 noon   Coffee Break
12.10 noon—2.00 p.m.   Pathology and Microbiology

Thursday, 3rd December, 1981
Cardiovascular System

8.00 a.m.—9.50 a.m.   Anatomy: Developmental—Gross and Microscopic
10.00 a.m.—11.00 a.m.   Biochemistry and Physiology
11.50 a.m.—12.10 noon   Coffee Break
12.10 noon—2.00 p.m.   Pathology and Microbiology

Thursday, 10th December, 1981
Respiratory System

8.00 a.m.—9.50 a.m.	Embryology: Development of Aortic Arches—Branchial apparatus and face Mouth, Nose-Larynx and Pharynx
10.00 a.m.—11.00 a.m.	Biochemistry—Introductory
11.50 a.m.—12.10 noon	Coffee Break
12.10 noon—2.00 p.m.	Pathology and Microbiology

Thursday, 17th December, 1981
The Genitourinary System

8.00 a.m.—9.50 a.m.	Anatomy: Developmental—Gross and Microscopic
10.00 a.m.—11.00 a.m.	Physiology
11.50 a.m.—12.10 noon	Coffee Break
12.10 noon—2.00 p.m.	Pathology and Microbiology

Thursday, 24th December, 1981
The Central and Autonomic Nervous System

8.00 a.m.—10.50 a.m.	Anatomy: Developmental—Gross and Microscopic
10.50 a.m.—11.10 a.m.	Coffee Break
11.10 a.m.—2.00 p.m.	Physiology

Thursday, 31st December, 1981
Endocrine, Metabolism and Bioenergetics

8.00 a.m.—2.00 p.m.	Physiology and Biochemistry

Thursday, 7th January, 1982

8.00 a.m.—9.50 a.m.	Behavioral Sciences
10.00 a.m.—11.50 a.m.	Biostatistics
11.50 a.m.—12.10 noon	Coffee Break
12.10 noon—2.00 p.m.	Immunology

81A—0905
English Language Course as a Preparatory Course for the Second V.Q.E. Course

Objectives: The course is to meet the needs of postgraduate doctors presently preparing for study abroad in the United States. The *immediate needs* of these postgraduate doctors is to raise their level of English to a standard which will enable them to pass the required examinations for admission to study abroad.

Place: Training Division, Ministry of Public Health.

Duration: 6 weeks, from 14th November, 1981 till 24th December, 1981.

Methodology: A language placement examination will be administered on Saturday, November 7, 1981.

Classes will begin on November 14, 1981.

Students will be divided into two groups on the basis of pretest results:

Group A: Those who perform below the mean score will meet three days a week — two hours each day.

Group B: Those who perform above the mean score will meet two days a week — two hours each day.

End of course evaluation will be carried out on Saturday, December 26, 1981.

Two language instructors (one for each group) will be needed. A third person will be asked to develop course materials before the beginning of the course. These materials will be taught together with the materials developed by the instructors during the course.

Organiser:	Training Division.
Programme Director:	Dr. Abdul Qayum Safi Centre for Evaluation and Measurement.
Participants:	Doctors who begin their course for V.Q.E. in January 1982.
Programme:	An intensive course stressing basic grammar review and exercises in the improvement of reading and listening skills, emphasizing listening and reading comprehension skills and the grammar for test-taking.

81A—01/12/23/33/3706
"Kuwait-Miami Comprehensive Medical Education Program"
Second V.Q.E. Course

Objectives: To prepare doctors for Visa Qualifying Examination.

Methods:

1. *Lectures*
Six (6) days—Saturday through Thursday.
5 hours daily, from 8.00 a.m. till 13.00 p.m. (30 hours per week), during 25 consecutive weeks, (750 hours per course).
Timing lectures. 45 minute lecture, 10 minute break after each lecture, one big break (50 minutes) during the day.
Postponement of Lectures: If for any circumstance a Visiting Professor is not able to travel to Kuwait on the dates of the schedule, the Program Director will immediately advise the Kuwait Office. For this unexpected event it is advisable to consider the possibility of extending the course after the closing session to re-schedule the lectures that were postponed.

2. *Other Educational Activities*
Shall be organised by the respective Coordinator from Kuwait as per subject being taught for the week.

3. *Basic Textbooks obligatory for the Course*
Preventive Medicine
Public Health and Preventive Medicine Review
(R. A. Penalver, Arco Publishing Co. N. Y. 1979)
Pharmacology
Handbook of Clinical Pharmacology by F. Bochner.
Medicine
Beeson, P. B. and McDermott, W., eds. Cecil-Loeb, *Textbook of Medicine,* 15th ed. Philadelphia, Saunders. 1979. 2 vol. ed.
Modern Practical Neurology by P. Scheinberg, 2nd ed.

Surgery
Principles of Surgery by Schwartz, in 2 vols.
Obstetrics and Gynaecology
Novak, E. R., Jones, G. S., and Jones, H. W. *Novak Textbook of Gynaecology,* 9th ed. Baltimore, Williams and Wilkins, 1975.
Obstetrics and Fetal Medicine by Stewart Taylor.
Paediatrics
Paediatrics by Mohsen Ziai.
Psychiatry
DSM III by the American Psychiatry Association, 1980.
Psychiatry-Pretest Self-Assessment by J. C. Nelson, 1977.
Behavioral Science in Medicine by H. R. Wiegfield.
General Review
Wright, Arthur W., Ed. *Rypin's Medical Licensure Examination,* 12th ed. Philadelphia, Lippincott, 1975.
Comprehensive—Medical   Examination/Review   Books, Vol. I, 1972.
A. *Text Books*—will be delivered to Kuwait prior to December 1, 1981. One set of text books for each registrant.
B. *Outline of Lectures*—The University of Miami Office of International Medical Education will deliver to Kuwait Airways in New York prior to December 1, 1981, outlines and handouts prepared by the faculty. Faculty members have been advised that it will not be possible to duplicate material for distribution in Kuwait.

Video recording:
Permission should be given for video recording of lectures and material for the Ministry, and the Ministry will guarantee that these will not be used except by consent of the Ministry of Public Health of Kuwait.

Duplication of Teaching Materials:
All materials brought by the faculty for the course, slides and other such teaching materials, will be made available for duplication in Kuwait. Three complete updated sets will be kept in the library of (Kuwait).

Preliminary and Final Examinations:
Each test will consist of 180 multiple-choice type questions. To be conducted during the first and last week of the course by the Programme Director.

Certificates:
Signed by His Excellency the Minister of Public Health of Kuwait and the Programme Director. Stating the number of credit hours, it will be presented at the closing session to registrants with an attendance at lectures and examinations of 75% or higher.

Programme Evaluating Criteria:
A. Individual performance of registrants: attendance, comparison of grades of preliminary and final examinations.

B. Guest Faculty performance, by subject-coordinator and registrants (to be performed during the last week of the course).

C. Program organisation (curriculum, audiovisuals materials distributed), by registrants, faculty and Programme Director.

Final Report:

To His Excellency the Minister of Public Health of the State of Kuwait and to the Vice President for Medical Affairs and Dean, University of Miami School of Medicine, the Programme Director will summarise the evaluations and formulate recommendations to strengthen and perpetuate the programme.

Memoirs:

To be printed in Miami prior to December 1982.

Place: Al Adan Hospital: Auditorium, Hospitals, Departments and Outpatients clinics.

Duration: 25 weeks, from January 9th, 1982 till July 20th, 1982.

Organiser:
a) Institute of International Medical Education, University of Miami School of Medicine.
b) The Joint Board of Postgraduate Medical Education, Kuwait.

Programme Director: Dr. Rafael Penalver (Miami University).

Registration for V.Q.E. Examination:

It is the personal responsibility of each applicant to register for the V.Q.E. Examination. According to the Educational Commission for Foreign Medical Graduates Regulations, the director of the programme will not assume any responsibility if for any reason the application form of the registrant is not accepted by the Educational Commission for Foreign Medical Graduates.

Faculty:

A. Guest Faculty—appointed by the Programme Director.

B. Local Faculty—Coordinators must be encouraged to gradually replace Guest Faculty starting in 1982.

Chief Coordinators in Kuwait:

Dr. Amin Maarafi and Dr. Mohammed Saad Almanee will jointly be the chief coordinators of the V.Q.E. Course. Their main task will be:

a) to coordinate between the local subject-coordinators and the visiting lecturers;

b) to take an interest in seeing that ultimately Kuwait will be able to take over the running of the V.Q.E. Course;

c) to see that the visitors are properly utilised during their two-week stay, especially with a programme for the second week (in continuing medical education activities), in consultation with the local subject-coordinators who have already been chosen by their respective disciplines.

Coordinators in Kuwait:
    Instructions for coordinators: see page 65

Executive Administration of the Course:
                    Mr. Raad Shakar Al-Tamimi.
                    The didactic area of the Al Adan Hospital belongs to the
                    Training Division. Mr. Sa'ed Al Nabhan, Asst. Head of
                    Administrative Affairs of the Training Division is in
                    change of this centre. This year as an administrator of the
                    didactic area of the Al Adan Hospital he nominated Mr.
                    Raad Shakar to look after and assist there with his team of
                    typists, clerks, public relations personnel (for transporta-
                    tion) and to comply with requests of the lecturers. The ca-
                    tering will be done by the hospital (Al Adan) itself.

The Role of the Training Division:
                    a) Dr. A. M. Abdel Malek, Assistant Head of the Training
                       Division, shall take care of academic activities for the
                       second V.Q.E. Course.
                    b) Dr. Sa'ed Al Nabhan will look after administrative af-
                       fairs of the V.Q.E. Course.

Participants: 25 Kuwaiti doctors who will finish two years of profession-
                    al training in December 1981.

                    Hassa Ali Yousef Al-Muzaini
                    Abdulla Haider Ben-Nekhi
                    Abdul Nabi Taher Mohamed Al Atar
                    Saleh Fahed Al Ateeqi
                    Siham Yousef Abdul Gha Four
                    Nail Subhi Nassar Al Ayoubi
                    Fawziyha A. A. Mandani
                    Wasmia Abdullah A. Al Quarani
                    Latifa Abdul Wahab Al Duaisan
                    Zahra Mohammad Ghollom Maddi
                    Khalil Abdulla Al-Awady
                    Ali Abdul Rahman A. Huwayel
                    Abdel Rashed Saleh Al Tawheed
                    Suad Ahm ed Al-Bussairi
                    Saleh Hamad Saleh Al Roomi
                    Ali Abdullah Zahir Al Hussaini
                    Jassim Mohammad Goloom Madi
                    Leila Abdullatif Al Fuza'e
                    Mohsen Abul Hassan Sadeq
                    Souad Mohamed Al Bahar
                    Masouma Habib
                    Iqbal Abdulla Al Aradi
                    Sabriya Al Langli
                    Sakina Ibrahim Haji Ibrahim
                    Abdulla Mansour.

Programme:

                    9th January—14th January, 1982
                    Introduction to the Programme
8.00 a.m.—13.00 p.m.   Opening Session

Multiple Choice Examinations in Medicine Foreign Medical Graduates in U.S.A.
Preliminary Examination

16th January—21st January, 1982

8.00 a.m.—13.00 p.m.   *Preventive Medicine*

Prof. Rafael A. Penalver, M.D.
Coordinator Dr. Ja'far Ezzat.

23rd January—4th February, 1982

8.00 a.m.—13.00 p.m.   *Physiology*

Prof. John Bullock, M.D.
Coordinator Prof. J. S. Juggy.

6th February—18th February, 1982

8.00 a.m.—13.00 p.m.   *Anatomy*

Prof. Humberto Valdes, M.D.
Coordinator Dr. Nabil A. Azzam

20th February—4th March, 1982

8.00 a.m.—13.00 p.m.   *Microbiology and Immunology*

Prof. Zigmund Kaminski
Coordinator Dr. T. D. Chugh

6th March—18th March, 1982

8.00 a.m.—13.00 p.m.   *Biochemistry*

Prof. Pamela Champe, M.D.
Coordinator Dr. Farida Mohamed Ahmed Al Awadi

20th March—1st April, 1982

8.00 a.m.—13.00 p.m.   *Pathology*

Prof. Latifa Ghandur, M.D.
Coordinator Dr. M. S. Al-Adnani

3rd April—15th April, 1982

8.00 a.m.—13.00 p.m.   *Pharmacology*

Prof. Kenneth F. Lampe, M.L.
Coordinator Prof. O. Thulesius

17th April—22nd April, 1982

8.00 a.m.—13.00 p.m.   *Gastroenterology*

Prof. Martin Kalser, M.D.
Coordinator Dr. Basil Al Naqeeb

24th April—29th April, 1982

8.00 a.m.—13.00 p.m.   *Respiratory Diseases*

Prof. Sami I. Said, M.D.
Coordinator Dr. R. Ellul-Micallef

1st May—6th May, 1982

8.00 a.m.—13.00 p.m.   *Paediatrics*

Prof. Akram Tamer, M.D.
Coordinator Dr. Promoda Mullick

8th May—13th May, 1982

8.00 a.m.—12.00 noon　*Cardiology*

Prof. Dorothy B. Linder, M.D.
Coordinator Dr. M. K. Emara

15th May—20th May, 1982

13.00 p.m.—17.00 p.m. *Haematology*

Prof. Adel Yunis, M.D.
Coordinator Dr. N. Hayat

22nd May—27th May, 1982

8.00 a.m.—13.00 p.m.　*Surgery*

Prof. Abdol Islami, M.D.
Prof. Joseph Timmes, M.D.
Coordinator Dr. Taiseer Abu N'ema

29th May—3rd June, 1982

8.00 a.m.—13.00 p.m.　*Endocrinology*

Prof. John M. McKenzie, M.D.
Coordinator Dr. A. Maarafi

5th June—10th June, 1982

8.00 a.m.—13.00 p.m.　*Neurology*

Prof. Nobel David, M.D.
Coordinator Dr. R. A. Shakir

12th June—17th June, 1982

8.00 a.m.—13.00 p.m.　*Radiology*

Prof. Edward Russell, M.D.
Coordinator Dr. Mohi Al Din Al Tamani

19th June—24th June, 1982

8.00 a.m.—13.00 p.m.　*Obstetrics and Gynaecology*

Prof. Allen McLeod, M.D.
Coordinator Dr. Ahmad Nabil Mustafa

26th June—1st July, 1982

8.00 a.m.—13.00 p.m.　*Toxicology*

Prof. Rafael A. Penalver, M.D.
Coordinator Prof. O. Thulesius

Closing Session 1st July, 1982 (Thursday)
Certificate of Attendance
　A certificate stating the number of credit hours, will be presented to registrants with an attendance at lectures of 80% or higher.

3rd July—8th July, 1982

8.00 a.m.—13.00 p.m.　*Immunology*

Dr. Scholtz
Coordinator

10th July—20th July, 1982

8.00 a.m.—13.00 p.m.　*Psychiatry and Behavioural Sciences*

Prof. Burton J. Goldstein, M.D.
Coordinator Prof. M. F. El-Islam

E.C.F.M.G. Examination—21st July, 1982

The examination of the Educational Commission for Foreign Medical Graduates (E.C.F.M.G.) is the screening examination for foreign trained physicians who wish to enter accredited graduate medical education programs in the United States. It is a one-day examination, administered in January and July of each year, consisting of 360 multiple-choice questions in Medicine, and a separate test of proficiency in the English language.

24th July—29th July, 1982

8.00 a.m.—13.00 p.m.   *Question Review*
Dr. Eric Reiss

V.Q.E. Examination—8th and 9th September, 1982

The Visa Qualifying Examination (V.Q.E.) is a two-day examination in medicine administered in *September* of each year. It was developed to meet the requirements of the 1976 and 1977 amendments to the U.S. Immigration and Nationality Act which affect the admission of alien physicians to the United States. The first day of the examination consists of questions from all major areas of the basic medical sciences. The second day is devoted to the clinical medical sciences.

Instruction
for Pleno Titulo Coordinators

General Terms

The V.Q.E. Course is conducted by a number of foreign lecturers from Miami University who come to Kuwait for two weeks. In the second week, the lecturer will be utilised for case studies, clinical rounds, lectures and other activities. To assure the success of the course and to create a good atmosphere, the guest lecturers should have their own constant partners from Kuwait as local coordinators of the teaching activities.

Because of the many subjects presented during the course, the lecturers coming from Miami will present different fields of medicine, surgery, and the basic medical sciences. The foreign lecturers may get proper contact and help from the local specialists of the given fields of medicine, surgery and sciences.

According to the agreement, the Guest Faculty (foreign lecturers) should also have educational activities during their stay in Kuwait. These should be conducted at hospitals, outpatient clinics, public health departments, industrial medicine clinics and so on, with active participation of the local faculty (coordinators) and local doctors. In this respect, the cooperation of the coordinator between the Kuwait Medical Faculty, the Chairman of the Discipline Committees and the foreign lecturers is most important.

Some of the local faculty (coordinators) may next year be the lecturers of this course, taking over the function of the foreign lecturers.

Instructions

The chief purpose of a coordinator is:

1. To create organisational conditions to satisfy the requirements of the foreign lecturer, allowing him in the most optimal way to realise the task given him by the programme director of the course.
2. To create conditions to fully utilise the wisdom of the foreign lecturer both for the Medical Faculty in Kuwait and the Hospitals of the Ministry of Public Health. To the duties of the coordinator belong creating the best didactic programme in his field of speciality for the Faculty of Medicine and other hospitals of the Ministry of Public Health. One of his final aims is to achieve the best results of training by doctors on the V.Q.E. Course.
3. To best prepare for his duties, the coordinator, after receiving information about the curriculum and topics of the coming foreign lecturers, must correspond with them personally in order to be well informed about their needs and requirements, and also for them to get acquainted with each other.
4. Before the arrival of the foreign lecturers, the coordinator should check with the Executive Administrator of the Course, so that all the needs and requirements, technical and didactical, of the foreign lecturers are fulfilled. He should also confirm the information about the doctor students concerning their proper preparation for the lectures.
5. It is most advisable that the coordinator should be present during the lecture or the visiting guest lecturer. Apart from the personal profits which he may have because of that, the basic objective is that later on he would be fully prepared for the tutor's functions in the post-course period, while the student doctors are preparing themselves for examinations.
6. The coordinator, in cooperation with the Training Division, and the Department of Public Health and Planning should prepare a programme of other educational activities to be conducted in hospitals and outpatient clinics etc., in order to get the most benefit from the contribution of the foreign visitors. Lectures and bedside practical activities have to find their proper proportion.
7. Foreign lecturers may also be used to lecture undergraduates of the Medical Faculty according to the agreement by the Dean of the Faculty.
8. One of the forms of utilisation of our esteemed foreign lecturers could be a conference or seminar which would allow a large number of doctors to hear and discuss the topics of common interest. This could also be done in cooperation with the Kuwait Medical Association.
9. Clinical rounds should be prepared in the departments of the Medical Faculty. But such teaching clinical rounds could also be arranged in some other hospitals if the coordinator found proper conditions for such an activity. In practical activities (bedside teaching, clinical rounds etc.) doctor-students of the V.Q.E. Course should also be involved. One should have in mind that this form should be used as often as possible. Practically, it means that after a theoretical lecture there should be some possibility of showing a practical approach to the problem.
10. The coordinator, having in mind a practical approach to the trainees, may also use the possibilities given by outpatient clinics. These didactic activities should be conducted, if possible, under the chairmanship of the foreign lecturer or conducted by the local doctors invited by the coordinator.
11. The coordinator should personally assist the foreign lecturers during his educational activities outside the curriculum of the course.

12. The coordinator, being the real host of the foreign lecturer in cooperation with the Training Division, may suggest a social program for him. The programme and its budget will be approved by the Civil Service Dept. of the Ministry of Public Health.

13. Finally, in his 2 weeks of cooperation with the foreign lecturer the coordinator should achieve personal professional success. He should assure the full use of the course by student doctors and other doctors in Kuwait, having in mind the labour of the whole system of national health care in Kuwait. At the end he should also make sure that the foreign lecturer is psychologically comfortable during his stay in Kuwait, and make him feel at home in cooperating with us.

14. To fulfil his duties, the coordinator should carefully read the curriculum of the course on the subject of his interest in order to write a proper programme of activities and to settle some details in advance with the foreign lecturer by correspondence.

1. Professional Training

b) Rotating Internship

First Year of Professional Training

Medicine includes dermatology, psychiatry and clinical laboratory medicine.
Surgery includes ophthalmology. E.N.T., Anaesthesiology and intensive care.

81A—12/56/61/66/7101
Medicine

General Clinical Experience During the First Year of Professional Training (Rotating Internship)

Objectives:	To train newly appointed residents in general medicine in order to:
	acquire further clinical skills and bedside techniques; undertake a number of practical procedures in history taking and general physical examination; improve his clinical knowledge; acquaint him with types of investigations and therapeutic approaches and the treatment of special diagnostic procedures.
Place:	Departments of Medicine in teaching hospitals.
Duration:	6 months.
Organiser:	The Area Executive Committee for Professional Training in collaboration with the Discipline Committee for Medicine.
Programme Director:	Head of Department of Medicine of the teaching hospital.
Participants:	Doctors appointed as Residents.
Programme:	In addition to rotations in various wards in general medicine, the candidate shall be exposed to one week in dermatology and special sessions in radiotherapy, and laboratory medicine.

The programme includes:

Clinical skills

History taking—general physical examination
Heart sounds, B.P., breath sounds, etc.
Specialised systemic physical examination
    Examination of Cardiovascular System
    Examination of Central Nervous System
    Examination of Gastrointestinal System
    Examination of the Unconscious Patient
    Examination of Respiratory System
Progress notes

Practical skills

    I.V. injection
    Veni puncture
    Drip infusion
    Blood transfusion
    Taking blood cultures

Bedside techniques

    E.C.G. recording
    Lumber puncture
    Circulation time measurement
    Hess test
    Bleeding and clotting time
    Prothrombin time
    Skin testing
    Fundoscopic examination
    Rectal examination

Special bedside techniques

    Mouth to mouth respiration
    Cardiopulmonary rescuscitation
    Nasogastric intubation and lavage

*Special Diagnostic Procedures*Paracentesis Abdominis
    Paracentesis Thoracis
    Aspiration of abscess
    Liver biopsy; attended only
    Bone marrow aspiration; attended only

Knowledge

    Diagnosis and management of the following acute medical emergencies:
    Coma
    Shock
    Haemorrhage
    Poisoning
    Cardiac failure
    Respiratory failure
    Acute renal failure
    Acute Abdomen

To learn special practical knowledge
   Reading normal E.C.G. and diagnosis of acute Myocardial Infraction
   Reading normal X-ray chest films, heart size, Pneumonia. (X-ray abdomen, Gall
   stones and renal stones)
   Interpretation of laboratory investigations
   Principles of prescribing drugs

Ward work

Punctuality
   Admission and regular in-hospital follow up of at least four beds. Participation
in all ward activities including the work rounds, teaching rounds, bed-side examinations and discussions, emergencies and outside consultations.
   Follow up of laboratory and radiology results of his/her patients in due time
and updating these results.
   Education of the patient or the family about the disease if deemed necessary by
the registrar or consultant.
   Participation in assuming night duties regularly as a member of the team, but
not assuming the final responsibility of making a disposition of the patient alone.
   Helping the nurses to handle difficult patients or procedures in the ward in the
best professional way he/she can.
   Immediate notification to a senior colleague of any serious development in the
clinical status of any ward patient.
   Preparation and submission in two copies of *at least one* well-written (or typed)
thorough review of a medical topic related to the problems of one patient worked
up by the resident during the rotation period. One copy of the report is given to and
discussed with any one of the consultants with whom the resident associates (but
prior to the evaluation time), and the other copy goes to the "Director of Education
for Medical Residents".

Other responsibilities

Attendance at all meetings scheduled for the residents' education programme.
Attendance at the departmental clinical meetings.

81A—56/1202
Dermatology

   Training in Medicine includes one week of training in Dermatology. This is to
be arranged locally by the Director of Education of the teaching hospital (see page
24) during the six months period of the training of Medicine (*attached*).

Objectives: To acquaint the residents with general clinical experience
                         in dermatology and venereology.
                         To deal with early diagnosis in these fields and to initiate a
                         proper treatment.
                         To learn how and when to seek the advise of a specialist.

Place: Dermatology Dept., Al Sabah Hospital.

Duration: One week sessions during each of the basic 6 months
                         courses of medicine.

Organiser: Area Executive Committee for Professional Training in collaboration with the Discipline Committee for Medicine.

Programme Director: Dr. Mohey El Din Selim, Head of the Department of Dermatology.

Participants: Doctors appointed as Residents (see page 24).

Programme:

Saturday: 1. Basic principles in dermatologic diagnosis (by the audio-visual aids of the American Association of Dermatology) including:
     a) How to examine a skin case.
     b) Primary cutaneous lesions (7.30—8.30).
 2. Lecture: General principles of Dermatologic therapy (by Dr. A. Rehak) (8.30—9.30).
 3. Clinical training in the outpatient clinic (9.30—1.30).

Sunday: 1. Lecture: Skin manifestations of systemic disease (by Dr. M. M. Selim) (7.30—8.30).
 2. Clinical training (8.30—12.30).
 3. Secondary cutaneous lesions (audio-visual) (12.30—1.30).

Monday: 1. Lecture: Cutaneous drug reactions (by Dr. El-Sayad) (7.30—8.30).
 2. Clinical training (8.30—9.30).
 3. Practical training in simple dermatologic interventions including:
     — Electro cautery,
     — Cryotherapy,
     — Intra lesional treatment
     — Pho chemotherapy (9.30—12.00)
 4. Popular eruptions (audio-visual) (12.00—1.30).

Tuesday: 1. Lecture: Potentially fatal skin diseases (by Dr. K. Abdul-Hafez) (7.30—8.30).
 2. Clinical training (8.30—10.30).
 3. Training in laboratory diagnostic procedures in Dermatology including:
     — Skin tests,
     — Examination of KOH preparations for fungi,
     — Microscopic examination of discharges,
     — Cytology for virus and bullous skin diseases,
     — Examination for Leishmania tropica,
     — Wood's light for diagnosis (10.30—12.30).
 4. Erythematous eruptions (audio-visual).

Wednesday: 1. Lecture on syphilis (by Dr. M. M. Selim) (7.30—8.30).
 2. Clinical training (8.30—12.30).
 3. Erythematous-squamous eruptions (audio-visual) (12.30—1.30).

Thursday: 1. Lecture: An introduction to Immunology as applied to Dermatology (by Dr. M. Derer) (7.30—8.30).
 2. Clinical training (8.30—12.30).
 3. Diseases of mucous membranes (audio-visual) (12.30—1.30).

81A—71/1203
Clinical Laboratory Medicine

Training in Medicine includes one month training in Clinical Laboratory Medicine. This is to be arranged locally by the Director of Education of the teaching hospital (see page 19) during the six month period of training of Medicine.

Objectives:	To expose residents to the types of work in Laboratory Medicine.
	To make them understand what is actually happening in the field of science.
	To get general knowledge of different branches of Laboratory Medicine, techniques and procedures.
	To get used to practice in Laboratory Medicine.
Place:	Department of Clinical Laboratory Medicine in teaching hospitals.
Duration:	One month during 6 months professional training in Medicine.
Organiser:	Area Executive Committee for Professional Training in collaboration with the Discipline Committee for Medicine and the Discipline Committee for Laboratory Medicine.
Programme Director:	Head, Department of Clinical Laboratory Medicine of the teaching hospital.
Participation:	Doctors appointed as Residents (see page 24).
Programme:	One week should be spent in one particular branch of laboratory medicine according to the choice of the candidate either in

      Histopathology
      Haematology
      Microbiology
      Biochemistry

The programme contains:
      A study of equipment and material used in the laboratory. Information regarding techniques and procedures. Demonstration of types of analysis carried on inside the laboratory. Observing, doing, reading and recording results.
      Practical lessons.

81A—23/45/47/51/6904
Surgery

General Clinical Experience During the First Year of Professional Training
(Rotating Internship)

Objectives:	The trainees in their first year of hospital practice are basically carrying out the duties and the responsibilities of the European House Surgeon or the North American Intern or First Year Resident. Consequently the objectives of this first period of exposure to surgery are to help the trainee recognise and manage common surgical problems and to understand the basic principles involved in surgical diag-

nosis and management, the indications, hazards, benefits and cost effectiveness of surgical therapy. In order to achieve these aims, the training programme during the first six months of attachment to various surgical services should be designed to cover the following three broad areas:
— Acquisition of knowledge
— Delivery of clinical care
— Acquisition of surgical skills (see programme).

Place: Departments of Surgery in teaching hospitals.

Duration: 6 months.

Organiser: Area Executive Committee for Professional Training in collaboration with Discipline Committee for Surgery.

Programme Director: Heads of the Departments of Surgery of the teaching hospitals.

Participants: Doctors appointed as Residents (see page 24).

Programme:
Acquisition of Knowledge
1. To learn how to gather accurate information and evidence of disease by good and complete history taking and thorough physical examinations. No short cuts.
2. To learn how to assemble the basic clinical data in a *problem oriented approach* in order to make intelligent surgical diagnosis. No snap diagnosis.
3. To learn to plan the appropriate investigation protocols that will help solve the patient's problems and make a more definitive diagnosis. No battery of routine investigations.
4. To learn to follow his patients hour by hour and day by day with diligence and curiosity and to be able to make objective and relevant progress reports. Surgical illness and surgical treatment are not static phenomena.
5. To learn to accept full responsibility for the physical and psychological welfare of all patients under his care.
6. To learn how to interpret the laboratory data and to relate this to the clinical problem at hand as a prelude to making intelligent surgical decisions.
7. To learn the methods and procedures required for the pre-operative preparation of patients for major surgical operations and to understand the value and the significance of good pre-operative care.
8. To understand basic physiological responses to trauma and to surgical operations and to learn how to render good postoperative care and to deal with common postoperative complications.
9. To learn how to show concern for his patients and their relatives and to handle them as fellow human beings with sympathy, tact and understanding.
10. To learn how to communicate clearly and appropriately with his patients, with his patients' relatives, with his colleagues and with his Chief and to feel and act as a responsible member of a surgical team.
11. To develop a critical mind and attitude towards all clinical problems and to learn to accept criticism of his own judgment and performance.

It is believed that the problem oriented method of medical recording is probably the best tool for helping to achieve the above objectives and it is strongly recommended that it be adopted as the standard procedure in the wards.

Delivering Good Clinical Care

The surgical trainee must learn from the start that surgical illness and surgical care have no time limits and that the work and the responsibilities of a surgeon, unlike those of a civil servant, do not stop at 1.00 p.m. but continue throughout the 24 hours. The trainee therefore must learn to visit his patients frequently and to remain within the hospital when his unit is on emergency call and to make himself available and to attend frequently to his patients whenever asked to do so by the nurse in charge or by any member of his surgical team.

Acquisition of Surgical Skills

The trainee must understand that during this stage of his surgical career he is not being trained to be a practising surgeon. When he decides to become a surgeon he will go through appropriate training for that speciality. However, he is expected to observe and participate in as many surgical procedures as his time allows and to be able to understand the anatomical, physiological and pathological basis for which these procedures are being carried out. In addition, he should learn to perform the following basic surgical skills which are part of the armamentarium of any good doctor:

1. Establishing a good intravenous line.
2. Carry out a cut down procedure.
3. Insertion of central venous catheter through peripheral vein and through subclavian vein and to understand the indications and hazards of all common intravenous fluids.
4. Asceptic catheterisation.
5. Routine scrubbing, gowning and assisting at surgery.
6. First aid, debridement, excision and dressing of wounds.
7. Splinting of fractures.
8. Indotracheal Intubation and cardio-pulmonary resuscitation.
9. The emergency management of trauma, shock and burns.
10. Protoscopy.
11. Indirect laryngoscopy.
12. Incision of an abscess.
13. Removal of superficial tumours.
14. The appropriate writing of preoperative and postoperative medications and orders.
15. Methods of wound closure and application of skin grafts.
16. Insertion of chest tubes, drainage of pleural and peritoneal fluids.
17. Supervision of surgical wounds and removal of sutures.
18. Towards the end of his surgical rotation, operations such as appendectomies may be performed under direct supervision of senior members of the staff.

Recommended Instructional Procedure and Protocols

In order to give the trainee the above knowledge and skills the following protocols are suggested:

1. Upon their joining the surgical services (and it is strongly recommended that all trainees join the service at the same time), the chairman or his designate meet the trainees to outline to them the objectives of their training, their responsibilities and to give them copies of this programme. Also, the programme of the department for clinical meetings, educational conferences, procedures, policies and do's and don'ts should be carefully outlined. This orientation and statement of purpose should take the greater part of their first day.
2. The trainees should be assigned to the various surgical wards by the chairman, taking into consideration the facilities and the staff available.

3. The chairman or his designate meet with the various consultants and the senior registrars on the surgical wards to outline and emphasize the objectives and the methods of this training programme.
4. The residents are given responsibility for the primary care of the patients in each of the wards. This should be under the supervision of the senior registrar and it should include being on call for that unit. It is recommended that for those trainees who have done six months medicine, they should be allowed to take full responsibilities including being first on call and the writing of medical orders one month after their joining the surgical service. For those trainees who have not done their medical rotation such responsibility should be given to them 2 months after their joining the surgical service. During this period of one to two months, the trainee should be accompanied by the Registrar when he is on call and all his medical orders be countersigned by his seniors.
5. The trainees in each unit will be placed under the responsibility of the senior registrar or the consultant who will be responsible for their training, conduct and evaluation.
6. The trainees will attend the surgical outpatients of their unit once per week and attend the operating theatre at least once per week.
7. The teaching programme should take the following form:
    a) Clinical and bedside teaching to be given by the consultant and/or the senior registrar in each unit twice weekly.
    b) Tutorial and/or group discussions prepared by the trainees on common surgical problems and illustrated by actual cases, once per week.
        In addition to teaching on specific cases, it is suggested that the following general topics be covered during the surgical rotation:
    a) Problem oriented medical recording,
    b) Preoperative care,
    c) Postoperative care,
    d) Use and misuse of antibiotic therapy,
    e) Treatment of wounds,
    f) Treatment of burns,
    g) Shock,
    h) Fluid and electrolyte therapy,
    i) Anaesthesia and Analgesia,
    j) Psychological and ethical problems,
    k) Abdominal trauma,
    l) Thoracic trauma,
    m) Skeletal trauma,
    n) Head and neck trauma,
    o) Surgical nutrition,
    p) Any other topic that is of special interest to a particular unit.
8. In order for the trainee to get the maximum amount of knowledge and acquire the optimal number of surgical skills, it is recommended that he should rotate through the following surgical services in addition to general surgery.

Accident and emergency	— 2 weeks
Anaesthesia	— 1 week
Intensive Care	— 1 week
E.N.T.	— 1 week
Ophthalmology	— 1 week.

While on this rotation the trainee should spend the day in one of the above services but should continue to take calls and be on night duty with his respective general surgical unit. It is recommended that in E.N.T. and Ophthalmology the majority of the time should be spent in the outpatient clinics with attendance at the ward rounds.

Evaluation

There should be 2 evaluations, one at three months and the other at six months, using the format now in existence. The evaluation should be carried out collectively with all the teaching staff on the department including the chairman, and after due discussion each candidate is called in and informed of his performance. At this time areas of improvement and other constructive criticism should be offered to the trainee. Only the results of the final evaluation are then communicated to the Division of Training in the Ministry of Health. It is recommended that in order to make the evaluation meaningful and be properly documented each trainee should have *one file* which should follow him throughout his period of training and all evaluation sheets and other comments and assessments should remain in that file at all times.

81A—54/2305
Ophthalmology

Objectives:	To expose the trainee to the speciality of Ophthalmology
	a) to create interest in the speciality so that he could choose it as a career;
	b) to expose him to the normal day-to-day work in the Eye department.
	To help him to understand and recognise the common Eye diseases which he is likely to meet as a General Practitioner in a clinic and to manage some of these simple conditions.
	Help him to recognise the Eye diseases which should be referred to the Eye department at the hospital without delay.
Place:	Department of ophthalmology in Ibn Sina Hospital.
Duration:	One week.
Organiser:	Area Executive Committee for Professional Training in collaboration with the Discipline Committee for Surgery.
Programme Director:	Head of the Department of Ophthalmology.
Participants:	Doctors appointed as Residents (see page 24).
Programme:	

Weekly Programme

1. *First day*
   a) Short lecture—"Diagnostic Methods"—30 minutes.
   b) Ward Round, diagnostic methods and squint clinic.

2. *Second day*
   a) Short lecture—"Red eye".
   b) General clinic or special clinic.

3. *Third day*
   a) Short lecture—"Visual Failure—Gradual, Sudden".
   b) General clinic or special clinic.

4. *Forth day*
   a) Short lecture—"Ocular Emergencies".
   b) Casualty.

5. *Fifth day*
   a) Short lecture—"Medical and Paediatric Ophthalmology".
   b) Operating theatre.

At the end of this period the trainee should be able to:

1. Understand and do the following examinations:
   a) Determine the visual acuity
   b) Rough field of vision
   c) Ophthalmoscopy — direct
   d) External examination of the eye by focal illumination corneal staining etc.

2. Familiarize himself with other ophthalmic diagnostic examinations:
   a) Slit lamp microscopy
   b) Recording intracular pressure
   c) Refraction-basic principles
   d) Indirect Ophthalmoscopy.

3. Casual visit to other specialised diagnostic and treatment sections:
   a) Ultra sonography
   b) Fluorescein Angiography
   c) Photocoagulation.

4. Recognise and manage ordinary casualties and ocular injuries.

5. Recognise the following common eye diseases:
   a) Squint
   b) Conditions causing red eye   — Inflammatory eye condition and glau-
                                             coma
   c) Conditions causing failure   — Cataract, external eye disease, retinal
      of vision   conditions
   d) Medical Ophthalmic problems   — Diabetes, hypertension, endocrine
                                             exophthalmos, neuro ophthalmos, op-
                                             tic atrophy and papilaodema.

6. Have some idea about the common ophthalmic operations.
   a) Cataract
   b) Glaucoma
   c) Squint.

7. Familiarize himself with the routine ward work by going on a ward round.

81A—47/2306
E.N.T.

Objectives: To acquaint the residents with general clinical experience
                     in ophthalmology.

Place: E.N.T. Department, Al Sabah Hospital.

Duration: One week.

Organiser:	Area executive Committee for Professional Training in collaboration with the Discipline Committee for Surgery.
Programme Director:	Dr. John McCallum F.R.C.S., Head of E.N.T. Dept. Sabah Hospital.
Participants:	Doctors appointed as Residents (see page 24).

Programme:

Before coming to the department they should prepare themselves by revising the formal lectures given during the undergraduate programme.

We must bear in mind that the objective is not towards training as E.N.T. specialists but to attempt to familiarise them with the common diseases in our speciality and how these should be treated.

To recognise E.N.T. conditions that require urgent referral or consultation.

As far as opportunity during this week allows, to demonstrate the management of E.N.T. emergencies such as laryngeal stridor, severe epistaxis, acute otitis media and swallowed foreign bodies.

Although in my opinion all their teaching to achieve these objectives should be in the outpatient department, to maintain their interest I will arrange one morning during this week to demonstrate minor and intermediate surgical procedures.

As more acute conditions tend to present themselves in the afternoon and evening, the trainees should spend two or three afternoons in the E.N.T. casualty department on days when they are not on emergency duty with their general surgery department.

General Programme:

On the first day they should report to the Head of the Department, who will give a short talk outlining the objectives of the week's programme.

They will then be attached to a senior member of the staff in the outpatient department. Unfortunately, because senior members of the staff spend part of their time in the new hospitals, it is impossible to arrange for the trainees to be with the same one every day.

Methods of examination of the upper respiratory tract will be demonstrated, but it is impossible to teach any one the use of the head minor in one week. They will, however, become familiar with the use of the electric otoscope, and by the end of the programme should become proficient in recognising a normal ear drum and obvious perforations.

Tutorial instruction will be given during the demonstrations on clinical cases by the doctor they are assigned to.

81A—69/45/2307
Anaesthesiology and Intensive Care

During a one month period the programme should include:
1. Teaching basic Anaesthesia.
2. Attending Theatre Sessions.
3. C.P.R. Training.
4. Attending Anaesthesia for Emergencies.

Introduction:

This training will take place in one of the general hospitals, and will give the trainee the opportunity to obtain training in different specialities, without the need for highly sophisticated anaesthetic techniques carried out in the specialised hospitals.

Duration of training: One continuous month to be specified for the speciality of anaesthesia and intensive care therapy; this month should not be included either in the surgery or medicine training periods.

Objectives of Training:
1. To attract newly qualified trainees to the art of anaesthesia and Intensive Care.
2. To introduce them to anaesthetic management, and choice of anaesthesia for surgical patients including preoperative and postoperative care.
3. To introduce them to the intensive care setup, the general principles of monitoring and the management of critically ill patients.
4. To train them in cardiopulmonary resuscitation including endotracheal intubation, cardiac compression, defibrillation, use of emergency drugs and the general setup of a proper resuscitation room.

Syllabus of Professional Training in Anaesthetics, Intensive Care and Resuscitation.
A.   *Anaesthetics:*
1* *Pharmacology:*
   a) Pharmacology of general Anaesthetic agents
      1. The anaesthetic gases.
      2. The volatile anaesthetic agents.
      3. Non-anaesthetic gases used in Anaesthesia.
      4. Intravenous anaesthetics.
   b) Pharmacology of muscle relaxants.
   c) Pharmacology of sympathomimetic agents and adrenergic blocking agents.

2* *Anaesthetic Machines and Apparatus:*
   a) Supply of Compressed Gases.
   b) Reducing Valves.
   c) Flow Meters.
   d) Vaporisers.
   e) Delivery of gases and vapours to the patient
      Magill attachment
      Non-return valve
      Closed circuit.

3* *Pre-Anaesthetic Examination and Therapy:*
   a) Anaesthesia out-patient clinic.
   b) Pre-anaesthetic examination.
   c) Preparation for anaesthesia and operation.
   d) Premedication: Reasons for premedication—pharmacology of premedication drugs.
   e) Identification of patient.

4* *Intravenous Therapy:*
   Apparatus and technique I.V. cannulation and C.V.P.
   Choice of infusion fluid.
   Blood transfusion.
   Estimation of blood loss.

5* *The Administration of a General Anaesthetic:*
   Induction of anaesthesia.
   The signs of anaesthesia.
   Maintenance.

6* *Endotracheal Intubation:*
Indications.
Anaesthesia for intubation.
Position for intubation.
Apparatus for intubation.
Technique of E.T.I.
Complications.

7* *The Prevention and Treatment of Complications during Anaesthesia:*
Complications during induction.
Complications during maintenance.

8* *Recovery Room—Aftercare of Patients:*
Criteria for Recovery.
Oxygen Therapy.
Management of complications.
Pain relief.
Restlessness.

9* *Anaesthesia for the Outpatient:*
Precautions before anaesthesia.
Anaesthetic techniques.

10* *Emergency Anaesthesia:*
Problems.
Anaesthetic management.

11* *Selected Local and Regional Techniques:*
Local analgesic agents with dosage, toxic effects.
Preparation for local analgesia.
Subarachnoid analgesic epidural analgesia.
I.V. regional analgesia.

12* *Mishaps and their Medico-Legal Aspects:*
Consent form.
Mishaps associated with injections.
Mishaps due to respiratory obstruction.
Vomiting and aspiration.
Peripheral nerve injuries.
Explosions—safety in operating theatres.

B. *Intensive Care:*
Introduction to general setups of an ideal intensive care unit.
Indications for admission to intensive care unit.
Monitoring—including interpretation of blood gas analysis.
Artificial ventilation and ventilators.
Indications for artificial ventilation.
Tracheostomy.

C. *Cardio-Pulmonary Resuscitation:*
a) Maintenance of clear air way.
b) Emergency drugs.
c) Cardiac compression procedure.
d) Defibrillation.
e) The general setup of a resuscitation room.

Control of Attendance and Final Evaluation:

1. A special card will be prepared for every trainee to be signed daily by the Consultant in charge.
2. During the month of training attendance should not be less than 75% of the total period or else the whole period should be repeated.
3. Final evaluation of the trainee will be carried out at the end of the training period by two consultants, the trainee should score not less than 70% on the evaluation test.

1. Professional Training

b) Rotating Internship

Second Year of Professional Training

During the second year of professional training the trainee will have to do the basic rotation of:

3 months in Gynaecology and Obstetrics
3 months in Paediatrics
2 months in Psychiatry
3 months in Community Medicine and Primary Health Care
1 month (optional) in Clinical Laboratory Medicine

81A—3308
Paediatrics

General Clinical Experience During the 2nd Year of Professional Training
(Rotating Internship)

Objectives:	To train residents in second year-clinical skills and experience in general paediatrics. To identify organ or system disturbance and congenital anomalies. To help him to manage and diagnose problems in infancy and childhood. To practise paediatric procedures and management of paediatric emergencies. To know nutritional requirements in infancy and childhood and management of nutritional deficiencies.
Place:	Paediatric department, Al Sabah Hospital.
Duration:	3 months.
Organiser:	Discipline Committee for Paediatrics.
Participants:	Doctors appointed as Residents.

Programme:

Rotation in general paediatric wards, neonatology and outpatient clinics, observe interpretation and participation in duties, clinical rounds meetings and lectures.

A group of residents will be divided into 4 subgroups: A, B, C, D, and will be attached as follows:

	General Paediatrics	Neonatology	Outpatient
3 weeks	A + B	C	D
3 weeks	A + B	D	C
3 weeks	C + D	A	B
3 weeks	C + D	B	A

General Paediatrics:

The resident will be attached in rotation to one of the paediatric consultants who will supervise his clinical training in paediatrics in wards. During these hours he/she will learn to observe and interpret alterations in sick children, and combine these data with the result of investigations to reach definite diagnosis and plan rational therapy.

The following points will be emphasized:

1. The gradual physiological maturation of different organs and systems which influence both host response to pathological situations and tolerance of therapeutic agents.
2. Points in history and examination which help to identify an organ or system which is disturbed.
3. Symptoms and signs of infection in infants and children.
4. Selection of proper investigatory procedures.
5. Recognition of life threatening congenital anomalies for which urgent attention is needed.
6. Nutritional requirements of infants and children and the management of the common nutritional deficiency states.
7. Interpretation of laboratory results and urgent radiological investigations.
8. Training in practical paediatric procedures such as venepuncture, venous cut-down, lumber puncture, resuscitation, etc.
9. Management of paediatric emergencies, e.g. acute abdominal trauma, poisonings, laryngeal obstruction, respiratory distress, heart failure, management of coma, convulsions, dehydration and acid/base disturbances.

Experience and knowledge gained in the ward will be supplemented by seminars and lectures on a twice weekly basis in addition to the weekly clinical paediatric meeting.

During the 3 week period the trainee doctor spends time getting some knowledge of neonatal problems. He will be trained to recognise, to initiate emergency care and to seek specialist consultation for the following neonatal conditions:

1. Birth injuries — traumatic and asphyxial
2. Respiratory distress
3. Major congenital malformations
4. Jaundice
5. Anaemia (acute and chronic)
6. Hypoglycaemia
7. Hypothermia
8. Infections: local and general
9. Hypocalcaemia
10. Seizures
11. Low birth weight babies (including preterm and late-for-date infants)
12. Infants of diabetic mothers
13. Infants born after difficult and prolonged labour

14. Assessment of babies admitted from outside the Maternity hospital. These above mentioned conditions will be made familiar to them through a series of didactic lectures, case demonstrations and follow-up examinations.

In addition to this the doctors will be made acquainted with the following procedures and techniques:

1. The art of history taking in a neonatal set-up.
2. Complete physical examinations including identification of above abnormal states/behaviour.
3. Normal newborn care in the delivery room and nursery including care of the skin, eyes and umbilical cord.
4. Technique of immediate postnatal assessment (Apgar scoring).
5. Resuscitation of newborn (principles and practice).
6. Venepuncture, labour puncture and cannulation of Umb. vessels.
7. Feeding practice: technique of breast feeding artificial feeding and orogastric and nasogastric feeding.

Paediatric Outpatient Training:

Doctors assigned to this subgroup will be attached to Consultants and Senior Registrars or specialist clinics during their consultation in order to gain experience in the management of chronic disorders such as asthma, nephrosis, epilepsy and chronic C.N.S. disorders, rheumatic and congenital heart disease endocrine disorders, etc.

They will also spend 2 days per week participating in the general outpatient reception service to learn the management of minor illnesses and the disposal of the critically ill child.

All doctors in these four subgroups will have to participate in the duty roster under the supervision of the doctor on call for the wards, and the Registrar on duty for the day.

81 A–3709
Gynaecology and Obstetrics

General Clinical Experience During the 2nd Year of Professional Training
(Rotating Internship)

Objectives:	To give residents in the second year exposure to gynaecology and obstetrics.
	To help him to recognise and manage gynaecological problems.
	To acquire skill in obstetric examination and normal delivery.
	To detect and manage an emergency, and first aid in gynaecology and obstetrics.
Place:	Maternity Hospital's various wards.
Duration:	3 months.
Organiser:	Discipline Committee for Gynaecology and Obstetrics.
Programme Director:	Head of the Dept. of Gynaecology and Obstetrics of the teaching hospital.
Participants:	Doctors appointed as Residents.

Programme:
Covers activities in reception room, labour room, operating theatre, clinics, gynaecology wards (with in-patients), formal lectures, rounds, seminars and clinical meetings.

Apart from weekly teaching rounds and weekly lectures, the residents also attend the other scientific hospital activities.

N.B. Lectures are not the main teaching medium, but small group contact.

1. *Fields of Training:*
   Reception room
   Labour room
   Operating theatre
   Clinic
   Ancillary Services
   Gynaecology and lying-in wards
   Lecture room

2. *Agents of Training:*
   Cognitive knowledge (lectures and introductory talk to items in "Fields of Training" (1) except "lecture room")
   Acquisition of psychomotor skills for items in "Fields of Training" (1) except "lecture room" (check list)
   Behavioural attitudes
   Evaluation

3. *Reception Room:*

The ethics and routine of patient reception	
History taking and recording	(do)
Gynaecological examination	(do)
Obstetric examination with aseptic precautions	(do)
The detection and management of an emergency— first aid—alerting other stations—recruiting blood donors	(do)
Referral procedure	(do)

4. *Labour Room:*

Intranatal care and record	(do)	
Conducting normal labour	(do)	
Episiotomy and repair	(do)	
Diagnosis of position and presentation	(do under supervision)	
Normal		
Abnormal		
Diagnosis of maternal and foetal well-being:		
Clinical Detection and management	clinicians	(do)
monitor- of the abnormal	residents	(watch)
ing		
Catheterisation	(do)	
Delivery by the ventouse	(under supervision)	
Forceps delivery	(assist)	
Caesarean section	(assist)	
Breach extraction	(assist)	
Managing the third stage	(do under supervision)	
The fourth stage	(do)	
Detection of puerperal trauma	(assist)	

Diagnosing and managing P.P.H.	(assist)
Toxaemia and Eclampsia management	(assist)
A.R.M.	(under supervision)
Oxytocic drip technique	(under supervision)
Immediate care of the newborn	(do with supervision)

5. *Operating Theatre:*

Theatre discipline	(know)
Scrubbing	(do)
E.U.A.	(do)
D and C	(do)
Evacuation	(do under supervision)
Minor vaginal operations	(do under supervision)
Major vaginal operations	(assist)
Laparotomy and Laparoscopy	(assist)
Documentation	(do)
Postoperative prescription	(do under supervision)
Venous cut down	(do under supervision)
Management of coagulopathy	(do under supervision)
Management of cardiac arrest	(demonstration and simulated practical)

6. *Outpatient:*

Case sheet record	(do)
Patient examination general	(do)
speculum	(do)
bimanual	(do under supervision)
Taking vaginal smear	(do)
Prescription	(do under supervision)
Cautery	(do under supervision)
Insufflation	(do under supervision)
Endometrial biopsy	(do under supervision)
Insert and remove intrauterine device	(do)
Surgical follow up	(do)
Antenatal care and diagnosis	(do)
Picking out the abnormal	(do under supervision)
Attending medical obstetrical clinic	(do)
Postnatal follow up	(do)
Referral to and from clinic	(do under supervision)

7. *Wards:*

Sheet and progressive notes	(do)
Clinical teaching rounds	(attend)
Pre- and postoperative care	(do under supervision)
Specimen collection	(do)
Aseptic dressing	(do)
Discharge documentation and instruction	(do under supervision)

8. *Ancillary Services:*

X-ray hystero salpinography	(do under supervision)
Cytology	(demonstration)
Pathology	(talk and demonstration)

9. *Lectures:*

Provisional, subject to continual review, suggested duration of lecture: 2 hours, two per week during working hours. Candidates will also attend the scientific programme of Uv. Hospital (conference and lectures, etc.)

Essentials of reproductive biology	Physiology of pregnancy
Genital inflammation	abortion
Congenital anomalies of genital tract	ectopic and molar pregnancy
Sterility and Family Planning	Haemorrhages of late pregnancy
Ethical and legal aspects of Ob. Gyn.	Toxaemia and eclampsia
Displacements	Medical diseases with pregnancy
Menstrual anomalies	Malpresentations
Tumours	Labour and its management
Laboratory aids in our work (by lab. staff)	Operative delivery
Electrolyte and fluid balance	
Shock	
Other topics	

81A—89/44/02/88/78/95/90/8610
Community Medicine and Primary Health Care

General Clinical Experience During the 2nd Year of Professional Training
(Rotating Internship)

Objectives: To acquaint the recently qualified doctors with the different disciplines of Community Medicine in theory, in its present practical application in Kuwait Society and in its adaptation to the changes that are taking place within the society which are effecting the disease patterns and the mechanisms of health delivery.

To get acquainted with disciplines of Community Medicine and practical applications.

To recognise factors affecting disease patterns and community studies.

To practice in primary health care centres.

Place: Department of External Health Services, Polyclinics, M.C.H. Centres and Preventive Divisions.

Duration: 3 months.

Organiser: Discipline Committee for Community Medicine and Primary Health Care.

Programme Director: Dr. Mustafa Sadek, Dr. Jaffar Ezzat.

Participation: Doctors appointed as Residents.

Programme: The 3 months course has been divided equally between Community Medicine and P.H. Care
6 weeks for Community Medicine (A) comprising Community Studies, Vital Health Statistics, Epidemiology and Disease Control and Occupational Health
6 weeks for Primary Health Care (B) covering work in Polyclinics. Maternity and Child Health Centres and Diabetes (C) Clinics

Community Medicine

Daily hours 7.30 a.m.—1.00 p.m.

Week 1

1. Concepts of Community Medicine
2. Social Medicine as applied to Kuwait
3. Biostatistics and Introduction to use of Computer
4. Vital Statistics
5. Introduction to Computer

Week 2

1. Epidemiology
2. Methods of Epidemiology
3. Applied Epidemiology

Week 3

1. Principles of Disease Control
2. Epidemiology of Infectious Diseases
3. Nesocomial Infection

Week 4

1. Epidemiology of Non-Communicable Diseases
2. Planning of Health Services
3. School Health

Week 5

1. Philosophy of Occupational Health
2. Occupational Diseases
3. Environmental Stress (Heat)
4. Environmental Pollution
5. Environment and Health
6. General Housing/Sanitation Problems
7. Food/Milk/Water Hygiene

Week 6

1. Port and Border Health
2. Tuberculosis Control Unit
3. Public Health Laboratories
4. Evaluation—Principles of Evaluation

Attachments:
There will be 36 hours of clinical attachment to the health centres and Infectious Diseases Hospital in the afternoon. A detailed time table will be issued at the beginning of the course.

Primary Health Care—Six Months

Primary Health Care is an integrated comprehensive service (curative and preventive) provided by a family physician and health team to the individual family and local community at the health centre peripheral level, incorporating the functions of the lower tier of the health care delivery system.

The primary care physician should have total responsibility for his practice population in the defined area of the health centre, and for a patient who is referred on a temporary basis until he goes back to his own primary physician for continuing care.

A health centre should be regarded as a unit with different and complementary functions which enable hospitals to be less overloaded and more efficient.

The family physician should not be regarded as a doctor treating minor illness (second class doctor), referring the patient to the hospital doctor (first class doctor).

The primary care physician and his team constitute the front line task force for providing community health care encompassing all medical specialities.

He should be trained as a specialist on his own merit; he should not be considered as taking care of simple problems and referring the more complex problems to a consultant specialist.

The family physician or primary care specialist must know enough about all health problems from the prespective of different specialists to enable him to make right decisions to meet the health needs of the community. This entails training him to be competent to handle all health problems at the local level efficiently.

The aim of this section of the course, the six-week programme in primary care, is to highlight certain clinical subjects as practiced in the context of primary care at the health centre level and to inculate certain desirable attitudes in the mind of the trainee.

This will be achieved by a panel of primary care physicians within the health service.

The trainees are attached to them for the whole six weeks spent as follows:

1- Four days a week participation in the daily work of the tutor at the health centre under his supervision
1-1 One week in the Child Welfare Centre
1-2 One week in the Mother Welfare Centre
1-3 One week in the Diabetic Centre
1-4 Three weeks in the Primary Health Care Centre
2- Two days a week of academic training *in the form of seminars* (39 1½ hour sessions at the rate of 4½ hours a day). All the tutors attend these sessions which take the form of:

i) Pre-selected reading material
ii) Prepared audio-visual material from the Audio-Visual Library of the Royal College of General Practice
iii) Group discussions with relevant specialists.

81A—6111
Psychiatry—2 Months

General Clinical Experience During the 2nd Year of Professional Training (Rotating Internship)

The resident doctor will work full time in the Psychological Medicine Hospital of Kuwait for a period of two months. His training will be based on the premise that he has had little instruction in the behavioural sciences or in psychiatry during his undergraduate years. It would therefore be necessary for the instructor to provide him with a minimal amount of pertinent information, laying special emphasis on those topics which are thought to be of particular relevance to their future assignments, e.g. general practice or specialist duties.

Training Schedule
I. *Lectures—Tutorials:*
   1. Three weekly lectures of 50 minutes each will be delivered with 10 minutes left for discussion. Audio-visual methods will be made use of as much as the facilities allow.
   2. The course will consist of 21 lectures covering the following general subjects:
   A. Introductory Part
   B. The Neuroses
   C. The Psychoses
II. *Clinical Training*
III. *Psychiatric procedures*

81A—7112
Clinical Laboratory Medicine

During the second year, any resident can arrange individually to spend his/her "optional month" in Laboratory Medicine. Such optional months can only arise in the periods, 16 May—15 June, 16 August—15 September, 16 November—15 December, or 16 February—15 March. Individual residents can apply to the Laboratory Medicine Dept., for such an attachment, and if the arrangement is made, the doctor's name should be passed to the Director of Hospitals Administration (so that they will know that such doctors are attending the Laboratory and not taking their optional leave at that time).

1. Professional Training

c) Assistant Registrarship

Third Year of Professional Training

81A—12/23/33/37/69/7113

1. General Idea of the Training

The third year of the professional training programme (Assistant-Registrarship) is in fact the first year of specialisation.

This year of training should be devoted to basic fields of medicine, such as

medicine (general)
surgery (general)
paediatrics
psychiatry
gynaecology and obstetrics
public health
laboratory medicine

Those doctors who have chosen their fields of subspeciality should be trained:

in *general medicine* if they intend to specialise in

internal medicine	12 months
cardiology	12 months
gastroenterology	12 months
pulmonology (including tuberculosis)	12 months
nephrology	12 months
endocrinology	12 months
haematology	12 months
metabolic diseases (including diabetology)	12 months
rheumatology	12 months
tropical medicine (including medical parasitology)	12 months
neurology	12 months
psychiatry	6 months
dermatology	6 months
anaesthesiology	3 months

in *general surgery* it they intend to specialise in

general surgery	12 months
cardio-vascular	12 months
orthopaedics	12 months
urology	12 months
neurosurgery	12 months
plastic	12 months
E.N.T.	6 months
ophthalmology	6 months
anaesthesiology	3 months

in *paediatrics* if they intend to specialise in

paediatrics	12 months

in *psychiatry* if they intend to specialise in

psychiatry	6 months

in *gynaecology and obstetrics*	12 months
in *public health*	12 months
in *anaesthesiology*	6 months
in *laboratory medicine*	12 months

2. Methodology

There is no detailed programme of lectures as such, but doctors should learn as they work. The third year of professional training is to give the doctor another opportunity to work in the basic fields of medicine and also to have him exposed to some of the subspecialities so that he is more able to make up his mind as to which of the sub-specialities he wishes to specialise in. It is also believed that this period of training will give the trainee a brief, informative and useful contact with other sub-specialities which is an important part of the training of any doctor. If any additional theoretical grounding is needed, this should be through one of the teaching programmes designed for that purpose, e.g. the introductory courses of D.M., M.R.C. or F.R.C.S. But the point should be made that each of these assistant registrars should participate more actively in the different scientific meetings and activities of the department.

During the third year of professional training (Assistant Registrarship) they will undertake one of the following attachments:

a hospital attachment, or
a general practice attachment, or
a basic medical science attachment.

In addition, a "primary type" basic medical science course will be offered annually by the Faculty of Medicine for those doctors who have successfully completed the first two years of the general training programme.

By the end of the year the resident should have taken part in all but the most extensive or complicated diagnostic and operative procedures, mainly assisting, but later assisted by, a senior colleague in some major but straightforward operations and professional activities. Residents should regularly attend a weekly departmental clinico-pathological conference to discuss cases of particular interest, morbidity, mortality and relevance to the routine of the work and modifications thereof. Each resident should prepare and present (singly or as a panel with two colleagues) a thesis including a full study of a topic chosen by his clinical supervisor and under his guidance.

Practicability of the Defined Objectives:

1. Candidates are to work full-time in the wards as assistant-registrars.
2. They should admit patients, take medical history, do clinical examinations and write case-sheets, order relevant investigations and institute treatment after consultation with a senior doctor.
3. They should present the case during ward rounds the following day and take part in the clinical discussion.
4. To follow up the patient until discharge and thereafter in the outpatient clinic.
5. To carry out practical procedures in the wards, like setting up I.V. drips, taking blood samples, doing lumber punctures, pleural aspirations, bone-marrow biopsy etc.
6. To observe and participate in as many surgical procedures as possible in order to learn to perform basic surgical skills.

7. To write and maintain proper clinical records.
8. To write a summary of each patient on discharge.
9. To take part in the outpatient clinic and examine new cases as well as follow up old ones under the guidance of a senior registrar or consultant.
10. To take part in emergency duties, including night duties by rotation.
11. To take part in ward seminars.

3. Laboratory Medicine—12 Months

The candidate should do rotational training in all subdivisions of pathology either by rotating for 3 months in each discipline or 6 months in two branches of Pathology according to the individual requirement.

4. Public Health—12 Months

Doctors who wish to work in future in the field of public health will have the third year of the professional training programme in the field of community medicine and primary health care. The one-year programme is divided into two periods each for 6 months.

I. *First Six Months:*
Community Medicine—Epidemiology
Biostatistics
Environmental Health
Occupational Health
Maternal and Child Health
Tuberculosis Control
Infectious Diseases Hospital
School Health
Nutrition Unit
Port and Border Health

II. *Second Six Months:*
Primary Health Care— General Medical Practice
Maternal and Child Health
Chronic Diseases (Diabetic Clinic)
School Health
X-ray
Laboratory

81B—1201
2. Speciality Training

Part I and II of the Course Preparing for the Examination for Membership of the Royal College of Physicians (M.R.C.P.—U.K.)

Objectives:	Course preparation for Mock examination towards Part I and Part II of the membership examination of the Royal College of Physicians (London).
Place:	Medical Wards of Al Sabah Hospital, Farwania Hospital, Ahmadi Hospital, Amiri Hospital and Adan Hospital.

Part I Course: Lectures will be held on Saturdays and Wednesdays in the Faculty of Medicine, Lecture Room 105.
Part II Course: The clinical sessions will be carried out on Thursdays.

Duration:	From 3. 1. 1981 till 15. 5. 1981.
Organiser:	Department of Medicine, University of Kuwait in collaboration with Ministry of Health, Kuwait.
Programme Director:	Professor F. F. Fenech.
Coordinator:	Dr. R. Shakir.
Participants:	21 doctors (for list of names see page 97).
Programme:	

Lectures and Clinical Sessions

a) The lectures will be held between 4.30 p.m. and 6.30 p.m. There will be a session on Tuesday, 24th February 1981.

b) The clinical sessions will be conducted between 10.00 a.m. and 12.00 noon.

Doctors are divided into two groups, A and B, and they will alternate on Thursday mornings. For the names for each doctors' group see page 97. Each Thursday two candidates have to come an hour before starting time of the clinical sessions to do long cases, at the end of which the cases will be discussed with them in the presence of the particular group. The names of each doctor and their dates are also attached.

Saturday, 3. 1. 1981	Applied pulmonary physiology—whole and regional lung function	Dr. Mustafa Khatem
	Pulmonary tuberculosis—concepts in management	Dr. M. Shaaban
Wednesday, 7. 1. 1981	Occupational allergic and non-allergic lung disease	Dr. M. Khogali
	Granulomatous and fibrosing lung disease	Dr. R. Ellul Micallef
Saturday, 10. 1. 1981	Thrombo-embolic pulmonary disease	Prof. F. F. Fenech
	Acute and chronic respiratory failure	Dr. E. Ellul Micallef
Wednesday, 14. 1. 1981	Clinical pharmacology of diuretics	Dr. N. Hayat
	Clinical pharmacology of B-Blockers	Dr. S. Bhatnagar
Saturday, 24. 1. 1981	Peptic ulcer and histamin H_2 antagonists	Dr. B. Naqeeb
	Inflammatory bowel disease	Dr. A. M. Dawson

Wednesday, 28. 1. 1981	Interpretation of liver function tests	Dr. M. Barakat
	Malabsorption	Dr. A. M. Dawson
Saturday, 31. 1. 1981	Disease of gall bladder and pancreas	Dr. B. Haqeeb
	Chronic hepatitis	Dr. A. M. Dawson
Wednesday, 4. 1. 1981	Diabetes mellitus I	Prof. F. F. Fenech
	Diabetes mellitus II	Prof. F. F. Fenech
5th February, 1981	Ward 1 Medical, Al Sabah Hospital	Dr. S. Bhatnagar
Saturday, 7. 2. 1981	Haemoglobinopathies	Dr. A. Hafez
	Iron deficiency and iron overload	Prof. J. Richmond
Wednesday, 11. 2. 1981	The leukaemias	Dr. S. Mutaweh
	Bleeding disorders— clinical and laboratory diagnosis	Prof. J. Richmond
12th February, 1981	Farwania Hospital	Prof. J. Richmond (Dr. Ashmawi)
Saturday, 14. 2. 1981	Megaloblastic anaemias	Dr. M. Hayat
	Polycythaemia and myeloproliferative disorders	Prof. J. Richmond
Wednesday, 18. 2. 1981	Investigate methods in cardiology	Dr. M. Nasser
	Valvular heart disease	Prof. J. Richmond
19th February, 1981	Ward 2 Medical, Al Sabah Hospital	Dr. Taha
Saturday, 21. 2. 1981	Congenital heart disease	Dr. Horky
	Newer concepts in heart failure management	Dr. M. Webb-Peploe
Tuesday, 24. 2. 1981	Remediable causes of hypertension	Prof. A. R. Yousof
	Anti-arrythmic drugs— classification and indications	Dr. W. Webb-Peploe
Saturday, 28. 2. 1981	Coronary care	Prof. A. R. Yousof
	Immune reactions and disease	Prof. M. Lessof
Wednesday, 4. 3. 1981	Basic cytogetics	Dr. Cuschieri
	Immune deficiency	Prof. M. Lessof

5th March, 1981	Ahmadi Hospital	Prof. M. Lessof (Dr. J. Lloyd)
Saturday, 7. 3. 1981	Genetic counselling	Dr. A. Cuschieri
	Bechet's disease and other connective tissue disease	Prof. M. Lessof
Wednesday, 11. 3. 1981	Investigation and diagnosis of inflammatory joint disease	Dr. N. Hayat
	Mental deficiency	Dr. P. Vassallo Aguis
12th March, 1981	Amiri Hospital	Dr. Basil Naqeeb
Saturday, 14. 3. 1981	Hypothalmic/pituitary disease	Dr. J. G. Lloyd
	Multiple sclerosis	Dr. I. T. Draper
Wednesday, 18. 3. 1981	Adrenal disorders	Dr. J. G. Lloyd
	Extrapyramidal syndrome	Dr. I. T. Draper
19th March, 1981	Ward 3 Medical, Al Sabah Hospital	Dr. I. T. Draper (Dr. Attia)
Saturday, 21. 3. 1981	Muscle disorders and myasthenia	Dr. I. T. Draper
	Thyroid disease— diagnostic and management aspects	Dr. M. N. Maisey
Wednesday, 25. 3. 1981	Fluid, electrolytes and acid base disorders	Dr. F. Woods
	Role of nuclear medicine	Dr. M. N. Maisey
26th March, 1981	Adan Hospital	Dr. M. N. Maisey (Dr. M. Emara)
Saturday, 28. 3. 1981	Urinary calculi	Dr. F. Woods
	Glomerulonephritis	Dr. C. Ogg
Wednesday, 1. 4. 1981	Urinary tract infection	Dr. A. Al-Rashid
	Acute renal failure	Dr. C. Ogg
2nd April, 1981	Amiri Hospital	Dr. C. Ogg (Dr. H. F. Wood)
Saturday, 4. 4. 1981	Chronic renal failure	Dr. C. Ogg
	Neonatal jaundice	Dr. L. Deverajan
Wednesday, 8. 4. 1981	Epilepsy and anticonvulsant drugs	Dr. R. Shakir
	Acute exanthemata	Dr. H. Majeed
9th April, 1981	Ward 5 Medical, Al Sabah Hospital	Dr. A. M. Karnik

Saturday, 11. 4. 1981	Neurological complication of systemic disease	Dr. R. Shakir
	New investigative techniques: ultrasound and SCAT	Dr. M. Bassiony
Wednesday, 15. 4. 1981	Neurological complications of alcoholism	Dr. R. Shakir
	Metabolic bone disease	Dr. M. Emara
16th April, 1981	Farwania Hospital	Dr. R. Naffessi
Saturday, 18. 4. 1981	Aetiology of psychiatric disorders	Prof. M. F. El-Islam
	Skin markers in internal malignant disease and skin lesions in rheumatic disease	Dr. M. Selim
Wednesday, 22. 4. 1981	Affective disorders	Prof. M. F. El-Islam
	Skin markers in endocrine and metabolic diseases	Dr. M. Selim
23rd April, 1981	Wards 1 and 12 Medical Al Sabah Hospital	Dr. N. Haya
Saturday, 25. 4. 1981	Medical eye disorders	Dr. M. Al-Shariff
	Management of anxiety and depression	Prof. M. F. Al-Islam
Wednesday, 29. 4. 1981	Diagnostic enzymes	Prof. K. Gumaa
	Organic psychiatric disorders	Prof. M. F. El-Islam
30th April, 1981	Wards 2 and 5 Medical, Al Sabah Hospital	Dr. Menon
Thursday, 14. 5. 1981	Mock examination (5.00—7.00 p.m.)	

Group 1 doctors will attend clinical sessions on the following days:

5th February, 1981
19th February, 1981
12th March, 1981
26th March, 1981
9th April, 1981
23rd April, 1981

Group 2 doctors will attend clinical sessions on the following days:

12th February, 1981
5th March, 1981
19th March, 1981
2nd April, 1981
16th April, 1981
30th April, 1981

Date	Long cases	Short cases
5. 2. 1981	Dr. Bader El-Shimali Dr. Nabillah Abdullah	Dr. Mubarek El-Daoob Dr. Ali Al-Aqid
12. 2. 1981	Dr. Rasheed Y. Al-Mussailam Dr. Hani Saba Al-Lidawi	Dr. Medhat M. Mokhtar Dr. Talal Abduo
19. 2. 1981	Dr. Mubarek El-Daoob Dr. Ali Al-Aqid	Dr. Bader El-Shimali Dr. Nabillah Abdullah
5. 3. 1981	Dr. Methat M. Mokhtar Dr. Talal Abduo	Dr. Rasheed Y. Al-Mussailam Dr. Hani Saba Al-Lidawi
12. 3. 1981	Dr. Awad Hassan El-Howlli Dr. Abdul El-Mowlah	Dr. Ibrahim Tarif Dr. Abdullah Saadeh
19. 3. 1981	Dr. Faleh Saleh Majid Dr. Abdul M. M. M. El-Sedawy	Dr. Nibal Katheh Dr. Mohamed Zaki Shafie
26. 3. 1981	Dr. Nassim Sami Faour Dr. Nail Mahmoud H. Shahtoo	Dr. Bader El-Shimali Dr. Nabillah Abdullah
2. 4. 1981	Dr. Yaser Khalil Abdel-Al Dr. Ghassan Husni Baidas	Dr. Rasheed Y. Al-Mussailam Dr. Hani Saba Al-Lidawi
9. 4. 1981	Dr. Bader El-Shimali Dr. Nabillah Abdullah	Dr. Mubarek El-Daoob Dr. Ali Al-Aqid
16. 4. 1981	Dr. Rasheed Y. Al-Mussailam Dr. Hani Saba Al-Lidawi	Dr. Medhat M. Mokhtar Dr. Talal Abduo
23. 4. 1981	Dr. Awad Hassan El-Howlli Dr. Abdul El-Mowlah	Dr. Ibrahim Tarif Dr. Abdullah Saadeh
30. 4. 1981	Dr. Faleh Saleh Majid Dr. Abdul M. M. M. El-Sedawy	Dr. Nibal Katheh Dr. Mohamed Saki Shafie

On the above dates candidates assigned to long cases are asked to come an hour earlier, i.e. at 9.00 a.m. to the ward as shown in the accompanying programme. They will take a medical history and do a complete physical examination for one hour, following which the case will be discussed with them by the two assessors.

Written examination

The following lectures, demonstrations and slide shows will be carried out on Monday evenings from 4.00—6.00 p.m. in the Faculty of Medicine Lecture Room 105. Each session will be for one hour and only those who have done Part I of the M.R.C.P. are allowed to attend.

2nd February, 1981	Cardiac catheterisation— data	4.00—5.00 p.m.
	Haematology—slides	5.00—6.00 p.m.
9th February, 1981	Haematology—data	4.00—5.00 p.m.
	Oral session—Prof. J. Richmond	5.00—6.00 p.m.

16th February, 1981	Radiology—contrast radiology	4.00—5.00 p.m.
	Hepatic data interpretation	5.00—6.00 p.m.
23rd February, 1981	Radiology—chest	4.00—5.00 p.m.
	Oral session—Prof. Webb-Peploe	5.00—6.00 p.m.
2nd March, 1981	Pulmonary function tests—data	4.00—5.00 p.m.
	Neurology slide show	5.00—6.00 p.m.
9th March, 1981	Dermatology—slide show	4.00—5.00 p.m.
	Oral session—Prof. Lessof	5.00—6.00 p.m.
16th March, 1981	Dermatology—slide show	4.00—5.00 p.m.
	Cardiology—E.C.G.s	5.00—6.00 p.m.
23rd March, 1981	G.I.T.—data	4.00—5.00 p.m.
	Neuroendocrinology— data (Dr. M. Maisey)	5.00—6.00 p.m.
30th March, 1981	Gray cases	4.00—5.00 p.m.
	Renal medicine—data (Dr. C. Ogg)	5.00—6.00 p.m.
6th April, 1981	Fundi—slide show	4.00—5.00 p.m.
	General radiology-bone	5.00—6.00 p.m.
13th April, 1981	Neuroradiology	4.00—5.00 p.m.
	Gray cases	5.00—6.00 p.m.
20th April, 1981	General medical slide show	4.00—5.00 p.m.
	Connective tissue diseases—data and slides	5.00—6.00 p.m.
27th April, 1981	Mock examination	

List of Doctors Attending the Course

Group 1

1. Dr. Bader El-Shimali	Ward 12, Al Sabah
2. Dr. Nabillah Abdullah	Ward 6, Al Sabah
3. Dr. Mubarek El-Daoob	Ward 6, Al Sabah
4. Dr. Ali Al-Aqid	Ward 3, Al Sabah
5. Dr. Awad Hassan El-Howlli	Farwania Hospital
6. Dr. Abdul El-Mowlah	Sulaibikhat Complex
7. Dr. Ibrahim Tarif	Adan Hospital
8. Dr. Abdullah Saadeh	Adan Hospital

9. Dr. Nassim Sami Faour   Farwania Hospital
10. Dr. Nail Mahmoud H. Shahtoo   Farwania Hospital

Group 2

11. Dr. Ghassan Husni Baidas   Ward 2, Al Sabah
12. Dr. Rasheed Yousuf Al-Mussailam   Amiri Hospital
13. Dr. Hani Saba Al-Lidawi   Amiri Hospital
14. Dr. Medhat Mahmoud Mokhtar   Amiri Hospital
15. Dr. Talal Abduo   Jahra Hospital
16. Dr. Faleh Saleh Majid   Amiri Hospital
17. Dr. Abdul Mowlah M. M. El-Sedawy   P. O. Box 31185, Sulaibikhat
18. Dr. Nibal Katheh (F)   Infectious Diseases Hospital
19. Dr. Mohamed Zaki Shafie   Cardiology Dept. Chest Hospital
20. Dr. Yaser Khalil Abdel-Al   P. O. Box 4369, Safat
21. Dr. Niazy Abu Farfakh   Adan Hospital

81B—1202
Part I and II of the Course Preparing for Examination for Membership of the Royal College of Physicians (M.R.C.P.—U.K.)

Objectives: A course preparing for the Mock examination towards Part I and Part II examination of the membership of the Royal College of Physicians (London).

Place: Medical wards of Al Sabah Hospital and Mubarak Al Kabir Hospital.
Lectures will be held on Saturdays and Wednesdays in the Faculty of Medicine Lecture Room 105, between 4.30 p.m. and 6.30 p.m. There will be a session on Sunday, 17th January, 1982.

Duration: From 2. 1. 1982 till 29. 4. 1982.

Organiser: Department of Medicine, University of Kuwait in collaboration with Ministry of Health, Kuwait.

Programme Director: Professor F. F. Fenech.

Coordinator: Dr. R. A. Shakir.

Participants: Candidates for Mock examination for M.R.C.P.

Programme:

2nd January, 1982 (Saturday)

4.30 p.m.   Basic cytogenetics
Dr. A. Cuscheri
5.30 p.m.   Pharmacokinetics
Prof. O. Thulesius

6th January, 1982 (Wednesday)

4.30 p.m.   Liver function
Dr. M. Barakat

5.30 p.m.   Applied pulmonary physiology
                             Dr. R. Ellul-Micallef

                             9th January, 1982 (Saturday)

4.30 p.m.   Prostaglandins—physiological and clinical applications
                             Prof. O. Thulesius
5.30 p.m.   Antibiotics—new and old rational use
                             Prof. F. F. Fenech

                             13th January, 1982 (Wednesday)

4.30 p.m.   Renal tubular disorders
                             Dr. A. Rashid
5.30 p.m.   Drugs and the kidney
                             Dr. M. K. Emara

                             17th January, 1982 (Sunday)

4.30 p.m.   Interstitial nephritis
                             Dr. H. F. Woods
5.30 p.m.   Disorders of fluid balance and acid-base abnormalities
                             Dr. B. Hoffbrand

                             20th January, 1982 (Wednesday)

4.30 p.m.   Acute and chronic renal failure
                             Dr. H. F. Woods
5.30 p.m.   Glomerulonephritis
                             Dr. B. Hoffbrand

                             23rd January, 1982 (Saturday)

4.30 p.m.   Metabolic and endocrine bone disease
                             Dr. B. Hoffbrand
5.30 p.m.   Interstitial and fibrotic lung disease
                             Prof. J. Howell

                             27th January, 1982 (Wednesday)

4.30 p.m.   Changes in patterns of bronchopulmonary infections
                             Prof. F. F. Fenech
5.30 p.m.   Respiratory failure—pathophysiology and management
                             Prof. J. Howell

                             30th January, 1982 (Saturday)

4.30 p.m.   Occupational allergic and non-allergic lung disease
                             Dr. M. Khogali
5.30 p.m.   Bronchial asthma
                             Prof. J. Howell

                             3rd February, 1982 (Wednesday)

4.30 p.m.   Drug interactions
                             Dr. R. Ellul-Micallef

| 5.30 p.m. | Gut hormones |
| | Dr. M. H. Barakat |

6th February, 1982 (Saturday)

4.30 p.m.	Medical aspects of treatment of peptic ulceration
	Dr. B. Naqeeb
5.30 p.m.	Inflammatory bowel disease
	Dr. T. J. Thomson

10th February, 1982 (Wednesday)

4.30 p.m.	Acute and chronic hepatitis
	Dr. B. Naqeeb
5.30 p.m.	Malabsorption
	Dr. T. J. Thomson

13th February, 1982 (Saturday)

4.30 p.m.	Pancreatic and gall bladder disease
	Dr. T. J. Thomson
5.30 p.m.	Complications of diabetes mellitus
	Dr. P. Watkins

17th February, 1982 (Wednesday)

4.30 p.m.	Hypoglycaemia
	Prof. F. F. Fenech
5.30 p.m.	Current therapy of diabetes mellitus
	Dr. P. Watkins

20th February, 1982 (Saturday)

4.30 p.m.	Salmonellosis
	Dr. M. H. Barakat
5.30 p.m.	Current concepts in therapy of tuberculosis
	Dr. N. Shaaban

24th February, 1982 (Wednesday)

4.30 p.m.	Malaria and schistosomiasis
	Dr. A. A. Wahab
5.30 p.m.	Immunisation update
	Dr. H. Majeed

27th February, 1982 (Saturday)

4.30 p.m.	Hypothalmic/pituitary disorders
	Dr. J. G. Lloyd
5.30 p.m.	Thyroid—pathophysiology and disorders
	Prof. F. F. Fenech

3rd March, 1982 (Wednesday)

| 4.30 p.m. | Normal hematopoesis and kinetics |
| | Dr. A. Hafez |

5.30 p.m.	Adrenals—pathophysiology and disorders Dr. J. G. Lloyd

6th March, 1982 (Saturday)

4.30 p.m.	The leukaemias Dr. S. Mutawa
5.30 p.m.	Macrocytic anaemia Dr. R. Hume

10th March, 1982 (Wednesday)

4.30 p.m.	Polycythaemia and myeloproliferative disorders Dr. R. Hume
5.30 p.m.	Lymphomas Dr. S. Mutawa

13th March, 1982 (Saturday)

4.30 p.m.	Haemoglobinopathies Dr. A. Hafez
5.30 p.m.	Investigation and management of thrombocytopenias Dr. R. Hume

17th March, 1982 (Wednesday)

4.30 p.m.	Poisoning Dr. J. G. Lloyd
5.30 p.m.	Strokes Dr. R. Shakir

20th March, 1982 (Saturday)

4.30 p.m.	Alcoholism Dr. R. Shakir
5.30 p.m.	Demylinating disease Dr. J. P. Ballantyne

24th March, 1982 (Wednesday)

4.30 p.m.	Epilepsy management Dr. R. Shakir
5.30 p.m.	Neuromuscular disorders Dr. J. P. Ballantyne

27th March, 1982 (Saturday)

4.30 p.m.	Extrapyramidal syndromes Dr. J. P. Ballantyne
5.30 p.m.	Neonatal Jaundice Dr. L. Devarajan

31st March, 1982 (Wednesday)

4.30 p.m.	Failure to thrive Prof. P. Vasallo Agius

5.30 p.m.   Mental deficiency
                           Prof. P. Vasallo Agius

                           3rd April, 1982 (Saturday)

4.30 p.m.   Applied physiology of the cardiovascular system
                           Dr. J. D. Stephens
5.30 p.m.   Indications for cardiac surgery in congenital heart dis-
                           ease
                           Prof. A. M. Yousof

                           7th April, 1982 (Wednesday)

4.30 p.m.   Cardiac arrhythmias—classification and therapy
                           Dr. J. D. Stephens
5.30 p.m.   Antihypertensive drugs
                           Prof. A. R. Yousof

                           10th April, 1982 (Saturday)

4.30 p.m.   Coronary artery disease—medical and surgery man-
                           agement
                           Prof. A. M. Yousof
5.30 p.m.   New aspects of treatment of congestive heart failure

                           14th April, 1982 (Wednesday)

4.30 p.m.   Newer diagnostic techniques—radiology
                           Dr. M. H. Bassiony
5.30 p.m.   Diagnostic enzymes
                           Dr. K. Gumaa

                           17th April, 1982 (Saturday)

4.30 p.m.   Mechanism of immunity and hypersensitivity
                           Dr. A. White
5.30 p.m.   Rheumatoid arthritis
                           Dr. H. Berry

                           21st April, 1982 (Wednesday)

4.30 p.m.   Immunodeficiency
                           Dr. A. White
5.30 p.m.   Sero-negative arthropathies
                           Dr. H. Berry

                           24th April, 1982 (Saturday)

4.30 p.m.   Gout
                           Dr. M. Sattar
5.30 p.m.   Clinical pharmacology of anti-rheumatic drugs
                           Dr. H. Berry

                           28th April, 1982 (Wednesday)

4.30 p.m.   Skin markers in endocrine and metabolic diseases
                           Dr. M. El Din Selim

5.30 p.m.   Depression
                                 Prof. M. F. El-Islam

1st May, 1982 (Saturday)

4.30 p.m.   Skin markers in malignant and connecative tissue
                                 diseases
                                 Dr. M. El Din Selim
5.30 p.m.   Psychotrophic drugs
                                 Prof. M. F. El-Islam

13th May, 1982 (Thursday)

5—7.30 p.m.   Mock examination

List of Lecturers

1. Professor P. Vasallo Agius, MD, FRCP, DCH, Professor of Paediatrics, University of Kuwait.
2. Dr. J. P. Ballantyne, Consultant Neurologist, Southern General Hospital, Glasgow, U.K.
3. Dr. M. H. Bassiony, Diagnostic X-ray Division, Al Sabah Hospital.
4. Dr. M. H. Barakat, MD, Associate Professor and Head, Gastroenterology Section, Mubarak Al-Kabir Hospital, Kuwait.
5. Dr. H. Berry, MA, DM, MRCP, Consultant, King's College Hospital London, U.K.
6. Dr. A. Cuschieri, MD, Ph.D., Associate Professor, Department of Anatomy, University of Kuwait.
7. Dr. L. Deverajan, MRCP (UK), DCH, Associate Professor, Department of Paediatrics, University of Kuwait.
8. Prof. M. F. El-Islam, MD, BCh., DPH, MRCP, MRC Psych., FRCP FRC Psy., Prof. of Psychiatry, Department of Medicine, University of Kuwait.
9. Dr. R. Ellul-Micallef, MD, Ph.D., Associate Professor, Department of Pharmacology, University of Kuwait.
10. Dr. M. H. Emara, MB, ChB., DN, DCVP, MRCP (UK), Associate Professor, Department of Medicine, University of Kuwait.
11. Prof. F. F. Fenech, MD, FRCP, FRCPE, Professor and Chairman, Department of Medicine, University of Kuwait.
12. Prof. K. Gumaa, MBBS, Ph.D., Professor and Chairman, Dept. of Biochemistry, University of Kuwait.
13. Dr. A. Hafez, MD, Ph.D., Consultant Haematologist, Amiri Hospital, Ministry of Health, Kuwait.
14. Dr. B. Hoffbrand, DM, FRCP, Consultant Physician, Whittington Hospital, London, U.K.
15. Prof. J. Howell, BSc., MB, Ph.D., FRCP, Dean, Southampton University Medical School, Southampton.
16. Dr. R. Hume, MD, FRCP, FRCP G, Consultant Physician and Haematologist, Southern General Hospital, Glasgow, U.K.
17. Dr. M. Khogali, MD, DPH, FFCh., Associate Professor, Department of Community Medicine, University of Kuwait.
18. Dr. J. G. Lloyd, MBBS, MRCP (UK), Senior Medical Specialist, Ahmadi Hospital, Kuwait.

19. Dr. H. A. Majeed, MRCP, DCH, Associate Professor, Department of Paediatrics, University of Kuwait.
20. Dr. S. Mutaweh, MD, FRCR, Consultant Radiotherapist, Ministry of Health, Kuwait.
21. Dr. B. Naqeeb, MD, Physician and Head, Gastroenterology Section, Sabah Hospital, Ministry of Health, Kuwait.
22. Dr. A. Rashid, MD, FRCP(1) DCH, Senior Consultant Paediatrician, Ministry of Health, Kuwait.
23. Dr. M. Sattar, MBBS, MRCP, Assistant Professor, Department of Medicine, University of Kuwait.
24. Dr. M. Selim, MD, Senior Consultant, Dermatologist, Ministry of Health, Kuwait.
25. Dr. M. Shaaban, MD, Director, Chest Hospital, Ministry of Health, Kuwait.
26. Dr. R. Shakir, MB, ChB, MRCP (UK), MSc., Assist. Professor Consultant Neurologist, Department of Medicine, University of Kuwait.
27. Dr. J. D. Stephens, MD, FRCP, Consultant Cardiologist, The London Hospital, London, U.K.
28. Dr. T. J. Thomson, O.B.E. FRCP Glasgow, Consultant Physician, Stobhill Hospital, Glasgow, U.K.
29. Prof. O. Thulesius, MD, Ph.D, Professor and Chairman, Pharmacology Dept., University of Kuwait.
30. Dr. P. Watkins, MD, FRCP, Consultant Physician and Diabetologist, King's College Hospital, London, U.K.
31. Dr. A. A. Wahab, Head of Internal Medicine Unit, Farwania Hospital, Kuwait.
32. Dr. A. White, BSc., Ph.D. Associate Professor, Department of Surgery, University of Kuwait.
33. Dr. F. Woods, MBBS, MRCP (UK), Consultant Nephrologist, Ministry of Health, Kuwait.
34. Professor A. M. Yousof, MB, ChD, FRCP, Ph.D., Professor of Cardiology, Dean, Faculty of Medicine, University of Kuwait.
35. Professor A. R. Yousof, MBBS, FRCPE, Professor of Medicine, University of Kuwait.

M.R.C.P. Part II Course

Written Examination

The following lectures, demonstrations and slide shows will be carried out on Monday evenings from 4.00—6.00 p.m. in the Faculty of Medicine Lecture Room 105. Each session will be for one hour and only those who have done Part I of the M.R.C.P. are allowed to attend.

18th January, 1982

4.00—5.00 p.m.	Calcium metabolism—data
	Dr. B. I. Hoffbrand
5.00—6.00 p.m.	Nephrology—slides
	Dr. B. I. Hoffbrand

25th January, 1982

4.00—5.00 p.m.	E.C.G.s
	Prof. J. B. L. Howell

5.00—6.00 p.m.	Oral session Prof. J. B. L. Howell

1st February, 1982

4.00—5.00 p.m.	Dermatology—slides
5.00—6.00 p.m.	Gray cases

8th February, 1982

4.00—5.00 p.m.	Radiology—chest
5.00—6.00 p.m.	Oral session Dr. T. J. Thomson

15th February, 1982

4.00—5.00 p.m.	Fundi—slides
5.00—6.00 p.m.	Diabetes—data Dr. P. Watkins

22nd February, 1982

4.00—5.00 p.m.	Dermatology—slides
5.00—6.00 p.m.	Radiology—general and bone

1st March, 1982

4.00—5.00 p.m.	Liver function—data
5.00—6.00 p.m.	Radiology—contrast

8th March, 1982

4.00—5.00 p.m.	General medical—slides Dr. R. Hume
5.00—6.00 p.m.	Oral session Dr. R. Hume

22nd March, 1982

4.00—5.00 p.m.	G.I.T.—data
5.00—6.00 p.m.	Gray cases

29th March, 1982

4.00—5.00 p.m.	Pulmonary function tests
5.00—6.00 p.m.	Endocrinology—data

5th April, 1982

4.00—5.00 p.m.	E.C.G.s Dr. J. D. Stephens
5.00—6.00 p.m.	Cardiac catheterisation—data Dr. J. D. Stephens

12th April, 1982

4.00—5.00 p.m.	Haematology—slides
5.00—6.00 p.m.	Haematology—data

19th April, 1982

4.00—5.00 p.m.	Rheumatology—data
	Dr. H. Berry
5.00—6.00 p.m.	Rheumatology—slides
	Dr. H. Berry

26th April, 1982

4.00—5.00 p.m.	Dermatology—slides
5.00—6.00 p.m.	Dermatology—data

3rd May, 1982

4.00—5.00 p.m.	Haematology—slides
	Dr. G. A. McDonald
5.00—6.00 p.m.	Haematology—data
	Dr. G. A. McDonald

M.R.C.P. Part II Course

Clinical Sessions

The Clinical Sessions for the Part II Course will be carried out as in the Programme below. The names in brackets shown with some of the sessions are those of our visiting professors and doctors who will participate in the clinical sessions. In addition there will be a further programme allocating faculty members to the clinical sessions at a later date.

Doctors in charge of the wards allocated in the following programme are asked to provide two long cases and at least six short cases on the day the clinical teaching is taking place in their particular ward. The short cases have to be varied and they should include at least two cardiology cases with heart murmurs and at least one neurology case. If there are any problems regarding the dates, cases or any other matter regarding the clinical sessions, please contact Dr. R. A. Shakir at the Department of Medicine in the Al Sabah Hospital or Mubarak Al Kabir Hospital.

21st January, 1982

Ward 16 and 18 Mubarak Hospital
Dr. B. I. Hoffbrand, Dr. A. M. Karnik

28th January, 1982

Farwania Hospital
Prof. J. B. L. Howell, Dr. Ashmawi A. Wahab

4th February, 1982

Ward 1 Medical, Al Sabah Hospital
Dr. T. H. Taha

11th February, 1982

Ahmadi Hospital
Dr. T. J. Thomson, Dr. J. Lloyd

18th February, 1982

Ward 2 Medical, Al Sabah Hospital
Dr. P. Watkins, Dr. Gassan Baidas

4th March, 1982

Ward 3 Medical, Al Sabah Hospital
Dr. M. R. Attia

11th March, 1982

Ward 18, Mubarak Hospital
Dr. R. Hume, Dr. A. K. Menon

18th March, 1982

Adan Hospital
Dr. J. P. Ballantyne, Dr. M. K. Emara

25th March, 1982

Amiri Hospital
Dr. H. F. Woods

1st April, 1982

Ward 5, Al Sabah Hospital
Dr. B. Al Naqeeb

8th April, 1982

Farwania Hospital
Dr. J. D. Stephens, Dr. R. Hafassi

15th April, 1982

Wards 1 and 2 Medical, Al Sabah Hospital
Dr. T. H. Taha

22nd April, 1982

Adan Hospital
Dr. F. Berry, Dr. M. K. Emara

29th April, 1982

Wards 16 and 18 Mubarak Hospital
Dr. G. A. McDonald, Dr. A. M. Karnik

M.R.C.P. Part II Course

Tutors for the Clinical Sessions will be as follows:

21st January, 1982

Dr. B. I. Hoffbrand
Professor F. F. Fenech

28th January, 1982

Professor J. B. Howell
Dr. R. A. Shakir

4th February, 1982

Professor A. R. Yousof
Dr. H. F. Woods

11th February, 1982

Dr. T. J. Thomson
Dr. J. Lloyd

18th February, 1982

Dr. P. Watkins
Dr. J. B. Johny

4th March, 1982

Professor F. F. Fenech
Dr. M. K. Barakat

11th March, 1982

Dr. R. Hume
Professor A. M. Yousof

18th March, 1982

Dr. J. B. Ballantyne
Dr. M. K. Emara

25th March, 1982

Professor A. R. Yousuf
Dr. R. A. Shakir

1st April, 1982

Professor F. F. Fenech
Dr. B. Al Naqeeb

8th April, 1982

Dr. J. D. Stephens
Dr. M. Sattar

15th April, 1982

Professor A. M. Yousof
Dr. J. G. Lloyd

22nd April, 1982

Dr. H. Berry
Dr. M. K. Emara

29th April, 1982

Dr. G. A. McDonald
Dr. R. A. Shakir

81B—23/0101
Part I (Basic Sciences) Course Preparing for Examination for Fellowship of the Royal College of Surgeons (F.R.C.S.—Dublin)

Objectives:	Course in basic sciences directed towards the Primary Fellowship of the Royal College of Surgeons in Ireland (Dublin).
Place:	Basic Science Building Faculty of Medicine, Kuwait.
Duration:	8 weeks, 31st January 1981—26th March 1981.
Organiser:	The Medical Faculty of the University of Kuwait and a visiting team of lectures from the Royal College of Surgeons in Ireland.
Programme Director:	Prof. S. Roy Choudhury.
Participation:	28 doctors selected.

Dr. P. D. Koshy
Dr. Riadh Ali Mohamed Sharif
Dr. Mahmoud Mohamed Abdul Rahman Al-Jabar
Dr. Mohammed Khairy Fares Lubbadeh
Dr. Abdul-Hamid A. M. Muhnna
Dr. Sami Babikir Awadalla
Dr. Mohammed Khalid Al-Mesh'aan
Dr. Samir Mohammed Fouad
Dr. Kamel Moustafa El Mellawani
Dr. Abdul Rahman A. Fatah Ateya
Dr. Nabil Mohammed Abdel Gawad
Dr. Mahmoud Samhan Aref Mohammed
Dr. Haitem Khalid Al-Hassan
Dr. Shakeel Sandozi
Dr. Nabil Mohamed Helmi Abdul Rahman
Dr. Abdul Wahid Hassan
Dr. Metwalli Afifi Mohamed El Sayed
Dr. Sheta Ali Gawdat El Sawi
Dr. Nidal Husni Saleh Khuffash

Dr. Mohamed Ashraf M. El-Saeed El-Naggar
Dr. Omer El Farouq Yousef Omer
Dr. Adnan Abdul-Rahman Zamil
Dr. Piyaray Mohan Dhar
Dr. Mohsen Abd El Monem El-Desoki
Dr. Hani Fayes Saad El Ahmed
Dr. Mohammad Milhim Masri
Dr. Nadar Ahmed Al-Safar
Dr. Mohamed Sharaf Mohsin Al-Khabbaz

Programme:

The Course is designed to cover the general background of Anatomy, Physiology and Pathology as these subjects relate directly to the clinical practice of surgery. All the lectures are very specifically slanted towards those aspects of the Sciences having such direct clinical relevance. The overall Course shall provide a comprehensive series of tutorials designed to prepare those on it for the Primary Fellowship Examination of this College, or any of the Royal Colleges.

There have been many alterations in the approach towards the Basic Sciences in the Primary Fellowship Examination over the past five years. The main function of this Course will be to orientate the students on it to current thinking in the Royal College in the United Kingdom, and to give them an organised technique of study and a properly orientated approach to the Examination.

Week 1

Saturday, 31st January, 1981

8.00 a.m.—11.00 a.m.	Introduction, objectives, terminology, the skull Prof. G. Lynch, RCSI
11.30 a.m.— 2.30 p.m.	Haematology I Dr. M. K. Y. Mustafa, Dept. Physiology

Sunday, 1st February, 1981

8.00 a.m.—11.00 a.m.	Haematology II Dr. M. K. Y. Mustafa, Dept. Physiology
11.30 a.m.— 2.30 p.m.	Cranial nerves, the meninges Prof. Lynch, RCSI

Monday, 2nd February, 1981

8.00 a.m.—11.00 a.m.	Haematology III Dr. M. K. Y. Mustafa, Dept. Physiology
11.30 a.m.— 2.30 p.m.	Intracranial hge. vertebrae, joints of skull and vertebrae Prof. Lynch, RCSI

Tuesday, 3rd February, 1981

8.00 a.m.—11.00 a.m.	Peripheral nerves and plexuses face, eyelids, lacrymal apparatus Prof. G. Lynch, RCSI
11.30 a.m.— 2.30 p.m.	Neuro-anatomy, bl. supply, brain sections Prof. S. R. Choudhury, Dept. Anatomy

Wednesday, 4th February, 1981

8.00 a.m.—11.00 a.m.	Anat. spaces, cervical fascia, side of neck Prof. G. Lynch, RCSI
11.30 a.m.— 2.30 p.m.	CNS—Introduction, spinal cord Prof. J. S. Juggi, Dept. Physiology

Thursday, 5th February, 1981

8.00 a.m.—11.00 a.m.	Test examination review Discussion.

Week 2

Saturday, 7th February, 1981

8.00 a.m.—11.00 a.m.	Solid organs, T.M. joint parotid gland, infratemporal and submandibular region Prof. G. Lynch, RCSI
11.30 a.m.—12.45 p.m.	Thyroid gland Prof. George Abouna, Dept. Surgery
1.00 p.m.— 2.30 p.m.	Nasal and paranasal sinuses Dr. Cuschieri, Dept. Anatomy

Sunday, 8th February, 1981

8.00 a.m.—11.00 a.m.	Cardiovascular physiology Prof. J. S. Juggi, Dept. Physiology
11.30 a.m.— 2.30 p.m.	The vessels of the neck cranial parasympathetic Prof. G. Lynch, RCSI

Monday, 9th February, 1981

8.00 a.m.—11.00 a.m.	Cardiovascular physiology Prof. J. S. Juggi, Dept. Physiology
11.30 a.m.— 2.30 p.m.	Orbit, eye ball, external ear Prof. G. Lynch, RCSI

Tuesday, 10th February, 1981

8.00 a.m.—11.00 a.m.	Cardiovascular physiology summary, discussions Prof. J. S. Juggi, Dept. Physiology
11.30 a.m.— 2.30 p.m.	Middle ear, larynx Prof. G. Lynch

Wednesday, 11th February, 1981

8.00 a.m.—11.00 a.m.	Renal physiology Dr. M. J. McBroom, Dept. Physiology
11.30 a.m.— 2.30 p.m.	Pharynx, revision Discussion Prof. G. Lynch, RCSI

Thursday, 12th February, 1981

8.00 a.m.—11.00 a.m.   Renal physiology
                       Dr. M. J. McBroom, Dept. Physiology

Week 3

Saturday, 14th February, 1981

8.00 a.m.—11.00 a.m.   Respiratory physiology
                       Prof. N. A. Mahmoud, Dept. Physiology
11.30 a.m.— 2.30 p.m.   Organisms of surgical importance
                       Prof. V. Bezjak, Dept. Microbiology

Sunday, 15th February, 1981

8.00 a.m.—11.00 a.m.   Organisms of surgical importance viruses and parasites
                       Drs. W. S. Al-Naqeeb and K. Behbehani, Dept. Micro-
                       biology
11.30 a.m.— 2.30 p.m.   Respiratory physiology
                       Dr. M. K. Y. Mustafa, Dept. Physiology

Monday, 16th February, 1981

8.00 a.m.—11.00 a.m.   Respiratory physiology
                       Dr. M. K. Y. Mustafa, Dept. Physiology
11.30 a.m.— 2.30 p.m.   Hospital infections
                       sterilisation, disinfection
                       Prof. T. D. Chugh, Dept. Microbiology

Tuesday, 17th February, 1981

8.00 a.m.— 9.15 a.m.   Immunology
                       Dr. A. White, Dept. Surgery
9.30 a.m.—11.00 a.m.   Antibiotics and chemotherapeutics
                       Prof. F. Fenech
11.30 a.m.— 2.30 p.m.   Skin, regulation of body temperature
                       Dr. N. S. Al-Zaid, Dept. Physiology

Wednesday, 18th February, 1981

8.00 a.m.—11.00 a.m.   Electrolyte and acid base balance discussions
                       Dr. M. J. McBroom, Dept. Physiology
11.30 a.m.—12.45 p.m.   Hypersensitivity
                       Dr. R. E. Micallef, Dept. Medicine
1.00 p.m.— 2.30 p.m.   Antibiotics and chemotherapeutic agents II
                       Prof. F. Fenech, Dept. Medicine

Thursday, 19th February, 1981

8.00 a.m.—11.00 a.m.   Principles of modern serological techniques, test M.C.Q.
                       Dr. W. S. Al-Naqeeb, Dept. Microbiology

Week 4

Saturday, 21st February, 1981

8.00 a.m.—11.00 a.m.   Cell structure and metabolism
                        Prof. G. Doyle, RCSI
11.30 a.m.— 2.30 p.m.   Abdomen—introduction
                        Lumbar. vert. and plevis abdominal wall. Inguinal region
                        Prof. W. N. Adams Smith, Dept. Anatomy

Sunday, 22nd February, 1981

8.00 a.m.—11.00 a.m.   Cell degeneration, necrosis
                        Prof. G. Doyle, RCSI
11.30 a.m.—12.45 p.m.   The peritoneum
                        Dr. W. N. Adams Smith, Dept. Anatomy
1.00 p.m.— 2.30 p.m.   The alimentary tract—general
                        Prof. G. J. M. Abouna, Dept. Surgery

Monday, 23rd February, 1981

8.00 a.m.—11.00 a.m.   Acute inflammation
                        Prof. G. Doyle, RCSI
11.30 a.m.— 2.30 p.m.   The stomach, spleen duodenum, small bowel, upper
                        branches of aorta
                        Prof. G. J. M. Abouna, Dept. Surgery

Tuesday, 24th February, 1981

Holiday

Wednesday, 25th February, 1981

Holiday

Thursday, 26th February, 1981

Holiday

Week 5

Saturday, 28th February, 1981

8.00 a.m.—11.00 a.m.   Chronic inflammation, chronic infective granulomata
                        Prof. P. Fitzpatrick, RCSI
11.30 a.m.— 2.30 p.m.   The liver gall bladder and biliary apparatus
                        Prof. G. Abouna, Dept. Surgery

Sunday, 1st March, 1981

8.00 a.m.—11.00 a.m.   Chronic infective granulomata, pathological calcification
                        and pigmentation
                        Dr. P. Fitzpatrick, RCSI
11.30 a.m.—12.45 p.m.   Portal venous system
                        Prof. G. Abouna, Dept. Surgery
1.00 p.m.— 2.30 p.m.   Post abd. wall, coelic plexus, sympathetic chain
                        Prof. W. N. Adams Smith, Dept. Anatomy

Monday, 2nd March, 1981

8.00 a.m.—11.00 a.m.	Regeneration and repair Dr. P. Fitzpatrick, RCSI
11.30 a.m.—12.45 p.m.	Kidneys and adrenals, vena cava Prof. G. Abouna, Dept. Surgery
1.00 p.m.— 2.30 p.m.	The diaphragm, lumbar plexus Dr. A. Cuschieri, Dept. Anatomy

Tuesday, 3rd March, 1981

8.00 a.m.—11.00 a.m.	Autoimmune diseases Dr. P. Fitzpatrick, RCSI
11.30 a.m.— 2.30 p.m.	The plevis pelvis fascia and floor scrotum, testes, perineal pouches Dr. A. Cuschieri, Dept. Anatomy

Wednesday, 4th March, 1981

8.00 a.m.— 9.30 a.m.	The uterus and broad ligaments Prof. Hathout
9.30 a.m.—11.00 a.m.	The lower branches of the aorta Prof. G. Abouna, Dept. Surgery
11.30 a.m.— 2.30 p.m.	Ischio-rectal fossa, male plevic organs, bladder, prostate, vas seminal vesicle, urets Dr. B. C. Bappna, Dept. Surgery

Thursday, 5th March, 1981

8.00 a.m.—11.00 a.m.	The colon and rectum, blood vessels of the pelvis Dr. K. K. Mahajan, Dept. Surgery
11.30 a.m.— 2.30 p.m.	MCQ, Discussions Dr. P. Fitzpatrick, RCSI

Week 6

Saturday, 7th March, 1981

8.00 a.m.—11.00 a.m.	Thrombosis, embolism Dr. P. Fitzpatrick, RCSI
11.30 a.m.— 2.30 p.m.	Metabolism, carbohydrate Dr. Jim Finucane, RCSI

Sunday, 8th March, 1981

8.00 a.m.—11.00 a.m.	Metabolism, fat, proteins Dr. Jim Finucane, RCSI
11.30 a.m.— 2.30 p.m.	Ischaemia, infarction, gangrene Dr. P. Fitzpatrick, RCSI

Monday, 9th March, 1981

8.00 a.m.—11.00 a.m.	Genetically determined disease Dr. P. Fitzpatrick, RCSI

11.30 a.m.— 2.30 p.m.   Metabolism, nucleic acids, vitamin, hypothalmic-pitui-
                         tary function
                         Dr. Jim Finucane, RCSI

Tuesday, 10th March, 1981

8.00 a.m.—11.00 a.m.   Hypothalmic-pituitary function, the thyroid
                        Dr. Jim Finucane, RCSI
11.30 a.m.— 2.30 p.m.   Plasma proteins—disorders
                        Dr. P. Fitzpatrick, RCSI

Wednesday, 11th March, 1981

8.00 a.m.—11.00 a.m.   Vitamin deficiency diseases
                        Dr. P. Fitzpatrick, RCSI
11.30 a.m.— 2.30 p.m.   The endocrine pancreas, adrenal gland
                        Dr. Jim Finucane, RCSI

Thursday, 12th March, 1981

8.00 a.m.—11.00 a.m.   MCQ, Discussions
                        Dr. P. Fitzpatrick, RCSI

Week 7

Saturday, 14th March, 1981

8.00 a.m.—11.00 a.m.   Gonadal function, regulation of menstrual cycle, para-
                        thyroids calcium and phos. metabolism
                        Dr. Jim Finucane, RCSI
11.30 a.m.— 2.30 p.m.   The thoracic cage, rib-movements of intercostal space
                        Mr. Hy Browne, RCSI

Sunday, 15th March, 1981

8.00 a.m.—11.00 a.m.   The pleura, mediastinum pericardium
                        Mr. Hy Browne, RCSI
11.30 a.m.— 2.30 p.m.   MCQ, Discussions
                        Dr. Jim Finucane, RCSI

Monday, 16th March, 1981

8.00 a.m.—11.00 a.m.   Gastrointestinal physiology, deglutition, oesophageal
                        motility and disorders
11.30 a.m.— 2.30 p.m.   Myocardium, conduction system bl. vs. great vessels,
                        lungs
                        Mr. Hy Browne, RCSI

Tuesday, 17th March, 1981

8.00 a.m.—11.00 a.m.   Neoplasia
                        Prof. M. Y. Ali, Dept. Pathology
11.30 a.m.— 2.30 p.m.   The upper GIT gastric secretion pylorus, pancreas, liver

Wednesday, 18th March, 1981

8.00 a.m.— 9.15 a.m.	The lower GIT Dr. M. Barakat, Dept. Medicine
9.30 a.m.—11.00 a.m.	Neoplasia Prof. M. Y. Ali, Dept. Pathology
11.30 a.m.— 2.30 p.m.	Trachea, bronchi, B. P. segments oesophagus. Vagus and phrenic nerves, sympathetic chain Mr. Hy Browne, RCSI

Thursday, 19th March, 1981

8.00 a.m.—11.00 a.m.	Bones of upper limb, shoulder girdle and joint, axilla upper arm Dr. P. K. Ray, Dept. Anatomy

Week 8

Saturday, 21st March, 1981

8.00 a.m.—11.00 a.m.	Spinal cord, tracts, sensation balance Prof. J. S. Juggi, Dept. Physiology
11.30 a.m.— 2.30 p.m.	Elbow and wrist joints. Forearm pronation, supination, carpal tunnel Dr. P. K. Ray, Dept. Anatomy

Sunday, 22nd March, 1981

8.00 a.m.—11.00 a.m.	The hand, palm and dorsum flexor tendons and sheath extensor mechanism Dr. P. K. Ray, Dept. Anatomy
11.30 a.m.— 2.30 p.m.	Cerebellum, tone. Posture, nasal ganglia, ventricles, intracranial pressure changes Prof. J. S. Juggi, Dept. Physiology

Monday, 23rd March, 1981

8.00 a.m.—11.00 a.m.	A.N.S. MCQ Discussions Prof. J. Juggi, Dept. Physiology
11.30 a.m.— 2.30 p.m.	Intravenous nutrition, fluid electrolyte balance Prof. G. Abouna, Dept. Surgery

Tuesday, 24th March, 1981

8.00 a.m.—11.00 a.m.	Lower limb—bones, hip joint gluteal region, femoral triangle ant. thigh, knee joint Mr. Hy Browne, RCSI
11.30 a.m.— 2.30 p.m.	Inner ear mechanism, hearing, vision, eye reflexes Dr. J. S. Juggi, Dept. Physiology

Wednesday, 25th March, 1981

8.00 a.m.—11.00 a.m.	Taste, smell, deglutition Review and discussion Dr. J. S. Juggi, Dept. Physiology
11.30 a.m.— 2.30 p.m.	Thigh-back, popliteal fossa leg—front and back, soleal pump, ankle joint Mr. Hy Browne, RCSI

Thursday, 26th March, 1981

8.00 a.m.—11.00 a.m.   The foot, review and discussion
                        Mr. Hy Browne, RCSI

81B-23/0102
Part I (Basic Sciences) Course Preparing for Examinations for Fellowship of the Royal College of Surgeons (F.R.C.S.—Dublin)

Objectives: Course on basic sciences directed towards the primary
                      fellowship of the Royal College of Surgeons in Ireland
                      (Dublin).
                      Course is designed to cover the general background of
                      anatomy, physiology and pathology as these subjects re-
                      late directly to the clinical practice of surgery. All the lec-
                      tures are very specifically slanted towards those aspects
                      of the sciences having direct clinical relevance, and the
                      overall course shall provide a comprehensive series of tu-
                      torials designed to prepare those on it for the Primary
                      Fellowship Examination of this college or any of the
                      Royal Colleges.

Methods: This course is full time and very intensive. The candi-
                      dates selected to attend the course are strongly advised to
                      do a period of preparatory study so that they will be in a
                      position to assimilate the teaching on the course at a very
                      intensive level. This will be particularly necessary for
                      those who, because of their work commitment, have been
                      out of touch with the academic aspects of these sciences
                      for a period of some years. There have been many alter-
                      ations in the approach towards the basic sciences in the
                      Primary Fellowship Examination over the past five years
                      and the main function of this course will be to orientate
                      the students on it to current thinking in the Royal Col-
                      leges in the United Kingdom and to give them an orga-
                      nised technique of study and a properly orientated ap-
                      proach to the Examination.
                      Any standard textbook in the appropriate Basic Sciences
                      constitutes acceptable reading material in preparation for
                      this course. The most popular texts in use in the Royal
                      Colleges at the moment are listed below and are recom-
                      mended by the panel of lecturers.

ANATOMY   *The system of anatomy* by Gray
                Anatomy descriptive and applied by Last

PHYSIOLOGY   *Textbook of physiology* by Guyton
                Clinical physiology by Campbell, Dicken-
                son and Slater

PATHOLOGY   *General pathology* by Walter and Israel
                Scientific foundation of surgery by Wells
                and Kyle

Any candidate who wishes to read a specific text in bio-chemistry is recommended to read the *Review of physiological chemistry* by Galong. This is probably not, in fact, necessary reading for the Examination.

Reading the course, a visiting lecturer from the Royal College of Surgeons in Ireland will be present in Kuwait most of the time. As much as possible, he or she will be available for discussion with the candidates on the course either singly or in groups. As will be seen in the programme, it is planned from time to time to run small assessment examinations and discussion periods with the candidates on the course, and this should be a great help to them in indicating how well they are keeping up with the material being presented.

Place (Venue):   All classes will take place in the Physiology Seminar Room, Faculty of Medicine.

Duration: 8 weeks, form Saturday, 30th January 1982, till Thursday, 25th March 1982. The Primary F.R.C.S. Examination will be held in Kuwait in late April, 1982.

Organiser: The course will be conducted jointly by the Medical Faculty of the University of Kuwait and a visiting team of lecturers from the Royal College of Surgeons in Ireland.

Programme Director: Professor S. Roy Choudhury
Coordinator, Primary F.R.C.S. Course Department of Anatomy, Faculty of Medicine, University of Kuwait.

Professor Gearoid Lynch
Dean of Postgraduate Surgical Studies R.C.S.I.

Participation: Doctors selected by the selection committee.

Programme:

Week 1

Saturday, 30th January, 1982

8.00 a.m.—11.00 a.m.   Introduction: Objectives, terminology; the skull
Prof. G. Lynch, RCSI

11.30 a.m.— 2.30 p.m.   Cardiovascular physiology
Prof. J. S. Juggi, Dept. Physiology

Sunday, 31st January, 1982

8.00 a.m.—11.00 a.m.   Cardiovascular physiology
Prof. J. S. Juggi, Dept. Physiology

11.30 a.m.— 2.30 p.m.   Cranial foramina, cr. nerves, meninges, venous sinuses
Prof. G. Lynch, RCSI

Monday, 1st February, 1982

8.00 a.m.—11.00 a.m.   CSF, intracranial hge, joints of skull and vertebrae
Prof. G. Lynch, RCSI

11.30 a.m.— 2.30 p.m.   Cardiovascular physiology
Prof. J. S. Juggi, Dept. Physiology

Tuesday, 2nd February, 1982

8.00 a.m.—11.00 a.m.	Neuroanatomy—surface topography blood supply Prof. S. R. Choudhury, Dept. Anatomy
11.30 a.m.— 2.30 p.m.	Cranial nerves, peripheral nerve plexuses, cervical plexus Prof. G. Lynch, RCSI

Wednesday, 3rd February, 1982

8.00 a.m.—11.00 a.m.	Face, cervical fascia, side of neck Prof. G. Lynch, RCSI
11.00 a.m.— 2.30 p.m.	Brain sections; cranial nerves—analysis Prof. S. R. Choudhury, Dept. Anatomy

Thursday, 4th February, 1982

8.00 a.m.—11.00 a.m.	MCQ Examination discussion Prof. G. Lynch, RCSI

Week 2

Saturday, 6th February, 1982

8.00 a.m.—11.00 a.m.	Parotid, thyroid glands, T. M. jt. inframtempo and submandibular region Prof. G. Lynch, RCSI
11.30 a.m.— 2.30 p.m.	Brain—introduction and functional areas, spinal cord

Sunday, 7th February, 1982

8.00 a.m.—11.00 a.m.	Sp. cord—coverings; afferent and efferent tracts
11.30 a.m.— 2.30 p.m.	Great vessels of neck, nasal and paranasal cavities Prof. G. Lynch, RCSI

Monday, 8th February, 1982

8.00 a.m.—11.00 a.m.	Orbit, eye ball, ext. ear Prof. G. Lynch, RCSI
11.30 a.m.— 2.30 p.m.	Cerebellum, tone posture and equilibrium

Tuesday, 9th February, 1982

8.00 a.m.—11.00 a.m.	Basal ganglia; ventricular system; C.S.F.
11.30 a.m.— 2.30 p.m.	Middle ear, larynx Prof. G. Lynch, RCSI

Wednesday, 10th February, 1982

8.00 a.m.—11.00 a.m.	Pharynx, revision and discussion Prof. G. Lynch, RCSI
11.30 a.m.— 2.30 p.m.	A.N.S.; inner ear mechanism and hearing

Thursday, 11th February, 1982

8.00 a.m.—11.00 a.m.	Vision; eye reflexes, taste and smell

Week 3

Saturday, 13th February, 1982

8.00 a.m.—11.00 a.m.	Skin; regulation of body temperature Dr. N. S. Al-Zaid, Dept. Physiology
11.30 a.m.— 2.30 p.m.	Basic immunology Prof. P. D. J. Holland, RCSI

Sunday, 14th February, 1982

8.00 a.m.—11.00 a.m.	Hypersensitivity Prof. P. D. J. Holland, RCSI
11.30 a.m.— 2.30 p.m.	Haematology I Prof. N. A. Mahmoud, Dept. Physiology

Monday, 15th February, 1982

8.00 a.m.—11.00 a.m.	Haematology II Prof. N. A. Mahmoud, Dept. Physiology
11.30 a.m.— 2.30 p.m.	Cell degeneration, necrosis Prof. P. D. J. Holland, RCSI

Tuesday, 16th February, 1982

8.00 a.m.—11.00 a.m.	Haematology III Prof. N. A. Mahmoud, Dept. Physiology
11.30 a.m.— 2.30 p.m.	Acute inflammation Prof. P. D. J. Holland, RCSI

Wednesday, 17th February, 1982

8.00 a.m.—11.00 a.m.	Chronic inflammation Prof. P. D. J. Holland, RCSI
11.30 a.m.— 2.30 p.m.	Disorders of plasma proteins Dr. M. S. Al-Adnani, Dept. Pathology

Thursday, 18th February, 1982

8.00 a.m.—11.00 a.m.	Chr. infective granuloma; pathological calcification and pigmentation

Week 4

Saturday, 20th February, 1982

8.00 a.m.—11.00 a.m.	Regeneration and repair Prof. P. D. J. Holland, RCSI
11.30 a.m.— 2.30 p.m.	Bones of abdomen and pelvis; the abdominal wall and inguinal region Mr. B. Lane, RCSI

Sunday, 21st February, 1982

8.00 a.m.—11.00 a.m.	Peritoneum; alimentary tract in general Mr. B. Lane, RCSI
11.30 a.m.— 2.30 p.m.	Autoimmune diseases Prof. P. D. J. Holland

Monday, 22nd February, 1982

8.00 a.m.—11.00 a.m.	Thrombosis. Embolism Prof. P. D. J. Holland, RCSI
11.30 a.m.— 2.30 p.m.	Stomach, duodenum and small gut. spleen, upper branches of aorta Mr. B. Lane, RCSI

Tuesday, 23rd February, 1982

8.00 a.m.—11.00 a.m.	The colon and rectum. Liver and biliary apparatus portal vein. Lower branches of aorta Mr. B. Lane, RCSI
11.30 a.m.— 2.30 p.m.	Vitamin deficiency diseases, MCQ examination Prof. P. D. J. Holland, RCSI

Wednesday, 24th February, 1982

8.00 a.m.—11.00 a.m.	Evaluation of MCQ examination; discussion Prof. P. D. J. Holland, RCSI
11.30 a.m.— 2.30 p.m.	Post. abd. wall; coelic plex., symp. chain; kidney and adrenals; vena cava Mr. B. Lane, RCSI

Thursday, 25th February, 1982

Holiday

Week 5

Saturday, 27th February, 1982

8.00 a.m.—11.00 a.m.	Diaphragm; lumbar plex/pelvic fascia, floor; genl. arrangement of pelvic viscera Mr. B. Lane, RCSI
11.30 a.m.— 2.30 p.m.	Metabolism, carbohydrate Dr. J. Finucane, RCSI

Sunday, 28th February, 1982

8.00 a.m.—11.00 a.m.	Fat and protein metabolism Dr. J. Finucane, RCSI
11.30 a.m.— 2.30 p.m.	Scrotum and testes; perineal pouches; ischio rectal fossa Mr. B. Lane, RCSI

Monday, 1st March, 1982

8.00 a.m.—11.00 a.m.	Male pelvic organs, bladder, prostate, vas, seminal ves. Mr. B. Lane, RCSI
11.30 a.m.— 2.30 p.m.	Nucleic acid and vitamin metabolism. Regulation of body temperature Dr. J. Finucane, RCSI

Tuesday, 2nd March, 1982

8.00 a.m.—11.00 a.m.	Hypothalamo-pituitary function Dr. J. Finucane, RCSI
11.30 a.m.— 2.30 p.m.	Pelvic ureter, urethra female pelvic organs uterus, ovary, broad lig. Mr. B. Lane

Wednesday, 3rd March, 1982

8.00 a.m.—11.00 a.m.	Female pelvic organs—contd. MCQ examination Mr. B. Lane
11.30 a.m.— 2.30 p.m.	Thyroid, endocrine pancreas Dr. J. Finucane, RCSI

Thursday, 4th March, 1982

8.00 a.m.—11.00 a.m.	Review of MCQ test Discussion

Week 6

Saturday, 6th March, 1982

8.00 a.m.—11.00 a.m.	Adrenal gland., gonadal function, menstrual cycle Dr. J. Finucane, RCSI
11.30 a.m.— 2.30 p.m.	Genetically determined diseases Prof. L. G. Lindberg, Dept. Pathology

Sunday, 7th March, 1982

8.00 a.m.—11.00 a.m.	Ischaemia, infarction, gangrene Dr. M. S. Al-Adnani, Dept. Pathology
11.30 a.m.— 2.30 p.m.	Parathyroid; calcium and phosphate metabolism Dr. J. Finucane, RCSI

Monday, 8th March, 1982

8.00 a.m.—11.00 a.m.	Respiratory physiology Dr. J. Finucane, RCSI
11.30 a.m.— 2.30 p.m.	Bones of upper limb; shoulder girdle and jt. axilla, arm Dr. P. K. Ray, Dept. Anaesthesiology

Tuesday, 9th March, 1982

8.00 a.m.—11.00 a.m.	Elbow and wrist joints; forearm-pronation/supination carpal tunnel Dr. P. K. Ray, Dept. Anaesthesiology
11.30 a.m.— 2.30 p.m.	Respiratory physiology Dr. J. Finucane, RCSI

Wednesday, 10th March, 1982

8.00 a.m.—11.00 a.m.	Respiratory physiology, MCQ examination Dr. J. Finucane, RCSI

| 11.30 a.m.— 2.30 p.m. | The hand, palm and dorsum, flexor tendons and sheaths, extensor mechanism
Dr. P. K. Ray, Dept. Anaesthesiology |

Thursday, 11th March, 1982

| 8.00 a.m.—11.00 a.m. | Review of MCQ test
Discussion
Dr. J. Finucane, RCSI |

Week 7

Saturday, 13th March, 1982

| 8.00 a.m.—11.00 a.m. | Thoracic cage; ribs and their movements; intercostal spaces
Dept. Anaesthesiology |
| 11.30 a.m.— 2.30 p.m. | Renal physiology I
Dr. J. McBroom, Dept. Physiology |

Sunday, 14th March, 1982

| 8.00 a.m.—11.00 a.m. | Mediastinum; the pleura and lungs, B.P. segments
Dept. Anaesthesiology |
| 11.30 a.m.— 2.30 p.m. | Renal physiology II
Dr. J. McBroom, Dept. Physiology |

Monday, 15th March, 1982

| 8.00 a.m.—11.00 a.m. | Physiology of GI tract. Deglutition. oesophageal motility and disorders
Dr. M. Barakat, Dept. Medicine |
| 11.30 a.m.— 2.30 p.m. | Pericardium. The heart, conduction system and bl. vs. of heart
Dept. Anaesthesiology |

Tuesday, 16th March, 1982

| 8.00 a.m.—11.00 a.m. | Neoplasia I
Prof. L. G. Lindberg, Dept. Pathology |
| 11.30 a.m.— 2.30 p.m. | The upper GI tract; gastric secretion pylorus; pancreas, liver
Dr. Barakat, Dept. Medicine |

Wednesday, 17th March, 1982

9.15 a.m.	The lower GI tract
9.30 a.m.—11.00 a.m.	Neoplasis II Prof. Ali, Dept. Pathology
11.30 a.m.— 2.30 p.m.	Fluid and electrolyte balance Dr. J. McBroom, Dept. Physiology

Thursday, 18th March, 1982

| 8.00 a.m.—11.00 a.m. | Trachea, bronchi; oesophagus, vagus, phrenic, sympathetic chain |

Week 8

Saturday, 20th March, 1982

8.00 a.m.—11.00 a.m.	Bones of lower limb; front of thigh; hip and knee joints; gluteal region
11.30 a.m.— 2.30 p.m.	Micro organisms of surgical importance Prof. E. Moorehouse, RCSI

Sunday, 21st March, 1982

8.00 a.m.—11.00 a.m.	Micro organisms of surgical importance Prof. E. Moorehouse, RCSI
11.30 a.m.— 2.30 p.m.	Thigh—back, popliteal fossa; leg front and back; soleal pump, ankle joint

Monday, 22nd March, 1982

8.00 a.m.—11.00 a.m.	The foot; review and discussion
11.30 a.m.— 2.30 p.m.	Hospital infections; carrier state Prof. E. Moorehouse, RCSI

Tuesday, 23rd March, 1982

8.00 a.m.—11.00 a.m.	Antibiotics and chemotherapeutic agents Prof. E. Moorehouse, RCSI
11.30 a.m.— 2.30 p.m.	Intravenous nutrition; fluid and electrolyte balance Prof. G. Abouna, Dept. Surgery

Wednesday, 24th March, 1982

8.00 a.m.—11.00 a.m.	Course evaluation Prof. Choudhury, Dept. Anatomy
11.30 a.m.— 2.30 p.m.	Defence mechanisms against infections Prof. E. Moorehouse, RCSI

Thursday, 25th March, 1982

8.00 a.m.—11.00 a.m.	Sterilization and disinfection Discussion and closure of course

81B—37/0101
Part I (Basic Sciences) Course Preparing for Examinations for Membership of the Royal College of Obstetrics and Gynaecology (M.R.C.O.G.—London)

Objectives:	Course in Basic Sciences directed towards Part I of the membership (M.R.C.O.G.) examination.
Methods:	This list of suggested text-books is for guidance only and is not compulsory reading. There are many other books, not listed here suitable for study purposes for the Part I Membership Examination.

Passnore, R., and Robson, J. S., eds. *A companion to medical studies.* 3 vols, in 4 parts. Oxford: Blackwell 1970. (General basis for study) (2nd edition of Vol. 1 now available—published 1976) (2nd edition of Vol. 2 due August 1978).

MacDonald, R. R. *Scientific basis of obstetrics and gynaecology.* 2nd ed. London: Churchill 1978.

Smout, C. F. V., et al. *Gynaecological and obstetrical anatomy.* 4th ed. London: Lewis 1969.

Gray, H. *Anatomy.* 35th ed. London: Longmans 1973.

Hytten, F. E., and Leitch, I. *The physiology of human pregnancy.* 2nd ed. Oxford: Blackwell 1971.

Bell, G. H., et al. *Textbook of physiology and biochemistry.* 9th ed. Edinburgh: Churchill Livingstone 1976.

Fox, H., and Langley, F. A., eds. *Postgraduate obstetrical and gynaecological pathology.* Oxford: Pergamon 1973.

Walter, J. B., and Israel, M. S. *General pathology.* 4th ed. London: Churchill Livingstone 1974.

Hamilton, W. J., Boyd, J. D., and Mossman, H. W. *Human embryology.* 4th ed. by W. J. Hamilton and H. W. Mossman. Cambridge: Heffer 1972.

Emery, A. *Elements of medical genetics.* 4th ed. Edinburgh: Churchill Livingstone 1975.

Gell, P. G. H., and Coombs, R. R., eds. *Clinical aspects of immunology.* 3rd ed. Oxford: Blackwell 1975.

Hall, R., et al. *Fundamentals of clinical endocrinology.* London: Pitman 2nd ed. 1974.

Hill, Sir Austin Bradford. *A short textbook of medical statistics.* London: Hodder and Stoughton 1977.

Parkinson, Joy. *A manual of English for overseas doctors.* 2nd ed. Edinburgh: Churchill Livingstone 1976.

Stewart, F. S., and Beswick, T. S. L. *Bacteriology and immunology for students of medicine.* 10th ed. London: Beilliere Tindall 1977.

Laurence, D. R. *Clinical pharmacology.* 4th ed. Edinburgh: Churchill Livingstone 1973.

Harper, H. A. *Review of physiological chemistry.* 16th ed. Lange 1977.

Ganong, W. F. *Review of medical physiology.* 8th ed. Lange 1977.

Shearman, R. P., ed. *Human reproductive physiology.* Oxford (etc.): Blackwell 1972.

Phillipp, E. E., et al. *Scientific foundations of obstetrics and gynaecology,* 2nd ed. London: Heinemann 1977.

Tindall, V. R. *MCO tutor: MRCOG part I. Basic sciences as applied to obstetrics and gynaecology.* London: Heinemann 1977 (available from the RCOG £ 3.75 or £ 4.75 overseas).

Place (Venue):   All classes will be held in the Physiology Seminar Room, Basic Sciences Building, Faculty of Medicine, Shuwaikh.

Duration: 4 weeks, from 2. 1. 1982 to 28. 1. 1982.
                               Part I MRCOG Examination will be held in Kuwait on
                               Monday, 1 March, 1982.
                               Application for the examination is to be submitted in
                               prescribed form directly to the Royal College of Obstetri-
                               cians and Gynaecologists, 27 Sussex Place, Regents Park,
                               London NWI 4 RG by December 1, 1981.

Organiser: Faculty of Medicine and Ministry of Public Health, Ku-
                               wait.
                               Institute of Obstetrics and Gynaecology, University of
                               London.
                               The Academic Department of Obstetrics and Gynaecolo-
                               gy, Middlesex Hospital, London.

Programme Director: Professor S. Roy Choudhury, Department of Anatomy,
                               Faculty of Medicine, P. O. Box 24923, Safat, Kuwait.
                               For examination particulars, please consult Professor
                               Hassan Hathout, Chairman, Department of Obstetrics
                               and Gynaecology, Faculty of Medicine, University of
                               Kuwait.

Participants: Application form and all relevant information regarding
                               the course and examination can be obtained from the
                               Secretary, Dept. of Anatomy.
                               Completed application form along with a recent photo-
                               graph and names and addresses of two referees should
                               be submitted not later than Wednesday, October 7, 1981.

Programme: As follows:

                               Saturday, 2nd January, 1982

                               Holiday

                               Sunday, 3rd January, 1982

8.00 a.m.—9.00 a.m.   Introduction and examination techniques
                               Sir J. Dewhurst, Institute
9.00 a.m.—10.00 a.m.   Multiple choice examination I
                               Sir J. Dewhurst, Institute
10.00 a.m.—10.15 a.m.   Break
10.15 a.m.—11.45 a.m.   Sex differentiation and its anomalies
11.45 a.m.—12.00 noon   Break
12.00 noon—1.15 p.m.   Cell structure and function
                               Dr. P. Sivandasingham, Dept. Anatomy
1.15 p.m.—2.30 p.m.   Cell damage, ionising radiation, isotopes
                               Prof. M. Y. Ali, Dept. Pathology

                               Monday, 4th January, 1982

8.00 a.m.—9.00 a.m.   Chromosome constitution and its anomalies I
                               Sir J. Dewhurst, Institute
9.00 a.m. — 10.00 a.m.   Chromosome constitution and its anomalies II
                               Sir J. Dewhurst, Institute
10.00 a.m. — 10.15 a.m.   Break

10.15 a.m.—11.45 a.m.	Inheritance of genetically determined abnormalities
11.45 a.m.—12.00 noon	Break
12.00 noon—1.15 p.m.	Puberty and menopause
	Sir J. Dewhurst, Institute
1.15 p.m.—2.30 p.m.	Enzymes
	Prof. K. A. Gumaa, Dept. Biochemistry

Tuesday, 5th January, 1982

8.00 a.m.—9.00 a.m.	Hypothalamo-pituitary-ovarian axis I
	Sir J. Dewhurst, Institute
9.00 a.m.—10.00 a.m.	Hypothalamo-pituitary-ovarian axis II
	Sir J. Dewhurst, Institute
10.00 a.m.—10.15 a.m.	Break
10.15 a.m.—11.45 a.m.	Genital tract-developmental abnormalities
	Sir J. Dewhurst, Institute
11.45 a.m.—12.00 noon	Break
12.00 noon—1.15 p.m.	Discussion and review session
	Sir J. Dewhurst, Institute
1.15 p.m.—2.30 p.m.	Metabolism of fat
	Prof. K. A. Gumaa, Dept. Biochemistry

Wednesday, 6th January, 1982

8.00 a.m.—9.00 a.m.	Antigen, antibodies and their reactions
	Dr. A. G. White, Dept. Surgery
9.00 a.m.—10.00 a.m.	Active and passive immunity
	Prof. T. D. Chugh, Dept. Microbiology
10.00 a.m.—10.15 a.m.	Break
10.15 a.m.—11.45 a.m.	Inflammation—acute
	Prof. M. Y. Ali, Dept. Pathology
11.45 a.m.—12.00 noon	Break
12.00 noon—1.15 p.m.	Inflammation—chronic
	Prof. M. Y. Ali, Dept. Pathology
1.15 p.m.—2.30 p.m.	Proteins and their metabolism
	Prof. K. A. Gumaa, Dept. Biochemistry

Thursday, 7th January, 1982

Holiday

Saturday, 9th January, 1982

8.00 a.m.—9.00 a.m.	Anaesthetics
	Prof. O. Thulesius, Dept. Pharmacology
9.00 a.m.—10.00 a.m.	Immunology of pregnancy, pregnancy test
	Prof. H. Hathout, Dept. Obstetrics and Gynaecology
10.00 a.m.—10.15 a.m.	Break
10.15 a.m.—11.45 a.m.	Carbohydrate metabolism
	Prof. K. A. Gumaa, Dept. Biochemistry
11.45 a.m.—12.00 noon	Break
12.00 noon—1.15 p.m.	CNS-afferent and efferent tracts
	Prof. S. R. Choudhury, Dept. Anatomy
1.15 p.m.—2.30 p.m.	Abdominal wall, inguinal and femoral regions

Sunday, 10th January, 1982

8.00 a.m.—9.00 a.m.	Breast Dept. Anatomy
9.00 a.m.—10.00 a.m.	Microorganisms—general characteristics Prof. T. D. Chugh, Dept. Microbiology
10.00 a.m.—10.15 a.m.	Break
10.15 a.m.—11.45 a.m.	Anticonvulsants, anticoagulants Prof. O. Thulesius, Dept. Pharmacology
11.45 a.m.—12.00 noon	Break
12.00 noon—1.15 p.m.	Vitamins Prof. K. A. Gumaa, Dept. Biochemistry
1.15 p.m.—2.30 p.m.	Autoimmune disease Dr. M. S. Al-Adnani, Dept. Pathology

Monday, 11th January, 1982

8.00 a.m.—9.00 a.m.	Wound infection Prof. T. D. Chugh, Dept. Microbiology
9.00 a.m.—10.00 a.m.	Antidiabetic drugs Prof. O. Thulesius, Dept. Pharmacology
10.00 a.m.—10.15 a.m.	Break
10.15 a.m.—11.45 a.m.	Histology of female genital tract Dept. Anatomy
11.45 a.m.—12.00 noon	Break
12.00 noon—1.15 p.m.	Iron metabolism Prof. K. A. Gumaa, Dept. Biochemistry
1.15 p.m.—2.30 p.m.	Degeneration Dr. M. S. Al-Adnani, Dept. Pathology

Tuesday, 12th January, 1982

8.00 a.m.—9.00 a.m.	Statistics I Prof. S. Jeffcoate, Institute
9.00 a.m.—10.00 a.m.	Reproduction physiology (excluding pregnancy) Prof. S. Jeffcoate, Institute
10.00 a.m.—10.15 a.m.	Break
10.15 a.m.—11.45 a.m.	Hypothalmo-pituitary-ovarian axis III Prof. S. Jeffcoate, Institute
11.45 a.m.—12.00 noon	Break
12.00 noon—1.15 p.m.	Thyroid gland Prof. S. Jeffcoate, Institute
1.15 p.m.—2.30 p.m.	Abdominal viscera—topography vascular and nerve supply Dept. Anatomy

Wednesday, 13th January, 1982

8.00 a.m.—9.00 a.m.	Adrenal glands I Prof. S. Jeffcoate, Institute
9.00 a.m.—10.00 a.m.	Adrenal glands II Prof. S. Jeffcoate, Institute
10.00 a.m.—10.15 a.m.	Break
10.15 a.m.—11.45 a.m.	Endocrine pancreas Prof. S. Jeffcoate, Institute

11.45 a.m.—12.00 noon	Break
12.00 noon—1.15 p.m.	Placenta—endocrine aspects
	Prof. S. Jeffcoate, Institute
1.15 p.m.—2.30 p.m.	Abdominal viscera—topography, vascular and nerve supply

Thursday, 14th January, 1982

8.00 a.m.—9.00 a.m.	Hospital infection, principles of control
	Prof. T. D. Chugh, Dept. Microbiology
9.00 a.m.—10.00 a.m.	Multiple choice examination II
	Prof. Hathout, Dept. Obstetrics and Gynaecology
10.00 a.m.—10.15 a.m.	Break
10.15 a.m.—11.45 a.m.	Statistics II
	Prof. S. Jeffcoate, Institute
11.45 a.m.—12.00 noon	Break
12.00 noon—1.15 p.m.	Statistics III
	Prof. S. Jeffcoate, Institute
1.15 p.m.—2.30 p.m.	Review and discussion
	Prof. S. Jeffcoate, Institute

Saturday, 16th January, 1982

8.00 a.m.—9.00 a.m.	Amniotic fluid
	Mr. S. J. Steele, Middlesex Hospital
9.00 a.m.—10.00 a.m.	Sedatives and analgesics
	Mr. S. J. Steele, Middlesex Hospital
10.00 a.m.—10.15 a.m.	Break
10.15 a.m.—11.45 a.m.	Hypotensive drugs and diuretics
	Mr. S. J. Steele, Middlesex Hospital
11.45 a.m.—12.00 noon	Break
12.00 noon—1.15 p.m.	Pelvis, pelvic wall, diaphragm
1.15 p.m.—2.30 p.m.	Calcium metabolism, rare metals
	Prof. K. A. Gumaa, Dept. Biochemistry

Sunday, 17th January, 1982

8.00 a.m.—9.00 a.m.	Uterine stimulants and inhibitors
	Mr. S. J. Steele, Middlesex Hospital
9.00 a.m.—10.00 a.m.	Pharmacology of ovulation
	Mr. S. J. Steele, Middlesex Hospital
10.00 a.m.—10.15 a.m.	Break
10.15 a.m.—11.45 a.m.	Contraceptives
	Mr. S. J. Steele, Middlesex Hospital
11.45 a.m.—12.00 noon	Break
12.00 noon—1.15 p.m.	Chemotherapeutic and antibiotic agents
	Prof. F. Fenech, Dept. Medicine
1.15 p.m.—2.30 p.m.	Repair and wound healing
	Dr. M. S. Al-Adnani, Dept. Pathology

Monday, 18th January, 1982

| 8.00 a.m.—9.00 a.m. | Prostaglandins |
| | Mr. S. J. Steele, Middlesex Hospital |

9.00 a.m.—10.00 a.m.	Cancer chemotherapy
	Mr. S. J. Steele, Middlesex Hospital
10.00 a.m.—10.15 a.m.	Break
10.15 a.m.—11.45 a.m.	Tranquilisers and antihistamines
	Mr. S. J. Steele, Middlesex Hospital
11.45 a.m.—12.00 noon	Break
12.00 noon—1.15 p.m.	Fetal skull and labour
	Dr. R. Dinwiddie, Institute
1.15 p.m.—2.30 p.m.	Fetal well being
	Dr. R. Dinwiddie, Institute

Tuesday, 19th January, 1982

8.00 a.m.—9.00 a.m.	Postnatal adaptation to life
	Dr. R. Dinwiddie, Institute
9.00 a.m.—10.00 a.m.	Fetal lung maturation
10.00 a.m.—10.15 a.m.	Break
10.15 a.m.—11.45 a.m.	Prematurity
11.45 a.m.—12.00 noon	Break
12.00 noon—1.15 p.m.	Contraceptives and sexual physiology
	Mr. S. J. Steele, Middlesex Hospital
1.15 p.m.—2.30 p.m.	Review and discussion
	Mr. S. J. Steele, Middlesex Hospital

Wednesday, 20th January, 1982

8.00 a.m.—9.00 a.m.	Fetal growth and nutrition
	Dr. R. Dinwiddie, Institute
9.00 a.m.—10.00 a.m.	Haemolytic disease of the new born
	Dr. R. Dinwiddie, Institute
10.00 a.m.—10.15 a.m.	Break
10.15 a.m.—11.45 a.m.	Viruses in obstetrics and gynaecology
	Dr. R. Dinwiddie, Institute
11.45 a.m.—12.00 noon	Break
12.00 noon—1.15 p.m.	Neoplasia I
1.15 p.m.—2.30 p.m.	Neoplasia II

Thursday, 21st January, 1982

8.00 a.m.—9.00 a.m.	Pelvic viscera I
	Prof. S. R. Choudhury, Dept. Anatomy
9.00 a.m.—10.00 a.m.	Microinvasive cancer, genital premalignancy
	Prof. L. G. Lindberg, Dept. Pathology
10.00 a.m.—10.15 a.m.	Break
10.15 a.m.—11.45 a.m.	Vaginal cytology
	Prof. L. G. Lindberg, Dept. Pathology
11.45 a.m.—12.00 noon	Break
12.00 noon—1.15 p.m.	Drug hazards, teratogenicity, fetal damage
	Dr. R. Dinwiddie, Institute
1.15 p.m.—2.30 p.m.	Review and discussion
	Dr. R. Dinwiddie, Institute

Saturday, 23rd January, 1982

8.00 a.m.—9.00 a.m.	Germ cells; gametogenesis and spermatogenesis Dr. J. Pryse-Davies, Institute
9.00 a.m.—10.00 a.m.	Fertilization, embedding and early embryogenesis Dr. J. Pryse-Davies, Institute
10.00 a.m.—10.15 a.m.	Break
10.15 a.m.—11.45 a.m.	General review of development Dr. J. Pryse-Davies, Institute
11.45 a.m.—12.00 noon	Break
12.00 noon—1.15 p.m.	Pelvic viscera II
1.15 p.m.—2.30 p.m.	Nutrition in pregnancy

Sunday, 24th January, 1982

8.00 a.m.—9.00 a.m.	Development and structure of placenta and fetal membranes Dr. J. Pryse-Davies, Institute
9.00 a.m.—10.00 a.m.	Development of cardiovascular system Dr. J. Pryse-Davies, Institute
10.00 a.m.—10.15 a.m.	Break
10.15 a.m.—11.45 a.m.	Development of G.I. and respiratory system Dr. J. Pryse-Davies, Institute
11.45 a.m.—12.00 noon	Break
12.00 noon—1.15 p.m.	Pelvic viscera III
1.15 p.m.—2.30 p.m.	Lactation—normal and abnormal

Monday, 25th January, 1982

8.00 a.m.—9.00 a.m.	Cell membrane and transport mechanisms Dr. M. de Swiet, Institute
9.00 a.m.—10.00 a.m.	Kidney Dr. M. de Swiet, Institute
10.00 a.m.—10.15 a.m.	Break
10.15 a.m.—11.45 a.m.	Acid base balance Dr. M. de Swiet, Institute
11.45 a.m.—12.00 noon	Break
12.00 noon—1.15 p.m.	Development of C.N.S. and musculoskeletal system Dr. J. Pryse-Davies, Institute
1.15 p.m.—2.30 p.m.	Development of urinary system and anomalies Dr. J. Pryse-Davies, Institute

Tuesday, 26th January, 1982

8.00 a.m.—9.00 a.m.	Assessment of fetal development malformations Dr. J. Pryse-Davies, Institute
9.00 a.m.—10.00 a.m.	Review and discussion Dr. J. Pryse-Davies, Institute
10.00 a.m.—10.15 a.m.	Break
10.15 a.m.—11.45 a.m.	Urogenital diaphragm, sacral plexus
11.45 a.m.—12.00 noon	Break
12.00 noon—1.15 p.m.	Circulation I Dr. M. de Swiet, Institute
1.15 p.m.—2.30 p.m.	Circulation II Dr. M. de Swiet, Institute

Wednesday, 27th January, 1982

8.00 a.m.—9.00 a.m.	Respiration I
	Dr. M. de Swiet, Institute
9.00 a.m.—10.00 a.m.	Respiration II
	Dr. M. de Swiet, Institute
10.00 a.m.—10.15 a.m.	Break
10.15 a.m.—11.45 a.m.	Fluid and electrolyte balance
	Dr. J. McBroom, Dept. Physiology
11.45 a.m.—12.00 noon	Break
12.00 noon—1.15 p.m.	G.I. tract physiology I
	Dr. M. Barakat, Dept. Medicine
1.15 p.m.—2.30 p.m.	G.I. tract physiology II
	Dr. M. Barakat, Dept. Medicine

Thursday, 28th January, 1982

8.00 a.m.—9.00 a.m.	Innervation of pelvic viscera. ANS
	Prof. S. R. Choudhury, Dept. Anatomy
9.00 a.m.—10.00 a.m.	Course evaluation
	Prof. S. R. Choudhury, Dept. Anatomy
10.00 a.m.—10.15 a.m.	Break
10.15 a.m.—11.45 a.m.	Genital infection and veneral diseases
	Prof. T. D. Chugh, Dept. Microbiology
11.45 a.m.—12.00 noon	Break
12.00 noon—1.15 p.m.	Placental transport
	Dr. M. de Swiet, Institute
1.15 p.m.—2.30 p.m.	Multiple choice examination III and course closure
	Dr. M. de Swiet, Institute

Monday, 1st March, 1982

Part I M.R.C.O.G. Examination will be held in Kuwait.

81B—69/0101
Course in Basic Sciences for Anaesthetists
Part I F.F.A.R.C.S. (England) Programme

Objectives:	Course in basic sciences directed towards preparation for sitting for the Part I F.F.A.R.C.S. (England) examination.
Place:	All classes will be held in the Amphitheatre 106 and the cafeteria, Faculty of Medicine, Shuwaikh, Kuwait.
Duration:	6 weeks, from 14th of April 1982 till 26th of May 1982, from 4.00 to 7.30 p.m. daily for 5 days, every week except Thursday from 4.00 p.m. to 6.00 p.m. (tutorials). Part I F.F.A.R.C.S. (England) examination will be in Kuwait on Saturday 19th of June 1982 in the premises of the Faculty of Medicine.

Organisers:	Ministry of Public Health Faculty of Medicine, Kuwait Welsh National School of Medicine
Programme Director:	Dr. M. M. I. Motaweh, Chairman, Anaesthesia Department, Sabah, Chest and Infectious Diseases Hospitals.
Assistant Coordinator:	Dr. Hussain A. E. F. Al-Yousof, Asst. Professor, Faculty of Medicine, Consultant Anaesthetist Mubarak Hospital.

Visiting

Lecturers:	MDV M. D. Vickers Professor of Anaesthetics WWM W. W. Mapleson Prof. of Physics Applied to Anaesthesia JNL J. N. Lunn Senior Lecturer in Anaesthetics JNH J. N. Horton Consultant Anaesthetist and Honorary Clinical Teacher MH M. Harmer Lecturer in Anaesthetics
Local:	OT Olav Thulesius Prof. and Chairman, Dept. of Pharmacology AA Abdulla Al-Khars Assistant Professor AE Abdulla Elkhawa Assistant Professor MA Maria Angelo-Khattar Assistant Professor MJM M. J. McBroom Associate Professor and Acting Chairman, Dept. of Physiology NAM N. A. Mahmoud, Professor KAG K. A. Gumaa, Professor JSJ J. S. Juggi, Professor KYM K. Y. Mustafa, Associate Professor ISA I. S. Aneja, Associate Professor
Participants:	All doctors Anaesthetists working in Kuwait. Six candidates from Gulf States, each State, one representative. The number of all candidates sitting for the course is 20 (twenty) doctors including the Gulf State representatives.
No. of candidates sitting for the examination	The number of candidates sitting for Part I of the F.F.A.R.C.S. (England) examination is unlimited. All candidates attending the course should sit for the 1st part of the examination.
Readings:	1. *Principles for clinical measurements* by Sykes, Vickers and Hull. 2. *The scientific foundations of anaesthesia* by Scurr and Feldman.

3. *Aids to anaesthesia* by Harrison, Healy and Thoronton.
   N. B. Read the physiology part only in this book.
4. *Drugs in anaesthetic practice* by Vickers, Wood-Smith and Stewart.
5. *Clinical pharmacology* by Lawrence.
6. *Applied cardiovascular physiology* by Prys Roberts.
7. *Applied respiratory physiology* by Nunn.
8. *Textbook of clinical pharmacology* by Rogers, Spector and Trounce.

This list of suggested textbooks is for guidance only and is not compulsory reading. There are many other books not listed here for study purposes for the 1st Part of the F.F.A.R.C.S. Examination.

Programme:

14th April, 1982 (Wednesday)

4.00—5.00 p.m.	Dimensions and S.I. units, WWM
5.00—6.00 p.m.	MCQ Test
6.30—7.30 p.m.	Mathematics 1, WWM

15th April, 1982 (Thursday)

4.00—5.00 p.m.	Optional
	Tutorial 1, MCQ results, MDV

17th April, 1982 (Saturday)

4.00—5.00 p.m.	Principles of measurement, WWM
5.00—6.00 p.m.	Local anaesthetics, MDV
6.30—7.30 p.m.	Mathematics 2, WWM

18th April, 1982 (Sunday)

4.00—5.00 p.m.	Transducers, MDV
5.00—6.00 p.m.	Gas laws, MMW
6.30—7.30 p.m.	Biological signals, MDV

19th April, 1982 (Monday)

4.00—5.00 p.m.	Gas storage, WWM
5.00—6.00 p.m.	Signal processing, MDV
6.30—7.30 p.m.	Gas flow, WWM

20th April, 1982 (Tuesday)

4.00—5.00 p.m.	Light etc., MDV
5.00—6.00 p.m.	Temperature and heat, WWM
6.30—7.30 p.m.	Tutorial: Essay results and volume measurement, MDV

21st April, 1982 (Wednesday)

4.00—5.00 p.m.	Vapours, WWM
5.00—6.00 p.m.	Sound and ultrasound, MDV
6.30—7.30 p.m.	Surface tension, WWM

22nd April, 1982 (Thursday)

Optional:
4.00—5.00 p.m.   Discussion of Maths. examples, WWM

24th April, 1982 (Saturday)

4.00—5.00 p.m.   Statistics I, MDV
5.00—6.00 p.m.   Diffusion and osmosis, WWM
6.30—7.30 p.m.   Statistics II, MDV

25th April, 1982 (Sunday)

4.00—5.00 p.m.   Gas analysis, WWM
5.00—6.00 p.m.   Statistics III, MDV
6.30—7.30 p.m.   Tutorial: Cardiac output, WWM

26th April, 1982 (Monday)

4.00—5.00 p.m.   Data processing, WWM
5.00—6.00 p.m.   Tutorial: Revision statistics, MDV
6.30—7.30 p.m.   Tutorial: Revision physics, WWM

27th April, 1982 (Tuesday)

4.00—5.00 p.m.   Clinical trials, MDV
5.00—6.00 p.m.   Uptake and distribution of anaesthetics, WWM
6.30—7.30 p.m.   Tutorial: Essay questions and discussion, MDV

28th April, 1982 (Wednesday)

4.00—5.00 p.m.   Cardiovascular physiology I (Kt), JSJ
5.00—6.00 p.m.   Pharmacology (Kt), AA
6.30—7.30 p.m.   Electricity I, JNH

29th April, 1982 (Thursday)

Optional:
4.00—5.00 p.m.   Tutorial: Ionizing radiation, JNH

1st May, 1982 (Saturday)

4.00—5.00 p.m.   Cardiovascular physiology 2 (Kt), JSJ
5.00—6.00 p.m.   Pharmacology 2 (Kt), AA
6.30—7.30 p.m.   Tutorial: Revision, JNH

2nd May, 1982 (Sunday)

4.00—5.00 p.m.   Cardiovascular physiology 3 (Kt), JSJ
5.00—6.00 p.m.   Pharmacology 3 (Kt), OT
6.30—7.30 p.m.   Electricity 2, JNH

3rd May, 1982 (Monday)

4.00—5.00 p.m.   Cardiovascular physiology 4 (Kt), JSJ
5.00—6.00 p.m.   Pharmacology 4 (Kt), MA
6.30—7.30 p.m.   Tutorial: Revision, JNH

4th May, 1982 (Tuesday)

4.00—5.00 p.m.	Neurophysiology 2 (Kt), ISA
5.00—6.00 p.m.	Pharmacology 5 (Kt), MA
6.30—7.30 p.m.	Electrical Safety, JNH

5th May, 1982 (Wednesday)

4.00—5.00 p.m.	Neurophysiology 2 (Kt), ISA
5.00—6.00 p.m.	Pharmacology 6 (Kt), OT
6.30—7.30 p.m.	Tutorial: Revision, JNH

6th May, 1982 (Thursday)

Optional:

4.00—5.00 p.m.	Discussion on written questions, JNH

8th May, 1982 (Saturday)

4.00—5.00 p.m.	Neurophysiology 3 (Kt), ISA
5.00—6.00 p.m.	Pharmacology 7 (Kt), OT
6.30—7.30 p.m.	Neonatal physiology, JNH

9th May, 1982 (Sunday)

4.00—5.00 p.m.	Neurophysiology 4 (Kt), OT
5.00—6.00 p.m.	Fluid and electrolytes 1 (Kt), MJM
6.30—7.30 p.m.	Obstetric physiology, JNH

10th May, 1982 (Monday)

4.00—5.00 p.m.	Neurophysiology 5 (Kt), ISA
5.00—6.00 p.m.	Fluid and electrolytes 2 (Kt), MJM
6.30—7.30 p.m.	Tutorial: Acid-base, JNH

11th May, 1982 (Tuesday)

4.00—5.00 p.m.	Cellular physiology 1 (Kt), KAG
5.00—6.00 p.m.	Fluid and electrolytes (Kt), MJM
6.30—7.30 p.m.	Tutorial: Revision

12th May, 1982 (Wednesday)

4.00—5.00 p.m.	Neuromuscular physiology 1 (Kt), KYM
5.00—6.00 p.m.	Anatomy Revision MH (Set Essays)
6.30—7.30 p.m.	Tutorial: Revision, JNH

13th May, 1982 (Thursday)

Optional:

4.00—5.00 p.m.	Lung function tests, MH

15th May, 1982 (Saturday)

4.00—5.00 p.m.	Neuromuscular pharmacology (Kt), AE
5.00—6.00 p.m.	Anti-emetics (Kt) OT
6.30—7.30 p.m.	Tutorial: Pharmacology of inhaled agents, MH

16th May, 1982 (Sunday)

4.00—5.00 p.m.	Neuromuscular physiology 3 (Kt), KYM
5.00—6.00 p.m.	Respiratory physiology I, JNL
6.30—7.30 p.m.	Tutorial: Muscle relaxants, MH

17th May, 1982 (Monday)

4.00—5.00 p.m.	IV induction agents (Kt), OT
5.00—6.00 p.m.	Endocrine system 1 (Kt), NAM
6.30—7.30 p.m.	Respiratory physiology 2, JNL

18th May, 1982 (Tuesday)

4.00—5.00 p.m.	Respiratory physiology 3, JNL
5.00—6.00 p.m.	Endocrine system 2, NAM
6.30—7.30 p.m.	Haematology 1, MH

19th May, 1982 (Wednesday)

4.00—5.00 p.m.	Respiratory physiology 4, JNL
5.00—6.00 p.m.	Tutorial: New agents, MH
6.30—7.30 p.m.	Respiratory physiology 5, JNL

20th May, 1982 (Thursday)

Optional:	
4.00—5.00 p.m.	Essay answers discussion, JNH and MH

22nd May, 1982 (Saturday)

4.00—5.00 p.m.	Respiratory physiology 6, JNL
5.00—6.00 p.m.	Haematology 2, MH
6.30—7.30 p.m.	Respiratory physiology 7, JNL

23rd May, 1982 (Sunday)

4.00—5.00 p.m.	MCQ paper, MH
5.00—6.00 p.m.	Tutorial: Revision, JNL
6.30—7.30 p.m.	MCQ results discussion, MH

24th May, 1982 (Monday)

4.00—5.00 p.m.	Trial vivas, JNL and MH, 12 candidates 15 minutes each

25th May, 1982 (Tuesday)

4.00—5.00 p.m.	Trial vivas, 8 candidates

26th May, 1982 (Wednesday)

4.00—5.00 p.m.	Revision Tutorials *2 groups,* JNL and MH Concentrating on physics and measurement.

Primary F.F.A.R.C.S. Examination in Kuwait
June, 1982
Revised Programme

(Arrangements for 37 candidates)

Saturday, 19th June *Multiple choice question paper* 9.00 a.m. to 12.00 noon
Presiding Examiners Prof. J. A. Thornton
Dr. I. T. Davie
Dr. G. W. Black

Sunday, 10th June *Essay paper* 9.00 a.m. to 12.00 noon
Presiding Examiners As above

Viva Voce Examinations

Tuesday, 22nd June	*Pharmacology and physiology*	8.00 a.m. to 12.30 p.m.
Wednesday, 23rd June		8.00 a.m. to 12.10 p.m.
Thursday, 24th June		
Saturday, 26th June	*Physics and*	8.00 a.m. to 12.30 p.m.
Sunday, 27th June	*clinical*	
Monday, 28th June	*measurement*	8.00 a.m. to 12.10 p.m.

Followed by *Report* (all Examiners) at the conclusion of the examination on Monday, 28th June.

Examiners

Pharmacology	Dr. I. T. Davie and Dr. G. W. Black
Physiology	Prof. J. A. Thornton and Prof. N. Mahmoud
Physics and	
clinical measurement	Prof. J. A. Thornton and Dr. I. T. Davie

81B—76 01 Course
Primary Dental Fellowship Course

Objectives:

The first Course in Basic Sciences directed towards the Primary Dental Fellowship of the Royal College of Surgeons in Ireland.

The course will be conducted jointly by the Medical Faculty of the University of Kuwait, The Ministry of Public Health of Kuwait, and a visiting team of lecturers from the Royal College of Surgeons in Ireland. It is designed to cover the general background of anatomy, physiology and pathology as these subjects relate directly to the clinical practice of dental surgery. The course will consist of an intensive series of tutorials and assessments with direct clinical relevance, designed to prepare those on it for the Primary Dental Fellowship Examination of this College or any of the Royal Colleges.

Methodology: The course is full time and very intensive. The candidates selected to attend the course are strongly advised to do a period of preparatory study so that they will be in a position to assimilate the teaching on the course at a very intensive level. This will be particularly necessary for those who, because of their work commitment, have been out of touch with the academic aspects of these sciences for a period of some years. There have been alterations in the approach towards the Basic Sciences in the Primary Fellowship Examinations over the past five years and the main function of this course will be to orientate the students on it to current thinking in the Royal Colleges in the United Kingdom and to give them an organised technique of study and a properly orientated approach to the examination.

During the course, there will be at most times a visiting lecturer from the Royal College of Surgeons in Ireland present in Kuwait. As much as possible, he or she will be available for discussion with the candidates on the course either singly or in groups. As will be seen in the Programme, it is planned from time to time to run small assessment examinations and discussion periods with the candidates on the course and this should be a great help to them in indicating how well they are keeping up with the material being presented.

Any standard text-book in the appropriate Basic Sciences constitutes acceptable reading material in preparation for this course. The most popular texts in use in the Royal College at the moment are listed below and are recommended by the panel of lecturers.

Anatomy
The System of Anatomy by Gray
Anatomy Descriptive and Applied by Last
Advanced Dental Histology, Advances in Dental Histology by Gaunt, Osborn and Ten Cate, Bristol. John Wright.

Physiology
Textbook of Physiology by Guyton
Clinical Physiology by Campbell, Dickenson and Slater
Introduction to Human Physiology by Green, Oxford University Press.

Pathology
General Pathology by Walter and Israel
Scientific Foundation of Dentistry Edited by Bertram *Cohen and I. R. H. Kramer* London, Willam Heinemann, Medical Books Limited.

Place (Venue):   All classes will take place in the Physiology Seminar Room, Faculty of Medicine.
Special Dental Lectures will be held at the Dental Centre, Kuwait.

Duration:	8 weeks, from 30th January, 1982 till 25th March, 1982.
Organiser:	Faculty of Medicine and Ministry of Public Health, Kuwait.
	Faculty of Dentistry, Royal College of Surgeons in Ireland, Ireland.
Programme Director:	Dr. Mahmoud Rajai in cooperation with the Training Division, Department of Public Health and Planning.
Coordinators:	Prof. M. Ragai Elmostehy, Coordinator of Postgraduate Dental Studies, Ministry of Public Health, Kuwait.
	Prof. S. Roy Choudhury, Coordinator, Primary F.R.C.S. Course, Department of Anatomy, Faculty of Medicine, University of Kuwait.
	Prof. Gearoid Lynch, Dean, Postgraduate Surgical Studies, RCSI.
Participants:	Dentists selected by the Selection Committee.
Programme:	

Week 1

Saturday, 30th January, 1982

8.00 a.m.—11.10 a.m.	Introduction: Objectives terminology, the skull Prof. G. Lynch, RCSI
11.30 a.m.— 2.30 p.m.	Cardiovascular physiology Prof. J. S. Juggi, Dept. Physiology

Sunday, 31st January, 1982

8.00 a.m.—11.10 a.m.	Cardiovascular physiology Prof. J. S. Juggi, Dept. Physiology
11.30 a.m.— 2.30 p.m.	Cranial foramina, cranial nerves, meniges, venous sinuses Prof. G. Lynch, RCSI

Monday, 1st February, 1982

8.00 a.m.—11.00 a.m.	CSF, intracranial hge, joints of skull and vertebrae Prof. G. Lynch, RCSI
11.30 a.m.— 2.30 p.m.	Cardiovascular physiology Prof. J. S. Juggi, Dept. Physiology

Tuesday, 2nd February, 1982

8.00 a.m.—11.00 a.m.	Neuroanatomy, surface topography, blood supply Prof. S. R. Choudhury, Dept. Anatomy
11.30 a.m.— 2.30 p.m.	Cranial nerves, peripheral nerve plexuses, cervical plexus Prof. G. Lynch, RCSI

Wednesday, 3rd February, 1982

8.00 a.m.—11.00 a.m.	Face, cervical fascia, side of neck Prof. G. Lynch, RCSI
11.30 a.m.— 2.30 p.m.	Brain sections: cranial nerves analysis Prof. S. R. Choudhury, Dept. Anatomy

Thursday, 4th February, 1982

8.00 a.m.—11.00 a.m.   MCQ examination discussion
                       Prof. G. Lynch, RCSI

Week 2

Saturday, 6th February, 1982

8.00 a.m.—11.00 a.m.   Parotid, thyroid gland TMJ. Infratempo and submandib-
                       ular region
                       Prof. G. Lynch, RCSI
11.30 a.m.— 2.30 p.m. Brain—introduction and functional areas, spinal cord
                       * Dept. Physiology

Sunday, 7th February, 1982

8.00 a.m.—11.00 a.m.   Spinal cord—coverings: afferent and efferent tracts
                       * Dept. Physiology
11.30 a.m.— 2.30 p.m. Great vessels of neck, nasal and paranasal cavities
                       Prof. G. Lynch, RCSI

Monday, 8th February, 1982

8.00 a.m.—11.00 a.m.   Orbit, eye ball, ext. ear
                       Prof. G. Lynch, RCSI
11.30 a.m.— 2.30 p.m. Cerebellum, tone, posture and equilibrium
                       * Dept. Physiology

Tuesday, 9th February, 1982

8.00 a.m.—11.00 a.m.   Basal ganglia, ventricular system, C.S.F.
                       * Dept. Physiology
11.30 a.m.— 2.30 p.m. Middle ear, larynx
                       Prof. G. Lynch, RCSI

Wednesday, 10th February, 1982

8.00 a.m.—11.00 a.m.   Pharynx, revision and discussion
                       Prof. G. Lynch, RCSI
11.00 a.m.— 2.30 p.m. A.N.S.: Inner ear mechanism and hearing
                       * Dept. Physiology

Thursday, 11th February, 1982

8.00 a.m.—11.00 a.m.   Vision; eye reflexes, taste and smell
                       * Dept. Physiology

----

* Name to be announced.

Week 3

Saturday, 13th February, 1982

8.00 a.m.—11.00 a.m.   Skin; regulation of body temperature
                          Dr. N. S. Al Zaid, Dept. Physiology
11.30 a.m.— 2.30 p.m.   Basic immunology
                          Prof. P. D. J. Holland, RCSI

Sunday, 14th February, 1982

8.00 a.m.—11.00 a.m.   Hypersensitivity
                          Prof. P. D. J. Holland, RCSI
11.30 a.m.— 2.30 p.m.   Haematology I
                          Prof. N. A. Mahmoud, Dept. Physiology

Monday, 15th February, 1982

8.00 a.m.—11.00 a.m.   Haematology II
                          Prof. N. A. Mahmoud, Dept. Physiology
11.30 a.m.— 2.30 p.m.   Cell degeneration, necrosis
                          Prof. P. D. J. Holland, RCSI

Tuesday, 16th February, 1982

8.00 a.m.—11.00 a.m.   Haematology III
                          Prof. N. A. Mahmoud, Dept. Physiology
11.30 a.m.— 2.30 p.m.   Acute inflammation
                          Prof. P. D. J. Holland, RCSI

Wednesday, 17th February, 1982

8.00 a.m.—11.00 a.m.   Chronic inflammation
                          Prof. P. D. J. Holland, RCSI
11.30 a.m.— 2.30 p.m.   Disorders of plasma proteins
                          Dr. M. S. Al Adnani, Dept. Pathology

Thursday, 18th February, 1982

8.00 a.m.—11.00 a.m.   Chr. infective granuloma path. calcification and pigmen-
                          tation
                          Prof. P. D. J. Holland, RCSI

Week 4

Saturday, 20th February, 1982

8.00 a.m.—11.00 a.m.   Regeneration and repair
                          Prof. P. D. J. Holland, RCSI

Sunday, 21st February, 1982

11.30 a.m.— 2.30 p.m.   Autoimmune diseases
                          Prof. P. D. J. Holland, RCSI

Monday, 22nd February, 1982

8.00 a.m.—11.00 a.m.   Thrombosis, embolism
                         Prof. P. D. J. Holland, RCSI

Tuesday, 23rd February, 1982

11.30 a.m.— 2.30 p.m.   Vitamin deficiency diseases, MCQ examination
                         Prof. P. D. J. Holland, RCSI

Wednesday, 24th February, 1982

8.00 a.m.—11.00 a.m.   Evaluation of MCQ test, discussion
                         Prof. P. D. J. Holland, RCSI

Thursday, 25th February, 1982
National holiday

Week 5

Saturday, 27th February, 1982

8.00 a.m.—11.00 a.m.   Neurophys. of mastic., speech and deglutition
                         Dr. F. Nally, RCSI
11.30 a.m.— 2.30 p.m.   Metabolism, carbohydrates
                         Dr. J. Finucane, RCSI

Sunday, 28th February, 1982

8.00 a.m.—11.00 a.m.   Fat and protein metabolism
                         Dr. J. Finucane, RCSI
11.30 a.m.— 2.30 p.m.   Physiology of facial pain
                         Dr. F. Nally, RCSI

Monday, 1st March, 1982

8.00 a.m.—11.00 a.m.   Neurology in relation, dent. surg.
                         Anaes. hypers. parasth. muscle tone, saliva
                         Dr. F. Nally, RCSI
11.30 a.m.— 2.30 p.m.   Nuclic acid and vitamin metabolism. Regulation of body
                         temp.
                         Dr. J. Finucane, RCSI

Tuesday, 2nd March, 1982

8.00 a.m.—11.00 a.m.   Hypothalomo-pituitary function
                         Dr. J. Finucane, RCSI
11.30 a.m.— 2.30 p.m.   Haematology, haemostasis, oral aspect
                         Dr. F. Nally, RCSI

Wednesday, 3rd March, 1982

8.00 a.m.—11.00 a.m.   Vitamins, oral aspects, review of MCQ and discussion
                         Dr. F. Nally, RCSI
11.30 a.m.— 2.30 p.m.   Thyroid, endocrine pancreas
                         Dr. J. Finucane, RCSI

Thursday, 4th March, 1982

8.00 a.m.—11.00 a.m.   Effects of radiation on tissue function. Review of MCQ
test
Dr. F. Nally, RCSI

Week 6

Saturday, 6th March, 1982

8.00 a.m.—11.00 a.m.   Adrenal gland, gonadal function, menstrual cycle
Dr. J. Finucane, RCSI
11.30 a.m.— 2.30 p.m.   Endocrinology, oral aspect
Dr. F. Nally, RCSI

Sunday, 7th March, 1982

8.00 a.m.—11.00 a.m.   Ischaemia, infection, gangrene
Dr. M. S. Al Adani, Dept. Pathology
11.30 a.m.— 2.30 p.m.   Parathyroid, calcium and phosphate metabolism
Dr. J. Finucane, RCSI

Monday, 8th March, 1982

8.00 a.m.—11.00 a.m.   Respiratory physiology
Dr. J. Finucane, RCSI
11.30 a.m.— 2.30 p.m.   Applied physiol. of tongue, O. M., healing of extr.
wound
Dr. F. Nally, RCSI

Tuesday, 9th March, 1982

8.00 a.m.—11.00 a.m.   Nerve impulse and local anaesthetics
Dr. F. Nally, RCSI
11.30 a.m.— 2.30 p.m.   Respiratory physiology
Dr. J. Finucane, RCSI

Wednesday, 10th March, 1982

8.00 a.m.—11.00 a.m.   Respiratory physiology, MCQ examination
Dr. J. Finucane, RCSI
11.30 a.m.— 2.30 p.m.   Trachea, branchi, oesoph., vagus, phrenic, sympathetic
chain
Dr. P. Sivandahsingham, Dept. Anatomy

Thursday, 11th March, 1982

8.00 a.m.—11.00 a.m.   Autoimmunity, oral aspects. Review of MCQ test and
discussion
Dr. F. Nally, RCSI

Week 7

Saturday, 13th March, 1982

8.00 a.m.—11.00 a.m.   Structure of a tooth germ and development of crown including pulp and dentin.
Dr. A. Hayward, RCSI

11.30 a.m.— 2.30 p.m.	Renal physiology I Dr. McBroom, Dept. Physiology

Sunday, 14th March, 1982

8.00 a.m.—11.00 a.m.	Structure and function of gingiva and junctional epithelium Dr. A. Hayward, RCSI
11.30 a.m.— 2.30 p.m.	Renal physiology II Dr. McBroom, Dept. Physiology

Monday, 15th March, 1982

8.00 a.m.—11.00 a.m.	Physiology of G.I. tract oesophagel motility and disorders Dr. M. Barakat, Dept. Medicine
11.30 a.m.— 2.30 p.m.	Structure and development of root-cementum and perio. ligament Dr. A. Hayward, RCSI

Tuesday, 16th March, 1982

9.00 a.m.—11.00 a.m.	Neoplasia I Prof. L. G. Lindberg, Dept. Pathology
11.30 a.m.— 2.30 p.m.	The upper G.I. tract, gastric secretion, pylorus pancreas, liver Dr. M. Barakat, Dept. Medicine

Wednesday, 17th March, 1982

8.00 a.m.— 9.00 a.m.	T.M.J. Dr. A. Hayward, RCSI
9.30 a.m.—11.00 a.m.	Neoplasica II Prof. M. Y. Ali
11.30 a.m.— 2.30 p.m.	Acid base balance Dr. J. McBroom, Dept. Physiology

Thursday, 18th March, 1982

8.00 a.m.—11.00 a.m.	Structure and development of bone, review of MCQ examination Dr. A. Hayward, RCSI

Week 8

Saturday, 20th March, 1982

8.00 a.m.—11.00 a.m.	Oral mucosa, structure and function including sensation Dr. A. Hayward, RCSI
11.30 a.m.— 2.30 p.m.	Micro-organisms of surgical importance Prof. E. Moorehouse, RCSI

Sunday, 21st March, 1982

8.00 a.m.—11.00 a.m.	Micro-organisms of surgical importance Prof. E. Moorehouse, RCSI
11.30 a.m.— 2.30 p.m.	Eruption, histological changes and mechanism Dr. A. Hayward, RCSI

Monday, 22nd March, 1982

8.00 a.m.—11.00 a.m.	Hospital infections; carrier state Prof. E. Moorehouse, RCSI
11.30 a.m.— 2.30 p.m.	Salivary glands, struct. functions, secretion of saliva. Occlusion Dr. A. Hayward, RCSI

Tuesday, 23rd March, 1982

8.00 a.m.—11.00 a.m.	Antibiotics and chemotherapeutic agents Prof. E. Moorehouse, RCSI
11.30 a.m.— 2.30 p.m.	Embryology and growth of face and jaws Dr. A. Hayward, RCSI

Wednesday, 24th March, 1982

8.00 a.m.—11.00 a.m.	Course evaluation Prof. S. R. Choudhury, Dept. Anatomy
11.30 a.m.— 2.30 p.m.	Defence mechanisms against infection Prof. E. Moorehouse, RCSI

Thursday, 25th March, 1982

8.00 a.m.—11.00 a.m.	Sterilization and disinfection, discussion and closure of course Prof. E. Moorehouse, RCSI

Report
on the Course Preparing for Mock Examination for Membership in the Royal College of Physicians

These are the comments I would like to make about the MRCP Courses which are held as part of the activities of the Area Executive Committee for Speciality Training and through the cooperation of the Ministry of Health and Department of Medicine of the Faculty of Medicine:

The attendance of the MRCP Part I Course has been quite satisfactory over the last 3 years with an attendance of over 100 and this applies to the attendance of the mock examination.

The Course content is more in the form of an up-date in the various fields of internal medicine and consists wholly of lectures. The mock examination helps us to identify the top 25 candidates who are then recommended to the Royal College of Physicians as being suitable to sit for the examination. The pass rate so far has been quite satisfactory varying from 33—53%. The attendance of Kuwaiti candidates leaves much to be desired and they seldom appear for the mock examination. In fact, for the mock examination held this year only 4 out of over a 100 candidates were Kuwaitis.

The MRCP Part 2 Course is tailored for the examination with practical and clinical sessions in which both local and visiting consultants participate. Since we have started this course three candidates seem to shy off from this course.

Professor F. F. Fenech

Report
on Primary Fellowship (F.R.C.S.—Dublin) Course and Examination

1. Preface

The Primary Fellowship programme completed its fourth successive year in '80—'81. This year saw the largest entry of candidates from all over the Gulf to the Primary Fellowship examination in Kuwait since its inception in '77—'78. However, the present year has been rather unglamourous from the point of view of examination results. The pass rate in the Kuwait centre dipped to its lowest ever in the last four years to 18%. Perhaps the only redeeming feature this year has been the appointment of two local examiners from the Kuwait Faculty of Medicine.

2. Planning

Planning started as early as April, 1980. A draft for the Primary Fellowship course was prepared after consultation with the relevant departments of the Faculty of Medicine and the Royal College of Surgeons in Ireland. Proposals concerning the Primary Fellowship course and examination were discussed in a meeting of the Postgraduate Committee, Faculty of Medicine on May 18, 1980.

A series of meetings followed in Dublin on September 8 and 9, 1980 between representatives of the Royal College of Surgeons in Ireland and the Kuwait Faculty of Medicine, represented by the undersigned. Arrangements for the Primary Fellowship examination and the course were finalized. Discussions also took place regarding appointment of local examiners. The Royal College extended examinership to Professor Nasr El Din A. Mahmoud and to the undersigned of the Kuwait Faculty of Medicine to act as examiners in Physiology and in Anatomy respectively. A case was made for the Professor and Chairman of Pathology, Kuwait Faculty of Medicine, to be considered for an examinership in Pathology. A detailed report of the Dublin meetings was submitted earlier on September 22, 1980.

To comply with the examinership regulations of the Royal College of Surgeons, Ireland, the undersigned and Professor Nasr El Din A. Mahmoud "sat in" the Primary Fellowship Examinations in Dublin (November, 1980) and in Dammam (January, 1981) respectively. The final draft of the Primary Fellowship course time table was submitted to the Chairman, Postgraduate Committee and to the Chairman, Joint Postgraduate Board on October 6, 1980.

3. Candidate Selection

A call for applications for the Primary Fellowship course was made in all leading Arabic and English dailies during the last week in August, 1980 with a closing date of October 8, 1980.

A total of 63 applications was received from Kuwait. Two candidates were nominated by the Ministry of Health, Bahrain. All applications were processed, documented and submitted to a selection panel comprising Professor A. M. Yousof, Dean, Faculty of Medicine; Dr. Nai'l A. Al-Naqeeb, Undersecretary, Ministry of Public Health; Professor A. R. Yousof, Chairman, Postgraduate Committee; Professor G. J. M. Abouna, Chairman, Department of Surgery; Professor N. A. Mahmoud, Professor of Physiology and Academic Vice Dean and Professor S. Roy Choudhury, Chairman, Department of Anatomy and Course Coordinator. Dr. S. F. Al-Ali, Vice Dean, Administration and Dr. Hilal Al-Sayer, Deputy Director, Amiri Hospital substituted for Professor A. M. Yousof and Dr. Nai'l A. Al-Naqeeb respectively on some sessions.

The selection was carried out in stages. In a shortlisting session on November 19, 1980, twentysix candidates were listed and the two applicants from Bahrain were selected without interview. The first interviews took place on December 2, 1980. Of the 26 candidates, 15 were accepted, 8 were rejected and 3 did not appear at the interviews. A second short list of 17 applicants was drawn up and the second interview session took place on December 14, 1980. Of the 17 candidates, 10 were accepted, 1 was rejected and 6 were absent. One candidate, whose name did not appear on the shortlist, was accepted as a special case by common consent. Thus, a total of 28 (2 from Bahrain + 15 selected at the first interview + 10 selected at the second interview + 1 selected without an interview = 28) candidates were selected.

The list of selected candidates is presented in *Appendix 1*.

One candidate (Dr. Abdul-Hamid A. M. Muhnna—Kuwaiti Doctor) passed the Pr. FRCS examination in January, 1981 from Dammam and did not attend the course.

The important criteria for selection were the candidate's age (below 30 preferred), academic and service record, extent of participation in ongoing educational activities and, above all, his level of knowledge in the applied basic sciences. The referee's evaluation also served as an important arbiter for selection. Everything being equal, Kuwaiti nationals were preferred.

4. The Primary Fellowship Course

a) The programme, venue and dates

A detailed course schedule was circulated to all selected candidates and tutors by December 15, 1980.

The Primary Fellowship course started on Saturday, January 31, 1981 and ended on Thursday, March 26, 1981. Classes were held in the Physiology Seminar Room, Basic Sciences Building and in the Anatomy Dissecting Room between 8.00 a.m. and 2.30 p.m. every Saturday through Wednesday and between 8.00 a.m. and 11.00 a.m. on Thursdays. There were no classes on February 24, 25 and 26, 1981 because of national holidays.

b) Tutors

Five visiting lecturers from the Royal College of Surgeons, Ireland, taught in the course, as follows:

Surgeon—Anatomists
Prof. G. Lynch
Mr. H. I. Browne

Pathologists
Prof. G. Doyle
Dr. P. Fitzpatrick

Clinical Physiologist

Dr. J. Finucane

The Kuwait Faculty of Medicine was represented by the following lecturers:

Clinical Anatomy

1. Prof. G. J. M. Abouna
2. Dr. T. Abu-Neema
3. Prof. W. N. Adams Smith
4. Dr. B. C. Bapna
5. Prof. S. R. Choudhury
6. Dr. A. Cuschieri
7. Prof. H. Hathout
8. Dr. K. K. Mahajan
9. Dr. P. K. Ray

Clinical Physiology

1. Dr. N. S. Al-Zaid*
2. Dr. M. H. Barakat
3. Prof. J. S. Juggi
4. Prof. N. A. Mahmoud
5. Dr. M. J. McBroom
6. Dr. K. M. Y. Mustafa

General Microbiology

1. Dr. W. S. Al-Naqeeb
2. Dr. K. Behbehani
3. Prof. V. Bezjak
4. Prof. T. D. Chugh
5. Prof. F. F. Fenech
6. Dr. R. E. Micallef
7. Dr. A. White

Pathology

1. Prof. M. Y. Ali

Three additional osteology tutorial sessions were conducted by Mr. Hugh G. Brown, Royal Victoria Infirmary, Newcastle upon Tyne on March 14, 15 and 18, 1981 by special arrangement (by courtesy of the Department of Surgery, Faculty of Medicine).

c) Course evaluation

At the end of the course, a comprehensive course evaluation was carried out. Twenty-six out of twenty-seven candidates returned the questionnaire. In general, the candidates preferred tutors who had had the experience of the Primary Fellowship Examination. Certain specific sections of the Physiology and Microbiology courses came under criticism. As regards Anatomy, the sections taught by local tutors were considered to be poorly taught, with some exceptions.

d) Public lectures by visiting tutors

The visiting tutors from the Royal College of Surgeons in Ireland presented the following public lectures at the Faculty of Medicine:

---

* Lectures were given by Dr. J. D. Welty, Dept. of Physiology, School of Medicine, University of South Dakota due to Dr. Al-Zaid's illness.

Name of speaker	Date and time	Topic
Prof. G. Lynch	February 2, 1981 1—2 p.m.	Reconstructive surgery of the breasts
Prof. G. Doyle	February 23, 1981 1—2 p.m.	Focal glomerulonephritis
Dr. P. Fitzpatrick	March 2, 1981 1—2 p.m.	Sarcoma of the uterus
Dr. J. Finucane	March 9, 1981 1—2 p.m.	Hyperlipaedimia in perspective
Mr. Hy Browne	March 18, 1981 1—2 p.m.	The management of chest injuries

The attendance at these lectures was generally poor.

e) Comments

i) Difficulty in candidate recruitment for the course:

For the first time in 4 years, difficulties were experienced in recruiting an adequate number of suitable candidates for the course. Another ominous trend was noted. A number of candidates did not present themselves at the interviews.

This probably reflects a phasic slump in the quality of candidates.

ii) Faculty participation:

The Faculty's participation in teaching rose to 55% in 1980—81. The following is a breakdown:

Kuwait Faculty 55%
RCS, Ireland   45%

Subject	Kuwait Faculty	RCS Ireland	Total hours
Anatomy	50% (51 hours)	50% (51 hours)	102 hours
Physiology	76% (64.5 hours)	24% (21 hours)	85.5 hours
Pathology	35% (22.5 hours)	65% (42 hours)	64.5 hours
			252 hours

iii) Criticism of the course:

This year the candidates have been critical of the course in general and of certain specific sections of the course in particular, as mentioned earlier. They also complained bitterly about the fact that one of the local professors did not fulfil his teaching commitments, which were substantial. The candidates were generally less receptive to the local lecturers who lacked the experience of the Primary Fellowship examination.

Admittedly some of the grievances are justified and because of their confidential nature, these are not reported here. The Dean of the Faculty of Medicine has been consulted on these issues and appropriate measures are being taken to prevent their recurrence. However, the stiff attitude of the candidates towards the local Faculty (particularly to the junior members) is utterly inappropriate.

iv) Museum facilities:

This year, all the candidates hat access to the dissection hall and the museum. Misuse of these facilities was much less (compared to the previous year) due to strict supervision.

v) Printing of the course time-table:

The responsibility for printing the time-table was given to the Royal College. The printed time-tables arrived very late (one day after the course started) and, hence, were of little use.

From next year on, the time-table will be printed locally.

5. The Primary Fellowship Examination

a) Application and fees

All candidates were required to apply directly to the Royal College of Surgeons in Ireland in prescribed form along with original certificates of graduation and internship. The last date for receiving applications was March 15, 1981. An examination fee of K.D 85 (an increase of K.D 10 over the previous year) had to be deposited with the Financial Department, Kuwait Ministry of Health.

All applications were processed in Dublin and a total of 91 candidates were provisionally listed.

b) Registration and issuance of admit cards

Seventy-eight candidates finally registered for the examination and were issued admit cards on April 25, 1981, by the Dean and Assistant Registrar of the Royal College.

c) The examination

The written examinations took place in the Testing Hall, Faculty of Arts, Shuwaikh. The time-table was as follows:

April 26, 1981: Sunday

8.00 a.m. to 8.50 a.m. — Anatomy MCQ
9.20 a.m. to 10.10 a.m. — Physiology MCQ
10.40 a.m. to 11.30 a.m. — Pathology MCQ
2.00 p.m. to 4.00 p.m. — Anatomy Paper

April 27, 1981: Monday

8.00 a.m. to 10.00 a.m. — Pathology Paper
10.30 a.m. to 12.30 p.m. — Physiology Paper

The orals took place in M.D.L. 1 (multidisciplinary laboratory) in the Faculty of Medicine. Examinations started on Tuesday, April 28, 1981 and concluded on Sunday, May 3, 1981 (no examinations on Friday, May 1, 1981). Fifteen candidates were admitted each day, except on Saturday, May 2, 1981, when 17 candidates were examined. One candidate did not appear for the orals. Thus, a total of 77 candidates completed the examinations.

The examiners were as follows:

Prof. S. Roy Choudhury
    (Fac. Med. Kuwait)   } Anatomy
Mr. Brian Lane (RCS, I)

Prof. N. A. Mahmoud
    (Fac. Med. Kuwait)   } Physiology
Mr. Anthony Walsh (RCS, I)

Prof. Patrick Holland (RCS, I)
Mr. R. J. McCormack
    (External from RCS, Edin-   } Pathology
    burgh)

The non-examining officials of the Royal College, Ireland were as follows:

Mr. James O'Connell   — President RCSI
Prof. W. A. L. McGowan   — Dean and Registrar, RCSI
Mrs. Angela Butler   — Asst. Registrar, RCSI

The following was the only observer from the Faculty of Medicine:

Prof. M. Y. Ali   — Pathology

The examination arrangements were assisted by Mr. Francis Victor Silvo and Miss Muyassar Gowhar Hussein of the Department of Anatomy, Faculty of Medicine.

d) The results

i) Overall results:

Seventy eight candidates sat for the written examinations and 77 completed their orals. Out of 78, 14 candidates passed (pass rate 18%).

ii) Results of course candidates:

Of the 27 course candidates, 5 did not appear. Out of 22, 6 passed (pass rate 27.3%).

e) Local examiners

For the first time, the examination team included two members from the Faculty of Medicine, Prof. Nasar El Din A. Mahmoud (Physiology) and Prof. S. Roy Choudhury (Anatomy), Prof. M. Y. Ali, Chairman of Pathology was newly appointed as an examiner in March, 1981. Next year ('81—'82), it is thus hoped that there will be three local examiners, one each in anatomy, physiology and pathology.

6. Comparative Data of the Past Four Years

i) Course applicants

	Number applied	Number selected	Number sat for exam.	Number passed	Success rate
1977—78	90	15	13	5	38.5%
1978—79	80	25	20	12	60 %
1979—80	62	28	27	10	37 %
1980—81	65	28	22	6	27.3%

ii) Kuwaiti candidates

Year	Number in the course	Number outside course	Total number sat for examination	Number passed	Success rate
1977—78	9		7	1	14.3%
1978—79	6		3	1	33.3%
1979—80	9	3*	9+3*=12	4+2*=6	50 %
1980—81	3	1*	3+1*= 4	0	0 %

* Candidates outside the course

iii) Examination results

Year	Number registered	Number completed exam.	Number passed	Success rate
1977—78	36	34	13	36 %
1978—79	58	57	22	37.9%
1979—80	76	69	23	30.3%
1980—81	78	77	14	18 %

iv) Faculty participation in teaching

Year	Hours taught	
	Kuwait Faculty	RCS, Ireland
1977—78	0	264
1978—79	21	243
1979—80	124.5	133.5
1980—81	138	144

7. Observations and Recommendations

Dissatisfaction with the course and a high failure rate at the examination were the keynotes of the Primary Fellowship Programme this year. The reasons for failure were discussed in the examiner's meeting on the last day in the presence of the

Dean and Vice Dean, Administration, Faculty of Medicine. It was felt that the high failure rate was contributed by a hard core of below-average calibre candidates, accumulated over the last few years. The Dean proposed the introduction of a screening test to sit for the Primary Fellowship examination.

On the basis of the foregoing report, the following recommendations are made:

a) To give candidates the maximum benefit from the course, selection of tutors is to be made with great care. Lecturers with adequate experience in postgraduate teaching should be used as far as possible. Tutor evaluation is to be conducted at the end of each course and this may be used as a guide for selection of tutors.

b) The possibility of introducing a screening test may be explored with the Royal College of Surgeons.

8. Vote of Thanks

The Ministry of Public Health is gratefully recognised for providing such unparalleled career opportunities for doctors in Kuwait as well as in the Gulf countries. Dr. Nai'l A. Al-Naqeeb, Undersecretary, Ministry of Public Health is particularly commended for his active support, advice and generous funding of the entire programme.

Sincere thanks are due to Professor A. M. Yousof, Dean, Faculty of Medicine, for his support, concern and guidance throughout the year. Thanks are also due to the University of Kuwait for funding trips for the local examiners to Dublin and Dammam.

All tutors of the Faculty of Medicine and Ministry of Health are recognised for their participation in the course. Hospital consultants have rendered invaluable support by providing references for applicants. The smooth running of the Primary Fellowship Programme has been largely due to the most efficient cooperation of the secretariat of the Ministry of Health, Mrs. Amal Harp in particular. Thanks are also due to Mr. James Almeida, Anatomy Department, for his expert secretarial assistance throughout the year.

Finally, heart-felt thanks are extended to all our beloved candidates, who have endured a lot and for whom the Primary Fellowship Programme has been really worthwhile.

Submitted by
S. Roy Choudhury
Professor & Chairman
Coordinator, Pr. FRCS Programme

Dated: May 20, 1981

Report on Primary F.F.A. Course and Examination

1. Preface

After the expansion of Anaesthetic Services in Kuwait and the presence of over one hundred anaesthetists all over the hospitals of Kuwait, the necessity to establish the F.F.A. Course and Examination arose.

2. Planning

Planning for the Primary F.F.A. Course and Examination started as early as April 1982. A preliminary programme was prepared by Professor Michael Vickers, Professor of Anaesthetics, Welsh National School of Medicine, and Dr. M. M. Motaweh.

The proposals were submitted to the Undersecretary of the Ministry of Public Health who supported the idea. The Chairman of the Postgraduate Joint Board approved it.

When presented with the draft, the Vice Rector and Dean of the Faculty of Medicine backed the suggestions. He advised a meeting with the chairmen of both the Pharmacology and Physiology Departments for fixing the dates, which took place accordingly.

The next stage in planning involved discussions in London between Dr. M. M. Motaweh and Professor Michael Vickers, as regards the final programme of the course which was submitted to all authorities.

The last stage in planning involved discussions between an official delegation from Kuwait headed by the Chairman of the Joint Board, the Chairman of the Discipline Committee of Anaesthesiology and Intensive Care, the Professor of Anatomy—the Faculty of Medicine, Kuwait, and the F.F.A.R.C.S. official in London in November 1981.

Earlier, in November 1981, a detailed report on the visit to London was submitted to the Ministry of Public Health and the Faculty of Medicine.

3. Candidate Selection

The call for applications for the Primary F.F.A. Course was made by a circular to all anaesthetists in Kuwait in Arabic and English during the 1st week of December 1981, giving the closing date as January 6th, 1982, for receiving the applications.

Letters were dispatched from the Chairman of the Joint Board to all Gulf States to nominate one candidate from every Gulf State to attend this course. There was only one candidate from Iraq.

A total of 30 applications was received. Unfortunately, not a single Kuwaiti candidate applied for the course.

All applications were processed, documented and submitted to a selection committee comprising Prof. A. M. Yousof, Vice Rector of Health Sciences Center and Dean—Faculty of Medicine; Prof. Olav Thulesius, Chairman Department of Pharmacology; Prof. S. Roy Choudhury, Chairman Department of Anatomy; Dr. M. M. Motaweh, Chairman, Discipline Committee for Anaesthesiology and Intensive Care and Course and Examination Coordinator, Dr. H. A. Youssof, Assistant Professor of Anaesthesia, and Assistant Coordinator.

Twenty candidates were selected. All the candidates had been interviewed except the Iraqi candidate making a total number of 21 candidates. The rest of them were advised to apply for the next course.

The list of selected candidates appears in *Appendix I*.

The important criteria for selection were the candidate's age, academic and service record, and his knowledge in the applied basic sciences. The referee's evaluation was taken into consideration.

4. The Primary F.F.A. Course

a) The time table, venue and dates

A detailed course schedule with the titles of lectures to be delivered was circulated to all selected candidates and tutors by the 6th of March 1982.

The Primary F.F.A. Course started on Thursday the 15th of April 1982 and ended on Wednesday the 26th of May 1982. The start of the course was postponed for one day due to a national strike on the 14th of April 1982.

. Classes were held in Amphitheatre 106, main building, Faculty of Medicine (daily) from 4.00 to 7.30 p.m. every day of the week except Thursday from 4.00 to 5.30 p.m. which was an optional tutorial session.

b) Tutors

The following 5 visiting lecturers from the Welsh National School of Medicine were involved in the course with the following schedule:

Prof. M. D. Vickers, Professor of Anaesthetics	from 13th April to 28th April
Prof. W. W. Mapleson, Professor of Physics Applied to Anaesthesia	from 13th April to 28th April
Dr. J. N. Lunn, Senior Lecturer in Anaesthetics	from 15th May to 27th May
Dr. J. N. Horton, Consultant Anaesthetist and Honorary Clinical Teacher	from 27th April to 13th May
Dr. M. Harmer, Lecturer in Anaesthetics	from 11th May to 27th May

The Kuwait Faculty of Medicine was represented by the following lecturers:

Pharmacology Department

Olav Thulesius	Professor and Chairman
Abdalla Al-Khars	Assistant Professor
Abdulla Elkhawad	Assistant Professor
Maria Angelo-Khattar	Assistant Professor

Physiology Department

M. J. McBroom	Associate Professor and Acting Chairman
N. A. Mahmoud	Professor
K. A. Gumaa	Professor
J. S. Juggi	Professor
K. Y. Mustafa	Associate Professor
I. S. Aneja	Associate Professor

The whole course included 90 periods, each period of one hour's duration. 66 periods were covered by overseas visitors and 24 hours by local tutors.

c) Course attendance

The attendance was very regular by all candidates, besides 7 to 15 listener visitors who attended regularly, daily.

However, one candidate Dr. Houssam Mohd Salah failed to attend the last 2 weeks due to a disc prolapse followed by an operation.

d) Course evaluation

The time of the course being in the afternoons was very convenient to most candidates. The overall opinion of the candidates about the topics covered by the overseas visitors was very satisfactory. Physiology topics covered by local Faculty was excellent but some lectures in pharmacology by local tutors came under criticism. This was covered by overseas tutors.

e) Course comments

Due to difficulties of the candidates in Part III, which includes physics and clinical measurements, it will be more convenient to expand the course from 6 to 7 weeks, covering nearly 110 periods.

There should be no haste in the replacement of overseas tutors by local Faculty especially in Part III.

5. The Primary F.F.A. Examination

a) Applications and fees

All examination entries were handled by the RCSE in London directly. Candidates were required to apply in a prescribed form along with original certificates of graduation, experience of 3 months in anaesthesia and 6 months in medicine, at least. The closing date of application was 31st March, 1982. Examination fees were estimated at KD. 80 per candidate and were deposited with the Financial Division, Department of Public Health & Planning, Ministry of Public Health, Kuwait. The original receipt was attached to the Examination Application Form.

A total of 37 candidates applied to sit for the examination. Besides candidates from Kuwait, the entries included 4 others from Iraq, Saudi Arabia and Bahrain.

b) Issuance of admit cards

All the admittance cards to those candidates in Kuwait were dispatched from the RCSE to the Coordinator of the Course where they were distributed locally. Those from the Gulf States received their registration cards directly from the officials of RCSE.

c) The examination and the examination board

The written examinations were held in the Amphitheatre 106, main building, Faculty of Medicine, Shuwaikh. The time table was as follows:

Saturday 19th June MULTIPLE CHOICE QUESTION PAPER
9.00 a.m. to 12.00 noon

Presiding Examiners { Prof. J. A. Thornton
Dr. I. T. Davie
Dr. G. W. Black

Sunday 20th June ESSAY PAPER — 9.00 a.m. to 12.00 noon

Presiding Examiners { Prof. J. A. Thornton
Dr. I. T. Davie
Dr. G. W. Black

Viva Voce Examinations

The VIVA examination took place in MDL I and MDL II (Multidisciplinary Laboratories), Faculty of Medicine, Shuwaikh, as follows:

Tuesday	22nd June	PHARMACOLOGY and PHYSIOLOGY	9.00 a.m. to 1.30 p.m.
Wednesday	23rd June		9.00 a.m. to 1.10 p.m.
Thursday	24th June		9.00 a.m. to 1.10 p.m.
Saturday	26th June	PHYSICS and	9.00 a.m. to 1.30 p.m.
Sunday	27th June	CLINICAL	9.00 a.m. to 1.10 p.m.
Monday	28th June	MEASUREMENT	9.00 a.m. to 1.10 p.m.

Examination Board

PHARMACOLOGY   Dr. I. T. Davie and Dr. G. W. Black
PHYSIOLOGY   Prof. J. A. Thornton and Prof. Nasr El Din Mah-
                      moud

PHYSICS and
CLINICAL MEASURE-   Prof. J. A. Thornton and Dr. I. T. Davie
MENT

Observer Examiners

Prof. Olav Thulesius   Chairman of Pharmacology Dept.
                          Faculty of Medicine;
Dr. M. M. Motaweh   Chairman of Discipline Committee for Anaesthe-
                          siology and Int. Care;
Dr. H. A. Yousof   Assistant Professor of Anaesthesia, Faculty of Medi-
                          cine.

d) The Results

Although 37 candidates were registered and had paid their fees, on the first day of the written examination only 34 of them attended. Candidate No. 16, Dr. Houssam Mohd Salah, from the course was one of them and he did not attend because he was operated upon. Another candidate outside the course was admitted to the Coronary Care Unit on the night of the examination. The third candidate from Saudi Arabia did not attend at all.

A list of the candidates as prepared by the RCSE in alphabetical order of the 37 registered is enclosed as *Appendix II.*

Nine of the 37 candidates were female. The final number who attended all the examinations were 26 candidates. Out of these, 6 candidates passed. All of them are from Kuwait except No. 5, Dr. Al Mazrooa Adnan Abdullah, who came from Saudi Arabia.

The total pass rate is 18% and the result of successful candidates from the course is 4, i.e. 20% of the total.

Details of the successful candidates are tabulated below:

Admit Card No.	Name	Course attended	Result	Remark
4.	Dr. Al-Alami Akram Mohamed	No	Passed	Palestinian
5.	Dr. Al Mazrooa Adnan Abdullah	No	Passed	Saudi Arabia
13.	Dr. Botrous Melad Saddeek	Yes	Passed	Egyptian
17.	Dr. Faraj Jaafar Hameed	Yes	Passed	Iraqi
24.	Dr. Metwali Kamal El-Din Hussien Ibrahim	Yes	Passed	Egyptian
32.	Dr. Sekar Muthukrishnan	Yes	Passed	Indian

e) Comments

i) Kuwait—the Gulf Centre

Kuwait will become the Gulf Centre for Primary F.F.A. examinations in the coming years. It is expected that the number of candidates sitting for the examination next year will grow increasingly. As a start 37 candidates applying for the first Primary F.F.A. examination in Kuwait is a very good record.

ii) Local examiners

One local examiner was included in the examination team in Physiology as well as 3 observer examiners from Kuwait.

iii) Pass rate

The total pass rate of 18% in the first Primary F.F.A. examination held in Kuwait is a rather good result, and with the passage of time the rate will be higher, due to the familiarity of the candidates with the procedures, and the type of these examinations. It is comparable to the pass rate in the United Kingdom which ranges from 15 to 25 percent.

The pass rate of 20% of those who attended the course is a considerably good result, and with the subsequent courses it is presumed that the pass rate will be higher.

In view of the fact that some candidates can appear at the examination without any screening procedure, the success rate of 18% may be looked upon favourably.

6. Observations and Recommendations

The comment from the tutor of the Welsh National School of Medicine as well as the examiners from overseas, was that the standard of the candidates in Kuwait is as good as any you would find in the United Kingdom. However, it was indicated by the tutors from the Welsh National School of Medicine that the standard of the candidates in Part III which includes clinical measurements and physics is a little bit lower than that in the United Kingdom due to education difficulties, especially in Secondary Schools, and the language barrier for terminology in physics and clinical measurements. Nevertheless, in order to achieve a better standard in Part III, it has been recommended that the course be prolonged by one week in order to cover most of the subjects concerned.

It is recommended that the Primary F.F.A. Course and the examination should be given active and continued support over the coming few years.

It is also recommended that the number of candidates sitting for the next course should be 20 plus those coming from the Gulf States.

7. Vote of Thanks

Sincere thanks are due to Dr. Nouri Al Kazemi, Chairman, Joint Postgraduate Board and Dr. Na'il Al Naqeeb, Undersecretary, Ministry of Public Health for their approval and generous funding of the programme. Professor A. M. Yousof, Vice Rector of the Health Sciences Center is gratefully commended for his advice, active support and guidance throughout the year.

All tutors from the Welsh National School of Medicine as well as local tutors from the Faculty of Medicine, and members of the Discipline Committee for Anaesthesiology and Intensive Care are thanked for their participation in teaching and their backing and help. So also all hospital consultants are commended for providing references for the candidates. Thanks are also given to Dr. Talib Astarabadi and Mr. Sa'ed Al Nabhan, Deputy Heads, Training Division.

Thanks are extended to Mrs. Amal Harb in particular, of the Secretariat, Ministry of Public Health, to Mrs. Nagah, Secretary in Dr. Nouri Al Kazemi's office and to the Secretary attached to the Discipline Committee for Anaesthesiology and Intensive Care. Heart-felt thanks are extended for the expert secretarial assistance rendered throughout the course and examination, and the smooth execution of the entire programme by Mr. Mohamed Kaleem Allah and Mr. Lawrence Rato.

Finally, thanks are extended to all our beloved candidates who have endured a lot and for whom all the efforts have been truly worthwhile.

Submitted by

Dr. M. M. Motaweh
Chairman, Discipline Committee
   for Anaesthesiology & Int. Care
Chairman Anaesthesia Departments
   Sabah, Chest Disease and Infectious
   Diseases Hospitals
Coordinator of Primary F.F.A.R.C.S.
Date: June 1982   Course & Examination in Kuwait

Appendix I
List of Selected Candidates for the Primary
F.F.A.R.C.S. Course in Kuwait 1981—1982

Sr. No.	Name	Nationality
1.	Dr. (Mrs.) Ekram M. El-Damhoughy	Egyptian
2.	Dr. (Mrs.) Hoda Mansour Ayoub	Egyptian
3.	Dr. (Mrs.) Elizabeth Philip	Indian
4.	Dr. (Mrs.) Nadia M. T. Kershah	Egyptian
5.	Dr. (Mrs.) Aida H. Hassan	Egyptian
6.	Dr. (Mrs.) Huda Daher Ismail Al-Shawi	Iraqi
7.	Dr. Jaafar Hameed Faraj	Iraqi
8.	Dr. Kamal Nassif Takla	Egyptian
9.	Dr. Malek Abdel Hamid Koheil	Egyptian
10.	Dr. Muthukrishnan Sekar	Indian
11.	Dr. Ziad Ragheb Awayes	Jordanian
12.	Dr. Ahmed Abdel Aziz Mohammed Abdel Maksoud	Egyptian

Sr. No.	Name	Nationality
13.	Dr. Syed Salahuddin Ahmed	Indian
14.	Dr. Melad Saddeek Botrous	Egyptian
15.	Dr. Ahamed Shamsuddin	Indian
16.	Dr. Houssam Mohd Salah	Egyptian
17.	Dr. El Sayed Mohd Abdel Monem Afifi	Egyptian
18.	Dr. Dasu Hari Rao	Indian
19.	Dr. Mohannad Mohd Bader El Rakshy	Egyptian
20.	Dr. Kamal El-Din H. I. Metwaly	Egyptian
21.	Dr. Samir Soliman Awad	Egyptian

Appendix II
List of Candidates Accepted for the Primary
F.F.A.R.C.S. Examination in Kuwait 1981—1982

	Admit Card No.	Name of doctor	Qualification/University	
	1.	Abdel Maksoud Ahmed Abdel Aziz Mohamed	MB BCh	Mansoura
	2.	Afifi El Sayed Mohamed Abdel Monem	–do–	Ain Shams
	3.	Ahmed Syed Salahuddin	MB BS	Madras
	4.	Al-Alami Akram Mohamed	MB BCh	Cairo
	5.	Al-Mazrooa Adnan Abdullah	–do–	Cairo
	6.	Al-Shawi Huda Daher Ismail	–do–	Basrah
w	7.	Aly Aida Mohamed Hassan	–do–	Ain Shams
w	8.	Ashgar Souad Taha	–do–	Baghdad
	9.	Awad Samir Soliman	–do–	Cairo
	10.	Awayes Ziad Ragheb Kasim	–do–	Alexandria
w	11.	Ayoub Hoda Mansour	–do–	Cairo
	12.	Barsoum Botrous Kamal Kamel	–do–	Ain Shams
	13.	Botrous Melad Saddeek	–do–	Ain Shams
w	14.	El-Damhougy Ekram Mahmood	–do–	Cairo
	15.	El Rakshy Mohannad Mohamed Bader El Din	–do–	Cairo
	16.	El Rayess Taher Mahmoud Soliman	–do–	Ain Shams
	17.	Faraj Jaafar Hameed	–do–	Baghdad
w	18.	Gerges Tereza Fahmy Farid	–do–	Cairo
	19.	Jokhio Raza Mustafa	MB BS	Sind
w	20.	Kershah Nadia Mohamed Tawfeek	MB BCh	Alexandria
	21.	Koheil Malek Abdel Hamid	–do–	Cairo
	22.	Kumar Manyam Ravi	MB BS	Osmania
	23.	Mannan Abdul	–do–	Punjab (Pak.)
	24.	Metwali Kamal El-Din Hussien Ibrahim	MB BCh	Ain Shams
w	25.	Mousa Ekhlas Ahmed Ali	–do–	Cairo
	26.	Nakhla Mansour Youssef Aziz	–do–	Alexandria
	27.	Nour-El-Din Ahmed Abdel Aziz Mohamed	–do–	Cairo

w = females

Admit Card No.	Name of doctor	Qualification/University	
w 28.	Philip Elizabeth	MB BS	Bangalore
29.	Rao Dasu Sri Hari	–do–	Osmania
30.	Saker Mohamed Medhat Abdul Aziz	MB BCh	Ain Shams
31.	Salah Houssam Mohamed	–do–	Cairo
32.	Sekar Muthukrishnan	MB BS	Poona
w 33.	Shamoun Evelyn Murad Younathan	MB BCh	Baghdad
34.	Shamsuddin Ahamed	MB BS	Andhra
35.	Singh Raj Kumar Achoubisana	–do–	Calcutta
36.	Takla Kamal Nassif	MB BCh	Ain Shams
37.	Vaidya Radhakrishnan Gopalkrishna	MB BS	Bombay

w = females

Report on Primary F.F.D. Course and Examination

I. Introduction

Circumstances giving rise to this report:

This overview of the evaluation of the Primary FFDRCSI Course, candidates, tutors, examination, overall comments and recommendations were undertaken by Dr. M. R. Elmostehy, Coordinator to the Primary FFDRCSI Course held in Kuwait from 30. 1. 82—25. 3. 82.

Up to that date, there was no dental course that could lead to a degree and hence considerations were given to start the F.F.D.R.C.S.I. (Dublin) program. This took several stages of preparation and several preliminary meetings and communications that started between the Ministry of Public Health, Faculty of Medicine and the Health Planning and Training Centre and the R.C.S. Dublin. The first actual step started when Dr. N. Al-Naqeeb, the Undersecretary, called upon Dr. M. R. Elmostehy to act as Coordinator of the Course of the Primary FFD. A proposed program was created after consultations with Prof. Roy Choudhury Coordinator of the Primary F.R.C.S. so that there was a dovetailing of both programs. It was thus put forward and submitted to Dr. Nouri Al-Kazemi, Dr. N. Al-Naqeeb and Dean, A. Mohsen Al-Yousef who consented to the idea that the course for the Primary FFD is the responsibility of the local authorities in Kuwait, and the examination should be under the direct supervision of the R.C.S. (Dublin). It was decided that the locally formulated course and examination regulations should be finalised with the R.C.S. Dublin and so Dr. Elmostehy and Prof. R. Choudhury, Coordinator to the Primary FRCS, were sent to Dublin. In the interview held on the 15th and 16th of September, '81 between the coordinators and the officials of R.C.S. Dublin a detailed program and examination regulations were discussed and finalized. A detailed report on this visit was submitted to the Ministry on 30. 9. 81.

II. Course

1. Candidate selection
2. General policy adopted in course construction
3. Tutors—dental and medical
4. Comments

1. Candidate selection

Information concerning launching a Pr. FFD Course, its starting date, applications and the name of the coordinator, were circulated to all dental personnel working in the Ministry of Public Health through a decree issued by the Undersecretary, Ministry of Public Health. 48 candidates (7 K and 41 NK) submitted applications to attend the course.

The completed files were sent to the selection committee headed by Prof. Abdul Razzak Al-Yousef, and the following members:

Prof. M. Al-Yousef, Dean, Faculty of Medicine
Prof. M. R. Elmostehy, Coordinator to Pr. FFD Course
Prof. Roy Choudhury, Coordinator to Pr. FRCS Course
Dr. A. Al-Jasem, Head of Dental Centre
Dr. I. A. Al-Yassin, Ass. Prof., Faculty of Medicine
Prof. J. S. Juggi, Physiol. Dept. Faculty of Medicine.

Due to lack of physical facilities the number of attendants at the dental course was limited to 12 candidates, thus the committee decided the following:

7 Kuwaiti candidates were accepted without an interview.
19 non-Kuwaiti candidates were accepted for a committee interview.
21 non-Kuwaiti candidates were rejected and 1 was asked to wait for one year.

In the interview performed by Dr. Elmostehy, Prof. Choudhury, Prof. Juggi, Dr. A. Al-Jasem, Dr. I. A. Al-Yassin, the final selection of 5 NK candidates was finalised. Thus the 12 candidates (7 K and 5 NK) were accepted to attend the 8-week course of the Primary FFD. The files containing the C.V.'s of the accepted candidates were submitted to Prof. A. Mohsen Al-Yousef, Dean of the Faculty of Medicine, Dr. Nouri Al-Kazemi, Chairman, Joint Postgraduate Board, Dr. N. Al-Naqeeb, the Undersecretary, M.P.H., Dr. Jassim Hussein, Director, Dept. of Dental and Paramedical Administration. Enclosed is a full list of the 12 accepted candidates.

File no.	Names of candidates
1	Dr. Saheb Qattan (K)
3	Dr. Hassan Sayegh (K)
4	Abbas Al-Yemah (NK)
5	Meha Kanaan (NK)
9	Kamal Shehab Eddeen (NK)
11	Mona Al-Busairi (K)
13	Chaneema Al-Dhakeel (K)
16	Suhail Al-Muhalhal (K)
30	Saleh Fameed (NK)
37	Mahmoud Ahmed Abo Mwais (NK)
43	Fareeda Al-Herz (K)
51	Raad Abdul Amir Hassan
	(Suhail 16 withdrew and the total number became 11)

2. General policy adopted in the construction of the course

The preliminary course of the Primary FFDRCS (Dublin) was proposed and discussed in its entirety with Prof. Choudhury, Coordinator of the Primary FRCS. Both coordinators agreed and discussed the detailed lectures and topics to be given to candidates of the Primary FFD. The proposed program was sent to Prof. M. Al-Yousef, Dean; Prof. McGowan (Registrar of R.C.S. Dublin), Dr. Hayward (Dental Anatomist), Dr. F. Nally (Dental Physiologist), Dr. W. Allwright (coordinator of dental studies, R.C.S.I.), Prof. Razzak Al-Yousef, Chairman, Internal Medicine Dept., and Dr. Nouri Al-Kazemi, Chairman, joint post-graduate board.

As mentioned before, the proposed program was constructed in a dovetailed manner with the program of the Primary F.R.C.S. so that general subjects (Anatomy, Physiology, Pathology) would be attended by candidates of both Primary FRCS and FFD in the Faculty of Medicine, while dental subjects (D. Anatomy and Dental Physiology) would be delivered in the dental centre.

The course started on 30. 1. 82 and ended on 25. 3. 82. Working hours were from 8 a.m.—2.30 p.m. except Thursdays from 8 a.m.—11 a.m.

3. Tutors participating in the primary FFD course, dental and medical

Because of the nature of the course being dovetailed with the Primary FRCS Course, the same tutors who lectured in the FRCS were informed that 11 dental candidates (last moment withdrawal of 1 candidate) would be attending the general lectures. In this respect, the course lectures were delivered by tutors from overseas (visiting) and by local staff from the Faculty of Medicine, Kuwait University.

Visiting tutors:

Anatomy	Mr. G. Lynch
	Mr. B. Lane
Oral and Dental Anatomy	Dr. A. Hayward
Physiology	Dr. J. Finucane
Dental Physiology	Dr. F. Nally
Pathology	Prof. P. Holland
	Prof. E. Moorehouse
Local Staff	Prof. R. Choudhury
	Prof. J. S. Juggi
	Dr. N. S. Al-Zaid
	Prof. N. A. Mahmoud
	Dr. M. S. Al-Adani
	Prof. L. J. Lindberg
	Prof. M. Y. Ali
	Dr. J. M. McBroom
	Prof. G. Abonna
	Dr. Aneja

4. Comments

1. It was felt that the course had shown an apparent difference in the levels between dental and medical candidates. Due to the lack of applied clinical knowledge observed in the dental candidates, there was a supremacy in the knowledge of the medical over the dental students (particulary in subjects of general physiology and

pathology). Due to the short time (8 weeks) allowed for both levels to assimilate the knowledge submitted, the dental candidates felt that a separate course for the dental purpose should be constructed, or a longer course spread over a greater number of weeks could be of help. (Comment of Coordinator: For the time being, the course should run as it is for a few years but general courses in anatomy, physiology and pathology should be furnished to the dental candidates long before the start of the condensed courses. Separation of the two courses, although not advisable this coming year, in long-term policy, is apt to happen.)

2. It was felt that the few oral pathology lectures given during this course were not of great value. Because oral pathology will be discussed in full detail in the final part of the FFD, it is advisable that such lectures be dropped from the course of the Primary FFD.

3. The dental candidates raised some comments in their course evaluation papers, and all indicated that the time was too short to prepare for the exams. They request that such a course be preceeded by thorough preparation of the assigned topics and run by members of the staff of the Faculty of Medicine. A detailed evaluation of the course by the coordinator has been submitted to the dean, Faculty of Medicine and Dr. Nouri Al-Kazemi. Because of the confidential nature of this evaluation, it will not be discussed here.

4. The coordinator suggests that dental candidates should see soft tissue specimens on Anatomy, Dental Anatomy and Pathology in the form of cadavers (head and neck), dental histological specimens and jars respectively, i.e. a procedure which was not persued during this course. This is anticipated to be conducted by the Faculty of Medicine and local members of the staff.

III. Primary F.F.D. Examination

1. Application for examination and date of examination

Applications to sit for the Primary FFD exams were delivered to all candidates attending the course. After the applications were filled out Prof. Lynch carried them to the Royal College of Surgeons in Dublin on his return there. Fees of KD. 100/- were paid by all candidates sitting for the exam. Candidates not attending the course and wishing to sit for the exam were advised to contact the registrar, RCS, Dublin directly so that their names could be included in the list of candidates sitting for the Primary FFD exam. It was decided that May 1st, 1982 will be the start of the examination of the Primary FFD (concurrently with that of FRCS) for the 1st 2 papers (Pathology and Physiology). 9. 5. 82 will be the date of the 3rd paper (Anatomy and Dental Anatomy).

2. Registration

On 29. 4. 1982, a registration committee from the Royal College of Surgeons, Dublin met with the candidates both for the Primary FFD and F.R.C.S. in the theatre, and 16 candidates received their registration cards and were informed as to the date, time and place of the examination. Two Kuwaiti candidates did not turn up for registration although they attended the 8 week course (Dr. Mona Al Busairi # 213 and Dr. Fareeda Ali Al-Herz, # 206).

3. Examination schedule

As said before, the examination was held in the Testing Hall, Kuwait University and started on 1. 5. 1982

1. 5. 82   10.30 a.m.—12.30 p.m.   Pathology written
            2.00 p.m.— 4.30 p.a.   Physiology written
9. 5. 82   8.00 a.m.—11.00 a.m.   Anatomy and Dental Anatomy.

The orals were held in the M.D.L., Faculty of Medicine starting at 8.00 a.m. and each candidate was given 20 minutes for each subject (Anatomy, Dental Anatomy, Physiology and Pathology).

15 started the written exams but only 12 finished to the last day of exams and took their viva.

4. Examiners

The following examiners were appointed by RCS, Dublin to act as examiners to the Primary FFD. From Kuwait 3 observers were appointed.

Prof. M. R. Elmostehy (Pathology)
Dr. A. A. Al-Jasem (Dental Anatomy)
Dr. I. A. Al-Yassin (Anatomy)

Pathology: 1. Mr. H. Browne
                    2. Prof. F. O'Brien (Oral Pathology)
Anatomy: 1. Prof. B. P. Rooney
                    2. Dr. A. Owen (Dental Anatomy)
Physiology: 1. Mr. D. S. Colbert
                    2. Prof. N. Mahmoud (Observer)

Also present was Prof. K. Healy (Dean, Faculty of Dentistry, RCS, Dublin).

Out of 12 candidates, one only satisfied the examiners in all subjects and this was Dr. M. Mosa Ahmed Abu Mwais who works in Salmieh Polyclinic, Nationality: Jordanian.

5. Comments

1. Some correspondence became confused regarding the date of the Anatomy Paper which indicated that it will be on 9. 5. 82. The registration committee informed the Primary FFD candidates that this paper is to be given on 2. 5. 82. This was not accepted either by the coordinator or students, and it was finally agreed that it would be held on 9. 5. 82 as indicated in the first information received through correspondence.

2. In the course of the examination, it was felt that the students should examine histological sections and diagnose them rather than see black and white photos of tissues as happened in the Dental Anatomy Oral Exams.

This also applies to Pathology specimens that the candidate should examine in jars and give his diagnosis.

3. The only candidate that satisfied the examiner was an unexpected "white horse". Yet two candidates were very near to making it (1 Kuwaiti and 1 Egyptian). As agreed by all examiners, those two candidates could have done it if they had been given enough time or coached properly prior to their condensed course. In this respect the examiners advised that dental candidates should be exposed to ex-

amination conditions in order to improve their ability to present their knowledge in a satisfactory manner.

Recommendations

One should stress that the recommendations to be contained in this report in most instances indicate the need for additional activity and study. To have the highest standards of excellence achieved in such a course, it is imperative that procedures be instituted which will enable students to reach the standards set by the Primary FRCS.

1. The course of the Primary FFD should continue as it was presented this year. In addition to the help given at birth, a new-born course as this should be assisted by all possible further amenities. Although the suggestion to separate the two courses was raised, it is the opinion of the coordinator that the course dovetailed with that of the Primary FRCS should be kept. It is in this respect that the assistance offered by the Faculty of Medicine, its Dean, Chairman of Post-Graduate Board and Coordinator of the Primary FRCS (Prof. Roy Choudhury) is greatly appreciated.

2. For such a condensed course to be fruitful, general comprehensive courses should be offered as early as possible to candidates wishing to sit for the Primary FFD exam. This is going to be the responsibility of the Faculty of Medicine, Kuwait University. A preliminary proposal will be offered to the Dean in due course by the coordinator.

3. It is advisable that the appointed observers to the Primary FFD exam should join the examination committee of the Primary FFD to be held in Dublin this sitting. They will indeed enjoy the advantage of not being biased by factors in the local situation which might have a personal effect on those within the local scene.

Epilogue

The author expresses his deep appreciation to: Dr. N. Al-Naqeeb, The Undersecretary, Ministry of Public Health, Prof. Abdul-Razzak Al-Yousef, Chairman of Internal Medicine Dept., Dr. Nouri Al-Kazemi, Chairman, Joint postgraduate board, and Dr. Jassim M. Hussein, Director, Dept. of the Dental and Paramedical Administration.

Without their kindness, consideration, helpfulness, enthusiasm, patience and support, it would have been impossible to bring a course and an examination of the Primary FFD to birth to be the first held in Kuwait.

My due thanks are offered to Prof. Roy Choudhury, Coordinator to the Primary FRCS whose help and support to the author solved several problems which assisted in achieving a goal in the advancement of dental studies in the State of Kuwait.

The creation of the Primary FFD Course and its examination is a great achievement and a credit to the dental profession in Kuwait, both by raising the general standard of dentists as well as a recognition of the Dental Services in Kuwait by a reputable institute such as the Royal College of Surgeons, Dublin.

Dr. M. Ragai Elmostehy F.D.S.
Periodontist

3. Continuing Medical Education

a) Local (In-Service) Continuing Medical Education
81C—1201

Sabah Hospital, Amiri Hospital, Farwania Hospital, Adan Hospital, In-Service Training in Medicine
October 1981—June 1982 Programme

Objectives: To check the advances in basic medical sciences and in clinical medicine.
To discuss the possibilities of implementing the advances of science into everyday practice.
To maintain good clinical relationships during the process of diagnosis and treatment of the patients.

Place: Sabah Hospital, Amiri Hospital, Farwania Hospital, Adan Hospital.

Duration: From October 1981 till June 1982, once a week in each hospital.

Organiser: Prof. F. F. Fenech, Chairman of the Department of Medicine, Sabah.

Program Director: Dr. S. Bhatnagar — Sabah Hospital
Dr. B. Naquib   — Amiri Hospital
Dr. Ashmawi   — Farwania Hospital
Dr. Emara   — Adan Hospital.

Participants: Local staff and visitors.

Programme: *Topics* shall be chosen by programme directors.
Forms: Bedside ward meetings, journals meetings (clubs), seminars, big bedside ward rounds, laboratory clinical seminars, specialised lectures in addition to daily rounds in different wards.

81C—1202
Amiri Hospital In-Service Training in Medicine
18. 4. 1981—6. 6. 1981 Programme

Objectives: To check advances in the basic medical sciences and in clinical medicine.
To discuss the possibilities of implementing the advances of science into everyday practice.
To maintain good clinical relationships during the process of diagnosis and treatment of the patients.

Place: Amiri Hospital

Duration: 18th April till 6th June 81.
All lecturers will start at 12 noon unless otherwise stated.

Organiser:	Director, Amiri Hospital	
Programme Director:	Dr. P. P. Boby	
Participants:	All trainee doctors are requested to attend the lectures without fail. Visitor doctors are also welcome to attend the lectures except radiology sessions.	

Programme:

Saturday, 18. 4. 1981	Differential Diagnosis of Chest Pain	Dr. P. P. Bobby
Sunday, 19. 4. 1981	Introduction to E.C.G. (1)	Dr. Ahmed Shawki
Tuesday, 21. 4. 1981	Radiology Session	Dr. Suraya, 8—9 a.m.
Wednesday, 22. 4. 1981	Acid-Base Balance and Electrolytic Imbalance	Dr. Woods
Saturday, 25. 4. 1981	Management of a Case of Bronchial Asthma	Dr. P. P. Boby
Sunday, 26. 4. 1981	Introduction to E.C.G. (2)	Dr. Ahmed Shawki
Tuesday, 28. 4. 1981	Epilepsy, its Diagnosis and Management	Dr. Abdul Rahman Khalifa
Wednesday, 29. 4. 1981	Etiology and Classification of Diabetes mellitus	Dr. Abdul Khader, 11—12 a.m.
Saturday, 2. 5. 1981	DVT and its Complications	Dr. Issam Sherbini
Sunday, 3. 5. 1981	Introduction to E.C.G. (3)	Dr. Ahmed Shawki
Tuesday, 5. 5. 1981	Management of Cardiac Arrest	Dr. Marwan
Wednesday, 6. 5. 1981	Diagnosis and Management of the Nephrotic Syndrome	Dr. Woods
Saturday, 9. 5. 1981	Radiology Session	Dr. Suraya, 8—9 a.m.
Sunday, 10. 5. 1981	Introduction to E.C.G. (4)	Dr. Ahmed Shawki
Tuesday, 12. 5. 1981	Diagnosis and Management of C.V.A. and T.I.A.	Dr. Abdul Rahman Khalifa
Wednesday, 13. 5. 1981	Diagnosis and Management of Acute Renal Failure	Dr. H. F. Woods
Saturday, 16. 5. 1981	Coma—D. D. and Management	Dr. Issam Sherbini
Sunday, 17. 5. 1981	Galls—Diagnosis and Management of Complications	Dr. Medhat Mukhtar
Tuesday, 19. 5. 1981	Radiology Session	Dr. Suraya, 8—9 a.m.

Tuesday, 19. 5. 1981	Investigation of a Case of Anaemia	Dr. Ahmed Hafez, 12 — 1 p.m.
Wednesday, 20. 5. 1981	Diagnosis and Management of Chronic Renal Failure	Dr. H. F. Woods
Saturday, 23. 5. 1981	Radiology Session	Dr. Suraya, 8 — 9 a.m.
Saturday, 23. 5. 1981	Investigation of a Case of Bleeding Disorders	Dr. Ahmed Hafez
Sunday, 24. 5. 1981	Introduction to Tropical Medicine	Dr. Ahmed Shawki
Tuesday, 26. 5. 1981	Management of Cardiac Arrhythmias	Dr. P. P. Boby
Wednesday, 27. 5. 1981	Management of Diabetes mellitus	Dr. Abdul Khader, 11 — 12 a.m.
Saturday, 30. 5. 1981	Inflammatory Bowel Disorders	Dr. Falah
Tuesday, 2. 6. 1981	Chronic Hepatitis	Dr. Medhat Mukhtar
Wednesday, 3. 6. 1981	Management of Peptic Ulcer	Dr. Georgetta
Sunday, 7. 6. 1981	Rheumatoid Arthritis and Related Disorders	Dr. Mohammed Sa'ade, 12 — 1 p.m.
Tuesday, 9. 6. 1981	Investigation and Management of a Case of Malabsorption Syndrome	Dr. Rashid

81C — 1203
Amiri Hospital In-Service Training in Medicine
28. 4. 1982 — 17. 6. 1982 Programme

Objectives: To check advances in the basic medical sciences and in clinical medicine.
To discuss the possibilities of implementing the advances of science into everyday practice.
To maintain good clinical relationships during the process of diagnosis and treatment of the patients.

Place: Amiri Hospital

Duration: 28th April till 17th June 1982. The teach-in session for trainee doctors will be held as usual on Wednesday at 12 noon.

Organiser: Director, Medical Education, Amiri Hospital.

Programme Director: Dr. P. P. Boby

Participants: All doctors are requested to read about the topic and attend the session. Visitor doctors are also welcome to attend the lectures.
The doctors have been divided into 3 groups.

Group I	Group II	Group III
Dr. Salim	Dr. Doulath	Dr. Talib
Dr. Iman Al-Garaf	Dr. Ibthesam	Dr. Iman Shahash
Dr. Nooriya	Dr. Nawal	Dr. Amad
Dr. Suheil	Dr. Mei	
Dr. Mohammed	Dr. Saad	

Radiology posting

Group I	1st May 1982— 6th May 1982
Group II	8th May 1982—13th May 1982
Group III	15th May 1982—20th May 1982

Nephrology posting

Group I	22nd May 1982—27th May 1982
Group II	29th May 1982— 3rd June 1982
Group III	5th June 1982—10th June 1982

Dr. Abdul Khader has agreed to teach the trainee doctors during his ward rounds on Sundays and Wednesdays from 9 a.m.—11 a.m. about the management of diabetes mellitus. The trainee doctors are requested to join him for the rounds.

Programme:

Wednesday, 28th April, 1982	Teach-in Session (Dr. P. P. Boby)	12.00 noon—1.00 p.m.
Thursday, 29th April, 1982	Introduction to ECG (1) (Dr. Ahmed Shawki)	12.00 noon—1.00 p.m.
Wednesday, 5th May, 1982	Teach-in Session (Dr. P. P. Boby)	12.00 noon—1.00 p.m.
Thursday, 6th May, 1982	Introduction to ECG (2) (Dr. Ahmed Shawki)	12.00 noon—1.00 p.m.
Monday, 10th May, 1982	Management of Diabetes mellitus (Dr. Abdul Khader)	8.00 a.m.—9.00 a.m.
Wednesday, 12th May, 1982	Teach-in Session (Dr. P. P. Boby)	12.00 noon—1.00 p.m.
Thursday, 13th May, 1982	Introduction to ECG (3) (Dr. Ahmed Shawki)	12.00 noon—1.00 p.m.
Sunday, 16th May, 1982	Acid Base Balance (Dr. Ghaze Kusma)	12.00 noon—1.00 p.m.
Monday, 17th May, 1982	Management of Diabetes mellitus (Dr. Abdul Khader)	8.00 a.m.—9.00 a.m.
Tuesday, 18th May, 1982	Management of Arrhythmia and Cardiac Arrest (Dr. Marwan)	12.00 noon—1.00 p.m.

Wednesday, 19th May, 1982	Teach-in Session (Dr. P. P. Boby)	12.00 noon—1.00 p.m.
Sunday, 23rd May, 1982	Management of Acute Renal Failure (Dr. Ghaze Kusma)	12.00 noon—1.00 p.m.
Monday, 24th May, 1982	Management of Diabetes mellitus (Dr. Abdul Khader)	8.00 a.m.—9 a.m.
Wednesday, 26th May, 1982	Teach-in Session (Dr. P. P. Boby)	12.00 noon—1.00 p.m.
Thursday, 27th May, 1982	Basics im Immunology (1) (Dr. Ahmed Shawki)	12.00 noon—1.00 p.m.
Sunday, 30th May, 1982	Renal Replacement Therapy (Dr. Ghaze Kusma)	12.00 noon—1.00 p.m.
Wednesday, 2nd June, 1982	Teach-in Session (Dr. P. P. Boby)	12.00 noon—1.00 p.m.
Thursday, 3rd June, 1982	Basics in Immunology (2) (Dr. Ahmed Shawki)	12.00 noon—1.00 p.m.
Saturday, 5th June, 1982	Bronchial Asthma and COAD (Dr. Issam Sherbini)	12.00 noon—1.00 p.m.
Wednesday, 9th June, 1982	Teach-in Session (Dr. P. P. Boby)	12.00 noon—1.00 p.m.
Thursday, 10th June, 1982	Heat Regulation, Heat Stroke and its Management (Dr. Ahmed Shawki)	12.00 noon—1.00 p.m.
Saturday, 12th June, 1982	Management of Congestive Cardiac Failure (Dr. Issam Sherbini)	12.00 noon—1.00 p.m.
Wednesday, 16th June, 1982	Teach-in Session (Dr. P. P. Boby)	12.00 noon—1.00 p.m.
Thursday, 17th June, 1982	Management of a Case of Acute Poisoning (Dr. Ahmed Shawki)	12.00 noon—1.00 p.m.

81C—3304
Sabah Hospital In-Service Training in Paediatrics
3. 2. 1982—2. 6. 1982 Programme

Objectives: To continue the process of learning and also to keep abreast of recent advances in all branches of paediatrics so as to increase one's knowledge.
To discuss complex problems and to elucidate them.
To present and discuss cases of clinical interest or diagnostic problems.

Place:	Al Sabah Hospital.
Duration:	Five months from 3rd Feb. 1982 till 2. 6. 1982.
Organiser:	Prof. Abdulla A. A. Al Rashid, Chairman of the Dept. of Paediatrics, Sabah Hospital.
Participants:	Local staff and D.C.H. candidates, visitors and residents.
Programme:	*Seminars and Clinical Sessions*

The seminars will be held between 8.30—9.30 a.m. on every Wednesday and Saturday.
Every Sunday from 8.00 a.m. to 9.00 a.m. there will be a journal club, where the important paediatrics journals will be reviewed.
On Thursdays there will be a clinical meeting at 11.30 a.m. (11.00 a.m. in summer). At these meetings clinical cases will be presented and their problems discussed. Doctors from other hospitals as well as visitors also participate in these meetings. The names of the speakers will be circulated a month in advance.

Lecture—Subject

Wednesday, 3. 2. 1982	Evaluation of child with anaemia
Saturday, 6. 2. 1982	Evaluation of proteinuria in children
Wednesday, 10. 2. 1982	Sickle cell disease in children
Saturday, 13. 2. 1982	Evaluation of haematuria in children
Wednesday, 17. 2. 1982	Thalassaemia syndrome
Saturday, 20. 2. 1982	Urinary tract infection in children
Wednesday, 24. 2. 1982	I.T.P.
Saturday, 27. 2. 1982	Nephrotic syndrome
Wednesday, 3. 3. 1982	A.L.L.
Saturday, 6. 3. 1982	Juvenile diabetes mellites
Wednesday, 10. 3. 1982	Haemophilia
Saturday, 13. 3. 1982	Acute glomerulonephritis
Wednesday, 17. 3. 1982	Auto-immune haemolytic anaemia
Saturday, 20. 3. 1982	Febrile convulsion
Wednesday, 24. 3. 1982	Red cell enzyme haemolytic anaemia
Saturday, 3. 4. 1982	Acute renal failure in children
Saturday, 27. 3. 1982	Haemolytic uraemic syndrome
Wednesday, 7. 4. 1982	Tetanus
Saturday, 10. 4. 1982	Acute gastroenteritis
Wednesday, 14. 4. 1982	Stridor in children
Saturday, 17. 4. 1982	Primary T. B.
Wednesday, 21. 4. 1982	Hypothyroidism
Saturday, 24. 4. 1982	Pneumonia
Wednesday, 28. 4. 1982	Infectious mononucleosis
Saturday, 1. 5. 1982	Rye syndrome
Wednesday, 5. 5. 1982	Rye syndrome
Saturday, 8. 5. 1982	Protracted diarrhoea
Wednesday, 12. 5. 1982	Bacterial meningitis
Saturday, 15. 5. 1982	Preterm, low birth weight baby
Wednesday, 19. 5. 1982	Rickets

Saturday, 22. 5. 1982   Rheumatic fever
Wednesday, 26. 5. 1982   Cystic fibrosis
Saturday, 29. 6. 1982   Enteric fever
Wednesday, 2. 6. 1982   Brucellosis

81C—6305
Mubarak Al-Kabir Hospital In-Service Training in Radiology

Organiser:	Prof. Dr. Leo Steinhart, Ph.D., D.B. Chairman, Radiology Department, Mubarak Hospital.
Participants:	Local staff and D.C.H. candidates, visitors and residents.
Daily: 7.30— 8.00	Urologic–Nephrologic–Radiologic meeting. Place: Consultant's area–Meeting room.
Weekly: Mondays	
7.30— 8.30	Orthopaedic–Path. Anat.–Radiologic: Bone and soft tissue tumors. Place: Consultants area–Meeting room.
8.30— 9.00	Surgical–Radiological meeting. Place: Consultant's area–Meeting room.
11.30—12.30	Medical–Radiological meeting. Place: Consultant's area–Meeting room.
Tuesdays	
12.00—13.00	Gastroenterological meeting. Medical–Surgical–Radiological. Place: Consultant's area–Meeting room.

81C—6306
Sabah Hospital In-Service Training in Radiology
1981—1982 Academic Year General Programme

Organiser:	Dr. M. H. Bassiony Chief Radiologist X-Ray Department, Sabah Hospital.
Participants:	Local staff and D.C.M. candidates, visitors and residents.

A list of the current activities of Sabah X-Ray Department

1. Departmental meeting every Thursday 8.00—9.30 a.m.
2. Continuous discussions of any difficult case on the spot.
3. Continuous practical training in general and special proceedings. The effect of 2 and 3 helped two colleagues to pass their Master's Degree of Radiology on first try, the last got it 15 months after joining us.
4. Interdepartmental meetings.
   a) Radio-orthopaedic meetings which have been going on for 21 years every alternative Monday in the Orthopaedic Hospital at 6.00 p.m.
   b) Sabah Oncology meeting every Thursday at 9.30—11.30.
   c) Radio-vascular Meetings:
      Used to be regular on Wednesday; stopped lately after Prof. Abouna moved to Mubarak Hospital.

The same thing happened for the conjoined Radio-gastroenterology and Urology meeting when the respective doctors concerned moved from Sabah Hospital.

d) Participation in the clinico-pathological meetings arranged by the Medical Department.

5. Participation in the activities of Professional Training:
Last year 5 lectures were given to the M.R.C.P. Candidates (enclosed is a copy of such programme).

81C—6307
Ibn Sina Hospital In-Service Training in Radiology
1981—1982 Academic Year General Programme

Organiser: Dr. M. Rudwan
Participants: Local staff and D.C.H. candidates, visitors and residents.

1. In spite of the shortage of senior radiologists I managed to train the two radiologists who are now performing all neuro-radiological and other procedures with competence, they are developing reasonable standards in interpretation. We are inviting a Paediatric Radiologist from the United States to help us in this field.

2. *Departmental Meetings.*
a) *Neuro-radiology Meeting:*   *Saturday 10.30—12.30*
This is an extremely regular meeting that has been going on for the past 7 years. It is attented by neurosurgeons and neurologists, both from the Ministry and from the University, including some medical students and neurological anaesthetists.
b) *Topic Discussions:*   *Thursday 8.00*
This is a joint meeting. So far it is not very regular because of the pressure of work, but hopefully it will be organised soon with the neurological staff.
c) *Daily Review of Cases:*   *12.30—1.30*
All special procedures and C.T. Scan are revised with the registrars before the reports are typed.

3. *Other Clinico-radiological Meetings.*
There are meetings with other disciplines in different hospitals like Orthopaedic and Oncology meetings, the details which will no doubt be given by other members of the Committee.

81C—6308
Farwania Hospital In-Service Training in Radiology
1981—1982 Academic Year General Programme

Organiser: Dr. Shafik, Head of Radiology Department.
Participants: Local staff and D.C.H. candidates and visitors and residents.

1. Radiologist's meeting daily from 7.00 to 8.00 a.m.
Place: Office of Head of Department.
Programme: Problem cases and demonstrations.

2. Weekly Sessions: Thursdays 7.30 to 8.30 a.m.
Place: Same as before.
Programme: Journal club
                   Tutorials presented by the staff
                   Preparing papers for publication.

3. Oncology Radiologic Meeting every Saturday 12.30 to 14.00
   Place: Ward 10
   Programme: Oncology cases
4. Paediatric Radiologic Meeting 3rd Monday of every month.
   Place: Lecture Room
   Programme: Paediatric cases
5. Radio-Orthopaedic Meeting every other Monday 18.00 to 20.00
   Place: Sulaibikhat Hospital Meeting Room
   Programme: Interesting orthopedic cases
   Problem cases.
6. Sharing in other departmental meetings whenever possible.

81C—6309
Jahra Hospital In-Service Training in Radiology
1981—1982 Academic Year Programme

Organiser: Dr. M. H. Zahran
Participants: Local staff and D.C.H. candidates, visitors and residents.

The following different activities are being carried out in the Department of Radiology.

I. *Meetings and Seminars.*
   a) Intradepartmental
      i. Daily case discussion
      ii. Weekly Journal Club every Thursday
   b) Interdepartmental
      Weekly combined clinico-radiological meetings with the Departments of Medicine and Surgery.
II. *Research Projects.*
   It is one of the main objectives of our department to carry out research. Some of the projects have already been completed and the others are underway.
III. *Invitation of External Visitors.*
   The following speakers were invited to deliver some lectures.
   a) Prof. Rafik Zaher Dean, Faculty of Medicine, Alexandria University (Medical versus Surgical Cholestasis)
   b) Prof. Effat Massanein, Prof. of Radiology and Vice Dean, Alexandria University (Role of P.T.C. in Obstructive Jaundice)
   c) Dr. Raymond Andreue, Ausconic University (Role of U.I. Octoson Ultrasound in Medical Diagnosis).

81C—6910
Sabah Hospital In-Service Training in Anaesthesia and Intensive Care
3. 9. 1981—8. 4. 1982 Programme

Weekly Scientific Meeting, Starting from 3rd September, 1981 till now

S. No.	Date	Topics
1.	3. 9. 1981	Premedication Rounds
2.	10. 9. 1981	Anaesthesia for Diabetic Patient
3.	17. 9. 1981	Anaesthetic Management of Hypertension
4.	24. 9. 1981	Opiate Receptors and Analgesia

S. No.	Date	Topics
5.	1. 10. 1981	Opiate Receptors and Analgesia
6.	8. 10. 1981	Opiate Receptors and Analgesia
7.	15. 10. 1981	Case Presentation:
		Volume Overloading during T.U.R.
8.	29. 10. 1981	Epidural Analgesia and Anaesthesia
9.	5. 11. 1981	Epidural Analgesia and Anaesthesia
10.	19. 11. 1981	Case Presentation:
		(Pulmonary Oedema during Upper Airway Obstruction)
		Anaesthetic Circuits
11.	26. 11. 1981	Shock Syndrome Introduction
12.	3. 12. 1981	Shock Pathophysiology
13.	17. 12. 1981	Shock Strategy for Treatment
14.	24. 12. 1981	Pharmacology of Autonomic Drugs.
15.	7. 1. 1982	Anaesthetic Vaporisers.
		Obesity and Anaesthesia.
16.	14. 1. 1982	Case Presentation:
		Some Mathematical Concepts.
17.	21. 1. 1982	Suxamethonium Apnea (case presentation and review of the literature)
18.	28. 1. 1982	Neuroleptanalgesia and Anaesthesia
19.	4. 2. 1982	Acid Base Balance
		Case Presentation
20.	11. 2. 1982	Post-operative Analgesia
		Self-administered Analgesia by Palliator Machine
21.	25. 2. 1982	Acid Base Balance:
		Case Presentation (Fatal Bronchospasm)
22.	4. 3. 1982	Sequential Clinical Trials
23.	11. 3. 1982	Acid Base Balance
		Anaesthesia for Micro Laryngeal Surgery
24.	18. 3. 1982	Oxygen: Its Physiological Role
		Oxygen: Use in Therapy
25.	25. 3. 1982	New Analgesic Drugs
26.	1. 4. 1982	Muscle Relaxants
27.	8. 4. 1982	Management of Patients with Coronary Artery Disease

Trainee Doctors

Name	Unit	Anaesthesia and I.C.U. One Week
1. Dr. Fawsia Al-Kandary	(E)	5. 9.—11. 9. 1981
2. Dr. Dina Jaber Ramadan	(F)	22. 8.—28. 8. 1981
3. Dr. Ekhlas Fatima	(C)	22. 8.—28. 8. 1981
4. Dr. Zohair Saleh	(F)	22. 8.—28. 8. 1981
5. Dr. Hanan Al-Hassouna	(A)	26. 9.— 2. 10. 1981
6. Dr. Moneeb M. Hamdan	(D)	31. 10.— 6. 11. 1981
7. Dr. Maher O. Mahmoud	(A)	31. 10.— 6. 11. 1981
8. Dr. Najeeba Al-Kattan	(C)	5. 9.—11. 9. 1981
9. Dr. Khalifa Al-Sakabi	(A)	5. 12.—18. 12. 1981
10. Dr. Ahlam Abdulla	(B)	5. 12.—18. 12. 1981

Name	Unit	Anaesthesia and I.C.U. One Week
11. Dr. Jamal Al-Diaj	(B)	7. 11.—20. 11. 1981
12. Dr. Wafaa Al-Shaygi	(C)	7. 11.—20. 11. 1981
13. Dr. Mossaed Al-Asfour	(F)	21. 11.— 4. 12. 1981
14. Dr. Asma'a Al-Tawari	(F)	5. 12.—18. 12. 1981
15. Dr. Mosaab Al-Saleh	(D)	21. 11.— 4. 12. 1981
16. Dr. A. Nasser Al-Othman	(E)	21. 11.— 4. 12. 1981
17. Dr. Laila Al-Jassem	(E)	21. 11.— 4. 12. 1981
18. Dr. Laila Bastaki	(E)	16. 1.—29. 1. 1982
19. Dr. Ali Al Arbash	(C)	16. 1.—29. 1. 1982
20. Dr. Mouna Al Khawari	(C)	2. 1.—15. 1. 1982
21. Dr. Adnan Al-Eidan	(F)	2. 1.—15. 1. 1982
22. Dr. Ibrahim A. Hadi	(E)	2. 1.—15. 1. 1982

81C—6911
Mubarak Hospital In-Service Training in Anaesthesia and Intensive Care
11. 2. 1982—11. 3. 1982 Programme

The Department of Anaesthesia conducts regular clinical meetings where both clinical and academic subjects are discussed. Further, clinical problems are discussed and analysed. As part of the postgraduate training activities the intern doctors are provided with intensive care and resuscitation training. Medical students are trained in the basics of anaesthesia and resuscitation. The anaesthetics staff is given intensive training and instruction in resuscitation and intensive care.

Weekly surgical mortality and morbidity meetings are conducted in association with surgical departments. Specialists in different fields attend these meetings and surgical and traumatology cases are discussed and analysed.

The department receives journals in Anaesthesia irregularly and will establish a library in due course.

Clinical Meeting

Place:	In Library room adjacent to theatre
Date:	Thursday, 11th February 1982, 8.30—9.30 a.m.
Organiser:	Dr. M. M. Yacoub, Head of Anaesthesia and ICU
Topic for Discussion:	Physiology of Diabetes, Diabetic Emergencies.

Clinical Meeting

Place (Venue):	Library room (adjacent to operating theatre)
Date:	18th February, 1982 (Thursday) 8.30 a.m.—9.30 a.m.
Organiser:	Dr. M. M. Yacoub, Head of Anaesthesia and ICU, Mubarak Hospital
Topics for Discussion:	
Clinical Case	Dr. Tayseer and Dr. Kamal—15 minutes (Collapse following Epidural Bupivacine)—Marcain
Lecture	Dr. Kamal—Physiology of Intracranial Pressure—30 minutes and effects of anaesthetic agents
Discussion:	15 minutes

Clinical Meeting

Place (Venue):	Library room
Date:	7th April 1982, 8.30 a.m.—9.30 a.m.
Organiser:	Dr. M. Yacoub, Head of Anaesthesia Dept.

Programme:	Talk by Dr. Mahannath El-Rakshi, followed by 15 minutes discussion
Topic	Synthetic Opiate Analgesics Endogenous Opiates and Endorphins

Clinical Meeting

Place (Venue):	Library Room
Date:	4th March 1982
Time:	8.30 to 9.30 a.m.
Programme:	1. *Chest X-Ray Slide Show*—22 minutes (Introduction)—to be continued) 2. *Physiology and Pharmacology* (30 minutes) Cerebral Circulation and Intracranial Pressure Dr. Rajkumar Singh (on 18. 3. 1982) Intracranial Effects of Anaesthetic Drugs, discussion 8 minutes

Clinical Meeting

Place (Venue):	Library Room
Date:	11th March 1982, 9.30—10.30
Organiser:	Dr. M. M. Yacoub, Head of Anaesthesia and ICU, Mubarak Hospital
Programme:	1. *Chest X-Ray Slide Show*—25 minutes (The large homogeneous or confluent shadow) to be continued. 2. Dr. Bader Al Raskhe Narcotic Analgesics / Endorphins

81C—6912
Farwania Hospital In-Service Training in Anaesthesia and Intensive Care
10. 9. 1981—18. 2. 1982

Organiser:	Dr. Khairy Naguid Chairman, Dept. of Anaesthesia and ICU
Participants:	Local staff and D.C.H. candidates, visitors and residents

Date	Topic	Speaker
10. 9. 1981	Morbidity and Mortality	Dr. Youssef Dr. Shams
17. 9. 1981	Septic Shock Slides	
24. 9. 1981	Electrical Hazards in Operating Theatre	Dr. Farouk
1. 10. 1981	Pharmacology of Local Anaesth. Agents Slides	
8. 10. 1981	Holiday	
15. 10. 1981	Muscle Relaxants	Dr. Shams
22. 10. 1981	Physiology of Aut. N.S.	Dr. William
29. 10. 1981	Short Acting Hypotensive Agents	Dr. William
5. 11. 1981	Carriage of CO_2 in the Blood O_2 Transport	Dr. Hussam
	O_2 Transport	Dr. Rao
	Journal Club	Dr. Zenab
12. 11. 1981	Local Anaest., Pharmacology and Anatomy	
	Pain Mechanism and Control	Dr. Philip

Date	Topic	Speaker
17. 11. 1981	Methods of Preservation of Blood	
	Significance of Changes in Stored Blood	Dr. Jan
	Complications of Blood Transfusion	Dr. Ashok
24. 11. 1981	Prolonged Ventilation	Dr. Khairy
	Ideal Ventilator	Dr. Karsk
31. 11. 1981	Pulmonary Circulation versus	Dr. Farouk
	Cerebral Circulation	
	Pulmonary Oedema	
	Morbidity and Mortality	
14. 1. 1982	Uptake and Distribution of Inhalation of	Slides
	Anaesthetic Agents	
	Tutorial—Principles of Cl. Measurements	
21. 1. 1982	Evaluation of Obst. Patient	Slides
	Pharmacology and Clinical Uses of Local	
	Anaesthetic Agents	Slides
28. 1. 1982	Pharmacology of Antiarrhythmic Drugs	Slides
	Parts I and II	
4. 2. 1982	Measurement of Flow	Dr. Jan
11. 2. 1982	Measurement of Pressure	Dr. Farouk
18. 2. 1982	Interpretation of Blood Gas Analysis	Dr. Shams

Journal Club

Date	Journal	Name
18. 4. 1981	Survey of Anaesthesiology	Dr. Rao
	No. 5 Oct. 1981	
25. 4. 1981	British Journal of Hospital Medicine	Dr. Asma
	24.5, November 1981	
2. 5. 1981	British Journal of Hospital	Dr. Karsk
	Medicine 24.5., Nov. 1980	
9. 5. 1981	Acta No. 3 June 1980	Dr. Ashok
16. 5. 1981	Acta No. 4 August 1980	Dr. Hussam
23. 5. 1981	B. T. A. No. 10 Oct. 1980	Dr. Farouk
30. 5. 1981	B. J. A. No. 11 Nov. 1980	Dr. Karsk
6. 6. 1981	Acta No. 6 Dec. 1980	Dr. Zenab
13. 6. 1981	B. J. A. No. 12 Dec. 1980	Dr. Sham
20. 6. 1981	Anaesth and Analgesia No. 11 Nov.	Dr. Moda
27. 6. 1981	Anaesth and ICU No. 4 Nov. 1980	Dr. Youssef

81C—6913
Sulaibikhat Hospital In-Service Training in Anaesthesia in Intensive Care
November 1981—March 1982 Programme

Organiser: Dr. Imran Qwaider, Head of Dept. of Anaesthesia Sulaibikhat Hospital.

Participants: Local staff and D.C.M. candidates, visitors and residents.

Topics	Speakers
1. Endo-Tracheal Intubation for the Surgeons of the Hospital	Dr. Imran
2. Blood Volume	Dr. Nadia
3. Peripheral Resistance	Dr. Takla
4. Sympathetic and Para-sympathetic Predominance during Anaesthesia	Dr. Malek
5. Acid-base	Dr. Ayham
6. Shock and Assessment of Blood Loss in Trauma and during Surgery	Dr. Basem
7. Drug Interaction	Dr. Sajed
8. I.V. Nutrition	Dr. Melko
9. Intensive Care Unit and Intensive Care Therapy	Dr. Ayham
10. Atropine—before, during and after Anaesthesia	Dr. Moneeb

81C—6914
Maternity Hospital In-Service Training in Anaesthesia and Intensive Care
1. 10. 1981—16. 6. 1982 Programme

Organiser: Dr. Okasha, Head of Anaes. Dept., Maternity Hospital
Date and Time: Every Thursday morning from 7.30 a.m to 9.00 a.m.
Participants: Local staff and visitors

Programme:

Date	Topics	Speakers
1. 10. 1981	Diagnosis and Management of Cardiac Arrest	Dr. Okasha
15. 10. 1981	Analysis for Normal Labour Part I	Dr. Okasha
22. 10. 1981	Analysis for Normal Labour Part II	Dr. Okasha
29. 10. 1981	Preoperative Assessment and Preparation of a Cardiac Patient	Dr. E. Kram
5. 11. 1981	Anaesthesia for Cardiac Patient	Dr. Cora
12. 11. 1981	Anaesthesia for Electrocanavalsive Therapy	Dr. Bashir
19. 11. 1981	Paediatric Anaesthesia Part I	Dr. Nadia
26. 11. 1981	Paediatric Anaesthesia Part II	Dr. Nadia
3. 12. 1981	Anaesthesia and Obst. Emergencies Part I	Dr. Mona
10. 12. 1981	Anaesthesia and Obst. Emergencies Part II	Dr. Mona
17. 12. 1981	Delayed Recovery	Dr. Bashir
24. 12. 1981	Drugs Acting on the Heart	Dr. Samir
31. 12. 1981	Muscle Relaxants Part I	Dr. Okasha
7. 1. 1982	Muscle Relaxants Part II	Dr. Okasha
14. 1. 1982	Drugs Interaction	Dr. Sayed
21. 1. 1982	Neonatal Asphyxia and Neonatal Respiratory Distress Syndrome	Dr. Leydia
28. 1. 1982	Policy in the Intensive Care Unit	Dr. Okasha
4. 2. 1982	Management of Chronic Intractable Pain and Theories of Pain	Dr. Cora
11. 2. 1982	Cardiac Arrest	Dr. Samir
18. 2. 1982	Surgery and Anaesthesia	
25. 2. 1982	Tranquilisers, Antidepressants and Sedatives	Dr. Laidi
11. 3. 1982	Monitoring of Critically Ill Patients	Dr. Okasha
18. 3. 1982	Blood Coagulation Defects and Anaesthesia Part I	Dr. Okasha

Date	Topic	Speaker
25. 3. 1982	Blood Coagulation Defects and Anaesthesia Part II	Dr. Okasha
1. 4. 1982	Mechanical Ventilators	Dr. E. Kram
8. 4. 1982	Mechanical Ventilators	Dr. E. Kram
15. 4. 1982	Oxygen Therapy	Dr. Laidi
22. 4. 1982	Body Response to Trauma	Dr. Sameer
29. 4. 1982	Intravenous Fluid Therapy	Dr. Leydia
6. 5. 1982	Intravenous Fluid Therapy	Dr. Leydia
13. 5. 1982	Coma	Dr. Sayed
20. 5. 1982	Extracorporeal Circulation	Dr. A. S. Okasha
27. 5. 1982	E.E.G. 7 ECG	Dr. Samir

Combined Anaesthesia with Gynaecology and Obstetrics

Date	Topics	Doctor's Name
13. 1. 1982	Intravenous Fluid Therapy	Dr. Okasha
17. 2. 1982	Drug Interaction	Dr. Sayed
17. 3. 1982	Anaesthesia in Obstetrics	Dr. Okasha
14. 4. 1982	Body Response to Trauma	Dr. Okasha
19. 5. 1982	Anaesthesia in Renal Failure	Dr. Okasha
16. 6. 1982	Analgesia for Labour	Dr. Okasha

Journal Club and Morbidity and Mortality

Date	Journal and care presentation	Doctor's name
1. 10. 1981	*Brit. J. Anaesth.* (August 1980)	Dr. Okasha
15. 10. 1981	*Anaesthesia J.* (August 1980)	Dr. Samir
22. 10. 1981	*Brit. J. Anaesth.* (September 1980)	Dr. Sayed
29. 10. 1981	*Anaesth. J.* (September 1980)	Dr. Nadia
5. 11. 1981	*Brit. J. Anaesth.* (October 1980)	Dr. Lydia
12. 11. 1981	*Anaest. J.* (October 1980)	Dr. Sayed
19. 11. 1981	*Brit. J. Anaesth.* (November 1980)	Dr. Cora
26. 11. 1981	*Anaesth. J.* (November 1980)	Dr. Okasha
3. 12. 1981	*Brit. J. Anaesth.* (December 1980)	Dr. Ekram
10. 12. 1981	*Anaesth. J.* (December 1980)	Dr. Mona
17. 12. 1981	*Brit. J. Anaesth.* (January 1981)	Dr. Yehia
24. 12. 1981	*Anaesth. J.* (January 1981)	Dr. Zaidi
31. 12. 1981	*Brit. J. Anaesth.* (February 1981)	Dr. Bashir
7. 1. 1982	*Anaesth. J.* (February 1981)	Dr. Okasha
14. 1. 1982	*Brit. J. Anaesth.* (March 1981)	Dr. Lydia
21. 1. 1982	*Anaesth. J.* (March 1981)	Dr. Samir
28. 1. 1982	*Brit. J. Anaesth.* (April 1981)	Dr. Mona
4. 2. 1982	*Anaesth. J.* (April 1981)	Dr. Nadia
11. 2. 1982	*Brit. J. Anaesth.* (May 1981)	Dr. Sayed
18. 2. 1982	*Anaesth. J.* (May 1981)	Dr. Cora
25. 2. 1982	*Brit. J. Anaesth.* (June 1981)	Dr. Ekram
11. 3. 1982	*Anaesth. J.* (June 1981)	Dr. Bashir
18. 3. 1982	*Brit. J. Anaesth.* (July 1981)	Dr. Yehia
25. 3. 1982	*Anaesth. J.* (July 1981)	Dr. Mona

Date	Journal and care presentation	Doctor's name
1. 4. 1982	*Brit. J. Anaesth.* (August 1981)	Dr. Sayed
8. 4. 1982	*Anaesth. J.* (August 1981)	Dr. Zaidi
15. 4. 1982	*Brit. J. Anaesth.* (September 1981)	Dr. Ekram
22. 4. 1982	*Anaesth. J.* (September 1981)	Dr. Okasha
29. 4. 1982	*Anaesth. J.* (September 1981)	Dr. Okasha
29. 4. 1982	*Brit. J. Anaesth.* (October 1981)	Dr. Samir
6. 5. 1982	*Anaesth. J.* (October 1981)	Dr. Lydia
13. 5. 1982	*Brit. J. Anaesth.* (November 1981)	Dr. Bashir
20. 5. 1982	*Anaesth. J.* (November 1981)	Dr. Yehia
27. 5. 1982	*Brit. J. Anaesth.* (December 1981)	Dr. Salwa
3. 6. 1982	*Anaesth. J.* (December 1981)	Dr. Okasha
10. 6. 1982	*Brit. J. Anaesth.* (January 1982)	Dr. Ekram
17. 6. 1982	*Anaesth. J.* (January 1982)	Dr. Cora
24. 6. 1982	*Brit. J. Anaesth.* (February 1982)	Dr. Zaidi

b) Nation-Wide (Institutional) Continuing Medical Education

81C—0201
Biostatistics for Clinical Use

Objectives: To understand the importance of medical statistics.
To become familiar with factors influencing medical statistics.
To learn statistical methodology for prospective or retrospective studies.
To undertake randomised clinical trials.
To evaluate and analyse statistical data.

Methods: Books:
1. Armitage, P. (1974) *Statistical Methods in Medical Research,* Blackwell Scientific Publications, London.
2. Daniel, W. (1978) *Biostatistics,* John Wiley and Sons, NY.
3. Fleiss, J. (1981) *Statistical Methods for Rates and Proportions,* John Wiley and Sons, NY.
4. Johnson, R. C., and Johnson, N. (1980) *Survival Models and Data Analysis,* John Wiley and Sons, NY.

Place: Department of Radiotherapy, Al Sabah Hospital.

Duration: 10 weeks—commencing on Sunday the 4th of October, 1981 at 7.30 a.m.

Organiser: Dr. Y.T. Omar, F.R.C.R., Chairman, Department of Radiotherapy, Al Sabah Hospital, Kuwait.

Programme Director: Dr. M. A. A. Moussa, Associate Professor, Dept. of Community Medicine, Faculty of Medicine, Kuwait University.

Participation: A course on medical statistics for the staff of the departments.

Programme:

1. Descriptive statistics.
2. Inferential statistics:
   Inference on one population means
   Inference on two population means
   Inference on more than two population means
   Inference on one population proportion
   Inference on two population proportions
   Inference on more than two population proportions
3. Determination of sample size to detect a proportion.
   Determination of sample size to detect a difference
   between two proportions.
4. Simple linear regression and correlation.
5. How to randomise.
6. Cross-sectional studies.
7. Prospective and retrospective studies.
8. Controlled comparative trials (case-control studies).
9. The analysis of data from matched samples.
10. Vital and health statistics—standardised rates.
11. Life tables—estimation of survival and hazard func-
    tions from grouped mortality data.

81C—0701
Some Clinical Aspects of Allergy and Immunology

Objectives:

The visit of Professor M. M. Lessof, MD, FRCP, Department of Medicine, Guy's Hospital Medical School,
London.
To teach recent advances in the field of allergy and immunology.

Place:

Department of Medicine, Al-Sabah Hospital Ahmadi
Hospital, Chest Hospital, Lecture Room 105, Faculty
of Medicine.

Duration:

10 days, from 28th February, 1981—8th March, 1981.

Organiser:

Ministry of Public Health.

Programme Director:

Professor F. F. Fenech, Chairman of the Department of
Medicine, Al-Sabah Hospital.

Participants:

Internists and training doctors in the above mentioned
hospital (MRCP Part I, Part II), attending lectures, clinical rounds and instruction sessions.

Programme:

Saturday, 28th February, 1981

10.00 a.m.   Teaching Round, Ward 2, Al-Sabah (Undergraduates)
              (Dr. Y. Killani)
5.30 p.m.   Lecture (MRCP Part I Course)
              Immune Reactions and Disease
              Lecture Room 105, Faculty of Medicine

Sunday, 1st March, 1981

10.30 a.m.   Visit to Ahmadi Hospital and Kuwait Oil Company Complex
                     Departure to Ahmadi at 10.30 a.m. and return in late afternoon
                     Lunch and Lecture at Ahmadi
                     (topic to be chosen by Professor Lessof)

Monday, 2nd March, 1981

9.00 a.m.   Visit to Kidney Transplant Unit, Chest Hospital
                     Visit to Immunology Laboratory, Chest Hospital
                     (Dr. A. White)
11.00 a.m.   Seminar on Coma
                     Chest Hospital
5.00 p.m.   MRCP Part II–Mock Viva Lecture Room 105, Faculty of Medi-
                     cine.

Tuesday, 3rd March, 1981

9.00 a.m.   Visit to Immunology Laboratory, Department of Medicine,
                     Al-Sabah Hospital
                     (Dr. A. Tahan)
10.00 a.m.   Teaching Round, Ward 3, Al-Sabah
                     (Dr. I. Abu Sabra)
12.00 noon   Clinical Meetings—Lecture Allergy and Bronchial Asthma Semi-
                     nar Room—Al-Sabah Hospital

Wednesday, 4th March, 1981

9.00 a.m.   Problem Cases Session
10.30 a.m.   Teach-in Session Immunosuppression and its Hazards, Seminar
                     Room, Dept. of Medicine, Al-Sabah Hospital
5.30 p.m.   Lecture (MRCP Part I Course)
                     Immune Deficiency
                     Lecture Room 105, Faculty of Medicine

Thursday, 5th March, 1981

10.00 a.m.   Clinical Session (MRCP Part II Course)
                     Ahmadi Hospital
                     Moch Clinicals at Ahmadi
                     (Dr. J. G. Lloyd and Dr. R. Shakir)

Saturday, 7th March, 1981

9.00 a.m.   Postgraduate Round, Ward 5, Al-Sabah Hospital
                     (Dr. M. H. Barakat)
5.30 p.m.   Lecture (MRCP Part I Course)
                     Bechet's Disease and other Connective Tissue Diseases
                     Lecture Room 105, Faculty of Medicine

81C—0702
Applied Immunology in Medicine

Objectives: To acquaint residents and registrars with the clinical ap-
                     plication of immunology.
                     To explore how and when to seek the advices of the im-
                     munologist.
                     To survey the recent advances in the field of immunology.

Place: In the main building of the Telecommunication Training Center, Shuwaikh.

Duration: 5 days, from 5th December to 9th December 1981.

Organiser: Discipline Committee for Clinical Laboratory Medicine.

Programme Director: Dr. Arthur G. White

Participants: Residents, registrars and specialists of various disciplines.

Programme:

Saturday, 5th December, 1981

8.30 a.m.— 9.30 a.m.	Development of Immunity Max Cooper
9.30 a.m.—10.30 a.m.	Immunoglobulins Keith James
10.30 a.m.—11.00 a.m.	Coffee
11.00 a.m.—12.00 noon	Non-Specific Immunity Arthur White
12.00 noon—1.00 p.m.	Cell-Mediated Immunity Keith James
1.00 p.m— 2.00 p.m.	Lunch
2.00 p.m— 3.00 p.m.	The Measurement of IgE Wilfried de Jong
3.00 p.m.— 3.30 p.m.	Tea
3.30 p.m.— 4.30 p.m.	The Natural Killer Cell Max Cooper

Sunday, 6th December, 1981

8.30 a.m.— 9.30 a.m.	Auto-Immunity Introduction James Irvine
9.30 a.m.—10.30 a.m.	The Complement System Ron Thompson
10.30 a.m.—11.00 a.m.	Coffee
11.00 a.m.—12.00 noon	Auto-Immunity and Endocrine Disease James Irvine
12.00 noon— 1.00 p.m.	Immune Mechanisms and Disease Ron Thompson
1.00 p.m.— 2.00 p.m.	Lunch
2.00 p.m.— 3.00 p.m.	Clinical Significance of Plasma Protein Determination in Hepatic and Renal Disease Wilfried de Jong
3.00 p.m.— 3.30 p.m.	Tea
3.30 p.m.— 4.30 p.m.	Immunology of Diabetes James Irvine

Monday, 7th December, 1981

8.30 a.m.— 9.30 a.m.	Tumour Immunology Keith James
9.30 a.m.—10.30 a.m.	Lymphoproliferative Disease Max Cooper
10.30 a.m.—11.00 a.m.	Coffee
11.00 a.m.—12.00 noon	Tumour Immunology Keith James
12.00 noon— 1.00 p.m.	Immuno-Therapy Ron Thompson
1.00 p.m.— 2.00 p.m.	Lunch
2.00 p.m.— 3.00 p.m.	Transplant Biology Arthur White
3.00 p.m.— 3.30 p.m.	Tea
3.30 p.m.— 4.30 p.m.	Immuno-Suppression George Abouna

Tuesday, 8th December, 1981

8.30 a.m.— 9.30 a.m.	Primary Immuno-Deficiency Ron Thompson
9.30 a.m.—10.30 a.m.	Secondary Immuno-Deficiency Max Cooper
10.30 a.m.—11.00 a.m.	Coffee
11.00 a.m.—12.00 noon	Phagocyte defects John Soothill
12.00 noon— 1.00 p.m.	Laboratory Investigation of Immune Status Ron Thompson
1.00 p.m.— 2.00 p.m.	Lunch
2.00 p.m.— 3.00 p.m.	Clinical Investigation in Immuno-Deficiency John Soothill
3.00 p.m.— 3.30 p.m.	Tea
3.30 p.m.— 4.30 p.m.	Radio Immuno Assay M. Awakati

Wednesday, 9th December, 1981

8.30 a.m.— 9.30 a.m.	Allergy John Soothill
9.30 a.m.—10.30 a.m.	Allergic Disease in Kuwait Roger Ellul-Micallef
10.30 a.m.—11.00 a.m.	Coffee
11.00 a.m.—12.00 noon	Factors Predisposing to Allergy John Soothill
12.00 noon— 1.00 p.m.	Immunogenetics Arthur White
1.00 p.m.— 2.00 p.m.	Lunch
2.00 p.m.— 3.00 p.m.	Immunology in Kuwait Arthur White, Ahmad Tahan
3.00 p.m.— 3.30 p.m.	Tea
3.30 p.m.— 4.30 p.m.	Closing Discussion

81C—0901
First Workshop on how to do Simple Illustrations Yourself

Objectives:	To teach how to do simple illustrations yourself. At the end of the workshop each participant should be able to do simple illustrations himself using the medical illustration kit provided in the resource room in his working place. The drawings provided would be legible according to rules he will learn in the workshop.
Place:	Al Adan Hospital, postgraduate teaching area.
Duration:	6 days, from 30th May 1981 till 4th June, 1981.
Organiser:	Training Division, Department of Public Health and Planning.
Programme Director:	Dr. Samir Wahdan, Head of Medical Illustration and Teaching Facilities Unit.
Participants:	10 consultants from different hospitals and different departments of the Ministry of Public Health.
Programme: *(General Outline)*	Introduction to basic rules of visual legibility. How to choose suitable media in teaching. Basic techniques of illustration. Introduction to the medical illustration kit. Practical training and doing simple illustrations.

81C—0902
Second Workshop on how to do Simple Illustrations Yourself

Objectives:	To teach how to do simple illustrations yourself. At the end of the workshop each participant should be able to do simple illustrations himself using the medical illustration kit provided in the resource room in his working place. The drawings provided would be legible according to rules he will learn in the workshop.
Place:	Al Adan Hospital, postgraduate teaching area.
Duration:	6 days, from 6th June 1981 till 11th June 1981.
Organiser:	Training Division, Department of Public Health and Planning.
Programme Director:	Dr. Samir Wahdan, Head of Medical Illustration and Teaching Facilities Unit.
Participants:	10 consultants from different hospitals and different departments of the Ministry of Public Health.
Programme: *(General Outline)*	Introduction to basic rules of visual legibility. How to choose suitable media in teaching. Basic techniques of illustration. Introduction to the medical illustration kit. Practical training and doing simple illustrations.

81C—0903
Third Workshop on how to do Simple Illustrations Yourself

Objectives:	To teach how to do simple illustrations yourself. At the end of the workshop each participant should be able to do simple illustrations himself using the medical illustration kit provided in the resource room in his working place. The drawings provided would be legible according to rules he will learn in the workshop.
Place:	Al Adan Hospital, postgraduate teaching area.
Duration:	6 days, from 13th June 1981 till 18th June 1981.
Organiser:	Training Division, Department of Public Health and Planning.
Programme Director:	Dr. Samir Wahdan, Head of Medical Illustration and Teaching Facilities Unit.
Participants:	10 consultants from different hospitals and different departments of the Ministry of Public Health.
Programme: (General Outline)	Introduction to basic rules of visual legibility. How to choose suitable media in teaching. Basic techniques of illustration. Introduction to the medical illustration kit. Practical training and doing simple illustrations.

81C—0904
Fourth Workshop on how to do Simple Illustrations Yourself

Objectives:	To teach how to do simple illustrations yourself. At the end of the workshop each participant should be able to do simple illustrations himself using the medical illustration kit provided in the resource room in his working place. The drawings provided would be legible according to rules he will learn in the workshop.
Place:	Al Adan hospital, postgraduate teaching area.
Duration:	6 days, from 20th June 1981 till 25th June 1981.
Organiser:	Training Division, Department of Public Health and Planning.
Programme Director:	Dr. Samir Wahdan, Head of Medical Illustration and Teaching Facilities Unit.
Participants:	10 consultants from different hospitals and different departments of the Ministry of Public Health.
Programme: (General Outline)	Introduction to basic rules of visual legibility. How to choose suitable media in teaching. Basic techniques of illustration. Introduction to the medical illustration kit. Practical training and doing simple illustrations.

Report by Antonia Land and Doig Simmonds, Royal Postgraduate Medical School, London on 4 Workshops on "How to do Simple Illustrations Yourself"

Introduction

In March / April 1980 the World Health Organisation Eastern Mediterranean Office invited Mr. D. Simmonds, Chief Medical Artist at the Royal Postgraduate Medical School London, to visit seven countries in the Middle East Region. The objective of this tour was to explore the possibility of introducing a do-it-yourself illustration system similar to that which now operates at the RPMS. It was felt that many simple illustrations for teaching or the publication of research papers could be made by medical authors and teachers without waiting for the establishment of medical illustration services and trained medical illustrators.

The Training Division of the Ministry of Health in Kuwait, directed by Prof. E. Ruzyllo, responded to the initial demonstration almost immediately following Mr. Simmonds' visit, and a series of workshops were arranged for July 1981.

As part of the development of facilities for the production of scientific illustrations in Kuwait, four workshops on "How to do simple illustrations in Kuwait" and four workshops on "How to do simple illustrations yourself" were held there in July 1981. On the average 12 people from various scientific backgrounds (doctors, technicians, nurses, dentists, etc.) attended each workshop.

The working language was English, and the principles and techniques taught were first developed at the Royal Postgraduate Medical School, Hammersmith Hospital, London, by Doig Simmonds.

Objectives:

That having attended the 6-day course, each participant would be able to produce simple illustrations using the medical illustration kit which will be provided at his place of work in the resource room.

That these illustrations would be legible when projected and acceptable for publication in the scientific press, the latter being particularly important.

Much first-class scientific data from the developing world is not published simply for want of illustrations of a statistical nature. This has given rise to an impression that medically significant material is non-existent in some institutions and this is not the case.

Place:

Postgraduate Medical Education Centre, Al-Adan Hospital, Kuwait.

Duration:

Four workshops of 6 days each were held.
Working hours were
9.30 a.m.—2.00 p.m. each day

Course 1: 4. 7. 1981— 9. 7. 1981
Course 2: 11. 7. 1981—16. 7. 1981
Course 3: 18. 7. 1981—23. 7. 1981
Course 4: 25. 7. 1981—30. 7. 1981

Organiser: Training Division, Department of Public Health and
                        Planning (Medical Illustration and Teaching Facilities
                        Unit)
                        Director: Professor E. Ruzyllo

Programme Director: Dr. Samir Wahdan, Head of Medical Illustration and
                        Teaching Facilities Unit.
                        Course Tutor: Antonia Lant, Royal Postgraduate Med-
                                      ical School, London
                                      Various ancillary staff

Participants: In spite of the fact that July 1981 was the month of
                        Ramadan, the workshops were heavily overbooked
                        three days after the initial announcements were made;
                        one institution alone wanted to send 66 persons to the
                        course!

The workshops were designed to be limited to 10 persons per 6-day period, making
a total of 40 persons in a month.

Course 1:

1. Dr. Rajai Al Mastehi   Dental Centre
2. Dr. R. Sridharan   Radiology—Farwania Hospital
3. Dr. Moustafa Helmy   Health Institute
4. Mrs. Salwa Beheiry   Health Institute
5. Mr. Soma Sundara Baskaran   Nursing Planning and Training Unit
6. Mrs. Annamma Jacob   Nursing Planning and Training Unit
7. Mr. Mustafa Al Dawi   Preventive Medicine
8. Dr. Mounir Guirgis   Preventive Medicine
9. Dr. Ahmed S. Teebi   Genetics Paediatrics
10. Dr. Sana Al Adawi   Laboratory / Maternity Hospital
11. Mr. Wa'el Rashed Abdalla   Hormone Lab., Sabah Hospital

Course 2:

1. Dr. Salem Mohammed Salem   Health Education
2. Ms. Soad Edward   Health Education
3. Mrs. Suzy Mathew   Nursing Planning and Training Unit
4. Dr. Joseph K. Cheriyan   Surgery—Al Adan Hospital
5. Dr. Ghaleb Al Galayini   Chest Disease Hospital
6. Dr. Ghassan Abu Al Naser   Dental—Al Adan Hospital
7. Dr. Janusz Matusik   Laboratory—Al Adan Hospital
8. Barbara Malkiewicz Wasowics   Laboratory—Al Adan Hospital
9. Dr. Mohsen Guirguis Mourad   Preventive Medicine
10. Mr. Said Ali Marmoush   Preventive Medicine
11. Dr. Mohamed Anis Helali   Surgery—Al Adan Hospital
12. Dr. Abdul Aziz Ali Al Sarraf   Paediatric—Al Adan Hospital

Course 3:

1. Mrs. Annamma Simon	Nursing Planning and Training Unit
2. Mr. Ghalib Azzam	Nursing Planning and Training Unit
3. Dr. Sayed Ahmed Seif el Din	Haematology—Al Adan Hospital
4. Mr. Kasi Mohamed Reda Shaber	Preventive Medicine
5. Mr. Abd Hussein Awda	Infectious Diseases Hospital
6. Dr. Ahmed Nabil Yousef	Maternity—Al Adan Hospital
7. Dr. Nelly Colaco	Nursing Planning and Training Unit
8. Dr. Azam Al Hambali	Dental—Al Adan Hospital
9. Mr. Ali Hameed Majeed	Laboratory—Mubarak Hospital
10. Dr. Amira Raghib	Paediatric—Mubarak Hospital
11. Mr. Nizar Yacoub	Laboratory—Al Adan Hospital
12. Dr. Alexander Celinski	Laboratory—Al Adan Hospital

Course 4:

1. Dr. Samir Kamel	Maternity—Al Adan Hospital
2. Dr. H. Youssef	Medical School
3. Dr. Majla Nouri	Paediatrics—Mubarak Hospital
4. Dr. Salim Youssef Ebeid	Maternity—Al Adan Hospital
5. Dr. Sayed Wajid	Paediatrics—Al Adan Hospital
6. Dr. Ziad Al Mograbi	Dental—Al Adan Hospital
7. Dr. Abdel-Munam Ebeid	Anaesthesia—Ibn Sina Hospital
8. Dr. Jassim Kamel	Radiotherapy—Al Adan Hospital
9. Dr. Sayed Kader Shah Sayeed	Anaesthesia—Al Adan Hospital
10. Mr. Abdul-Majid Saadi	Nursing Education—Mubarak Hospital
11. Mrs. Sarala Mammen	Community Health
12. Dr. Medhat Mohamed Farghaly	Surgery—Al Adan Hospital
13. Dr. Amin Maarafi	Medical—Al Adan Hospital

Programme

The following timetable is meant only as a guide to the topics covered in the workshop. It was liable to vary according to the individual needs of the participants.

Day 1: a) A general introduction stressing the importance of shape and size of art work and their relationship to the legibility of the final product.
   b) Care and use of technical pens.
   c) Familiarisation with other items in the kit.

Day 2: a) Producing lettering for drawings using both lettering guides and dry transfer.
   b) Working method for producing charts and graphs.

Day 3: a) Consideration of the special limitations on art work produced for slides as apposed to publication.
   b) Tables and use of the typewriter in this respect.
      (The typewriter exercises were minimised to one exercise per participant to overcome the lack of English typists.)
   c) Critical group discussion of the work produced to date.

Day 4: a) Ways of introducing colour into artwork; diazo, hand-coloured negative, coloured tape, colour overlay, coloured paper, etc.

   b) Limitations of colour.
   c) Curves: Flexible curves, French curves, flexible tape.

Day 5: a) Survey of copyright law.
   b) Using the rotoboard to make a simple black and white line drawing
      from a complex colour slide.
   c) Free-hand drawing with technical pens.

Day 6: a) Final critical analysis of work produced during the week.

Opinions:

A questionnaire was circulated on the last day of each workshop and was completed by all participants (Appendix II). This provided helpful information for the
organisers which will affect the planning and running of future courses. The outcome of the questionnaire over the four weeks was as follows:

All participants found the course helpful to their specialities:

46% found it useful for research.
71% found it useful for lectures.
43% found it useful for public presentation.
72% found it useful for publishing scientific data.

One person found it useful for preparing books for publication.

95% of the participants found that the course attained its objectives.
87% found it satisfying for their particular needs in illustration.

One person found it satisfied only 60% of his particular needs in illustration.

80% of the participants had no previous experience of the techniques taught at
   the workshop.
96% found the workshop properly organised.
55% learnt from the lecturers.
94% learnt from practical demonstration.
49% learnt from audio/visual means.
45% learnt through self-gained experience.

In the second workshop the majority of them said that individual supervision
and help from tutors aided learning.

94% think the course should be repeated.
45% think this should happen once a year.
18% think this should happen twice a year.
19% think this should happen every 2—4 months.

Most of the participants found the lecturers and auxiliary personnel very helpful, although some found that the typing service was inadequate.

All of them used the facilities provided and most found them up to their expectations.

In the four weeks, 48 participants produced a total of 320 illustrations—an average of 7 illustrations per person per week.

The least number produced by any one person per week was 1 and the maximum was 25. 86% think they gained enough experience to do it themselves. Most of
the participants think that each workshop should run for a longer period—e.g. 2
weeks—and should include some photography. One of the non-Muslim participants expressed dissatisfaction at the workshop being held during Ramadan, especially as it ran through late hours.

Equipment

At every workshop, each participant was supplied with a medical illustration kit, comprising technical pens, lettering devices, paper, etc. Although most people were initially unfamiliar with items in the kit and some of the technical terms used, by the end of the course they felt confident about producing illustrations at their place of work using the same equipment.

Problems with Equipment

A "package" of equipment comprising specific makes of all the necessary items had been recommended for these workshops by Mr. Simmonds.

The contents of this "package" had all been previously tested in the RPMS art studio (Appendix I).

Because the recommended "package" was not completely adhered to during the purchasing of the Kuwait Medical kit, some items caused problems, in particular the following:

a) *The Cumberland flexible ruler* was not flexible enough, and should be replaced by a flexicurve minor, or similar.

b) *The Stanopen set* contained a 0.25 mm pen, when a 1.0 mm pen would be more useful. There was no place in the set for resting pens in the upright position whilst working. The pens "blobbed" significantly more than Mars Staedtler 700 pens, particularly in the larger nib widths. The elaborate compasses are not necessary in a kit for simple illustrations—a Harling Multipurpose Compass is adequate and much cheaper.

c) *The French curves* should have a stepped edge on both sides, such as in Rotring primus, so that they can be used in both directions.

d) *UHU glue sticks* are a poor substitute for Pritt sticks. The former have an inadequate "wind-up" device and are less adhesive.

e) *Poster paint* is less opaque and wetter than Q-white.

f) *A letraset 5 cabinet* is inappropriate for the materials that need to be stored at each workplace. Rather than drawers, "pockets" are better for storing Rapiscience and paper. A small tray is needed for holding those items which get lost amongst other, i.e. blue pencil, sharpener, rubber, scalpel and burnisher. A larger tray would hold masking tape, tissue paper, Pritt, scissors, ruler and lettering guides.

Recommendations

Copiers:

The most pressing need is for a quick copying device which will convert original black and white artwork with corrections into a perfect black and white print. This obviates the need for perfect artwork when intending to add colour. It also provides prints of sufficient quality for editors, so that originals can be kept by the author. The best copiers of this type use the Agfa Gevaert Copyrapid and Copyproof systems. The Copyproof system provides better quality prints but the paper is less suitable for the application of colour either in the form of film or crayon than Copyrapid paper.

Reducing and enlarging:

It is essential to be able to reduce drawings. During the workshops a photocopier provided this service. However, a device which could both reduce and enlarge would be of greater use. On some occasions this could be done on the Copyproof, but a Copyscanner, or photocopier with an enlarging cassette would cover all needs.

Desks:

Round tables are unsuitable to work at. We understand that desks will soon be provided with suitable storage space for paper, transfers, pens, etc.

Typewriters:

Large-face typewriters should be provided and the best replacement for the now obsolete IBM Executive range is the IBM 82C with the "Orator Presentor" golf ball using carbon ribbon IBM T III.

Assessment

Numbers of participants:

It is not possible for 1 tutor to teach more than 10 people at a time. When the groups during the workshop were 12 or 13 it was difficult to give each person sufficient attention each day. In future there should be a maximum of 10 people in each workshop.

Bringing work:

Participants who benefited most from the workshops were those who brought their *own* work. This was converted into drawings suitable for publication or slides which would later be used by the participant for lecturing.

It is very important that in the future each prospective participant bring their own work to the workshop, and an advisory letter should be circulated to each person to this effect, together with a guide on the best draft size for illustrations.

Photography:

During the recent courses no full-time photographers were present (volunteer help provided slides only during the first and second weeks). This lack meant that proper discussion of work produced could not take place during the last two workshops.

As the essence of the workshops is to teach participants the relationship between the size of their original drawing and its legibility when projected or published, slides must be produced during the workshops to illustrate the relationship.

It is necessary therefore to run the workshops with the cooperation of a photographic department with at least one photographer permanently available.

Participants often suggested in their questionnaires that more aspects of photography should be explained during the courses. In our opinion it would be beneficial if an additional day or half-day were spent demonstrating photographic copying, processing, printing, lighting, etc. However, any more elaborate study of photography would have to be part of a separate course.

Length of the workshops:

Each workshop ran for 6 days. Most of the participants stated in their questionnaires that workshops should run for longer than this—a period of 2 weeks was often mentioned. We still feel, however, that 6 days is sufficient to cover the relevant facts and techniques, but additional time is necessary for practising, of course.

In the long-term, four 6-day workshops should be run each year to keep up standards and build on the experience gained on this occasion.

Staff:

From our experiences at Al Adan we can now say that to run workshops of this kind a minimum of the following staff is required:

1 Programme director
1 Course tutor

1 Photographer (see Section 12.4)
1 Receptionist / Librarian
2 English typists
1 Driver + car

Cleaning and portering staff

A librarian is necessary to help participants who require books on their subjects, recent periodicals, etc.

During the recent workshops only 1 English typist was available from 9.30 a.m.—12.30 p.m. each day. It was impossible for her to keep up with the work load of tables, graphs, "word" slides, etc. and this resulted in some tension.

A driver is essential for immediate collection of supplies, replacement equipment, etc., especially bearing in mind the distance between the Al Adan Postgraduate Centre and Kuwait City.

It was found important to have name plates for each participant on his individual desk. This helps both participants and course organiser to communicate.

As the end of the month an exhibition was arranged of all participants' work, and certificates of attendance were given out (Appendix II) in a final ceremony. This was an important function as it gave a certain dignity to the experience and each participant felt that something tangible had been achieved.

Antonia Lant found that at the start of each day a synopsis of the work to be attempted had to be made. This gave the participants a feeling that they were on a "structured course".

Summary:

The opinions of the other organisers, the participants and the visitors to the final exhibition confirm our view of the overall success of the courses.

There is certainly a need for further workshops of this type in Kuwait both to consolidate and increase the knowledge and skills of those who attended the recent courses, and to introduce the techniques and ideas to those who have not yet had the opportunity to attend.

Four workshops of 6 days each should be held each year, with no more than 10 participants at each one if only one tutor is present (see Sections 12.1 and 12.4). Section 12.2, 12.3 and 12.5 should also be adopted concerning:
  a) notification that participants should bring their own work (12.2);
  b) photographers (12.3);
  c) back-up staff (12.5).

In a country where training and education in the life sciences are of paramount importance every means for improving these areas should be welcomed. When doctors, nurses, dentists, technicians and others can control and produce their own illustrations for teaching and research this will be an immense advantage.

It is obvious that it is necessary to develop back-up support for the workshop idea. Film strips, tape slide programmes and notes in Arabic will give continued support to those who may need reminding of the various techniques. It is vital not to let this become a "one-off" experience which will sink into oblivion if neglected.

It is particularly important to support the package or "kit" idea. In spite of its apparent cost it works better than obtaining local substitutes which have not stood the test of lengthy trials.

Acknowledgements (by Doig Simmonds):

I am particularly grateful to Dr. M. A. C. Dowling and Dr. A. H. Taba who made my introductory visit to the EMRO region possible and who organised it with such care. Professor E. Ruzyllo of the Training Division welcomed the idea of a workshop in Kuwait—the first country to respond to the idea initiated by the WHO Eastern Mediterranean Region. The organisation and success of this experiment depended in the main on Dr. Samir Wahdan who provided the drive and enthusiasm necessary to make it all work.

I am particularly grateful to Antonia Lant for the hard work she put into each workshop. We owe the success of the courses very much to her ability to communicate techniques and this is all the more remarkable for a young lady working in a Moslem country during the month of Ramadan.

81C—1301
Cardiology

Objectives:	The visit of Dr. M. M. Webb-Peploe, FRCP, MD Consultant Cardiologist, St. Thomas' Hospital, London. To teach advances in cardiology.
Place:	Department of Medicine, Al-Sabah Hospital, Cardiology Department, Chest Hospital.
Duration:	7 days, from 21st till 27th February 1981.
Organiser:	Ministry of Public Health.
Programme Director:	Professor F. F. Fenech, Chairman of the Department of Medicine, Al-Sabah Hospital.
Participants:	Internists and Cardiologists. The lectures are also conducted for the MRCP Part I Course.

Programme:

Saturday, 21st February, 1981

9.45 a.m.   Teaching Round
                   (Professor A. R. Yousof)
5.30 p.m.   Lecture (MRCP Part I Course)
                   Newer Concept in Heart Failure Management
                   Lecture Room 105, Faculty of Medicine

Sunday, 22nd February, 1981

9.00 a.m.   Out-patient session, Al-Sabah Hospital
                   (Professor A. R. Yousof)

Monday, 23rd February, 1981

9.00 a.m.   Session in Cardiology Department, Chest Hospital
                   (Professor A. M. Yousof)
5.00 p.m.   MRCP Part II Course, Mock Vivas
                   Lecture Room 105, Faculty of Medicine

Tuesday, 24th February, 1981

9.00 a.m.   Postgraduate Round at C.C.U.,
                   Al-Sabah Hospital
12.00 noon   Clinical Meeting—Lecture Cardiomyopathy
                   Al-Sabah Hospital, Nursing Institute

5.30 p.m.   Lecture (MRCP Part I Course)
                             Anti-arrhythmic drugs—classification and indications
                             Lecture Room 105, Faculty of Medicine

81C—1302
Cardiomyopathies

Objectives: To refresh the knowledge of the structure of the heart
                             muscle and its physiology in the light of present ad-
                             vances of the science.
                             To learn the advances in clinical procedures with car-
                             diomyopathies and methods of diagnosis.
Place: Chest Hospital.
Duration: 2 weeks, from October 10, 1981 till October 23, 1981.
Organiser: Prof. A. M. Yousof M.B., Ch.B., Ph.D., F.R.C.P. (Glas).
                             Dean of the Faculty of Medicine.
Programme Director: Prof. A. M. Yousof.
Participants: The course is aimed at cardiologists and doctors work-
                             ing in the field of medicine and surgery.

Programme:
There will be six lectures on the topic of Cardiomyopathies each lasting 45 mi-
nutes with 15 minute discussion and clinical sessions.
The lectures will be held on 12th, 13th and 17th October at 4 p.m. at the Chest
Hospital.
Following the lectures on the 13th, there will be an echocardiography demon-
stration.

Lectures

Monday, 12th October 1981, 4 p.m.

Anatomy and Physiology of the Heart Muscle.   Prof. Yousof, A. M.
Classification of Cardiomyopathies   Dr. Ruzyllo, W.

Tuesday, 13th October 1981, 4 p.m.

Clinical Features and Diagnosis of Cardiomyopathies. Prof. Yousof, A.R.
Cardiac Catheterisation and Angiocardiography in   Dr. Ruzyllo, W.
Cardiomyopathies

Saturday, 17th October 1981, 4 p.m.

Myocardial Biopsy and Histopathology in Cardio-   Dr. Ruzyllo, W.
myopathies
Medical und Surgical Therapy for Cardiomyopathies.   Prof. Yousof, A. M.

81C—1303
Seminar on Cardiology

Objectives: The visit of Dr. J. D. Stephens, M.D., MRCP, Consult-
                             ant Cardiologist.
                             The London Hospital (Whitechapel), Whitechapel,
                             London, U.K.

Place:	Mubarak Al Kabir Hospital, Sabah Hospital, Chest Disease Hospital, Ahmadi Hospital.
Duration:	3rd—10th April, 1982.
Organiser:	Discipline Committee for Medicine.
Programme Director:	Prof. F. F. Fenech.
Participants:	The seminar is aimed at physicians attending the MRCP Part I Course and Physicians interested in the topic.

Programme:

3rd April, 1982 (Saturday)

9.00 a.m.	Meeting with Prof. F. F. Fenech, Department of Medicine Mubarak Al Kabir Hospital
11.30 a.m.	Meeting with Prof. A. R. Yousuf Sabah Hospital
4.30 p.m.	Lecture (MRCP Part I Course) Topic: Applied Physiology of the Cardiovascular System.

4th April, 1982 (Sunday)

9.30 a.m.	Meeting with Prof. A. R. Yousuf Sabah Hospital
10.00 a.m.	Visit to C.C.U.—Sabah Hospital
12.00 noon	Teaching Round—Ward 1 Sabah Hospital

5th April, 1982 (Monday)

9.00 a.m.	Meeting with Prof. A. M. Yousuf Chest Disease Hospital
4.00—6.00 p.m.	Lecture (MRCP Part II Course) E.C.Gs. Cardiac Catheterisation-data

6th April, 1982 (Tuesday)

10.00 a.m.	Visit to Ahmadi Hospital and Kuwait Oil Company complex Departure to Ahmadi at 10.00 a.m. and return in late afternoon Lunch and Lecture at Ahmadi—topic to be chosen by Dr. D. J. Stephens

7th April, 1982 (Wednesday)

9.00 a.m.	Meeting with Prof. F. F. Fenech Department of Medicine Mubarak Al Kabir Hospital

12.00 noon	Clinical Meeting, Mubarak Al Kabir Hospital, topic to be chosen by Dr. J. D. Stephens
4.30 p.m.	Lecture (MRCP Part I Course) Topic: Cardiac Arrhythmias— Classification and Therapy

8th April, 1982 (Thursday)

9.00 a.m.	MRCP Part II Course, Clinical Session, Dr. Sattar and Dr. R. Hafassi Farwania Hospital

10th April, 1982 (Saturday)

9.00 a.m.	Meeting with Prof. A. R. Yousuf Sabah Hospital
11.00 a.m.	Teaching Round—Ward 5, Sabah Hospital
5.30 p.m.	Lecture (MRCP Part I Course). Topic: New Aspects of Treatment of Congestive Heart Failure

81C—1304
Seminar on Cardiology

Objectives:	The visit of Dr. D. B. Linder, Miami University. To teach recent advances in the field of Cardiology.
Place:	Al Sabah Hospital, Mubarak Hospital, Farwania Hospital, Jahra Hospital.
Duration:	6 days, 15th May, 1982 till 20th May, 1982.
Organiser:	Training Division in cooperation with the Office of International Medical Education, University of Miami.
Programme Director:	Dr. M. K. Emara.
Participants:	The course is aimed at cardiologists and doctors interested in cardiology.
Programme:	

Saturday, 15th May, 1982

9.00 a.m.	To meet Prof. F. Fenech, Chairman of Medicine, Mubarak Hospital
10.00 a.m.	Clinical Session, Mubarak Hospital

Sunday, 16th May, 1982

10.00 a.m.	Clinical Session, Mubarak Hospital with Dr. M. K. Emara

Monday, 17th May, 1982

9.00 a.m.	To meet Prof. A. R. Yousof, Head of the Department of Medicine, Al Sabah Hospital

| 10.00 a.m. | Clinical Session, Al Sabah Hospital |
| 12.00 noon | Dr. Dorothy B. Linder, lecture on: Cardiology |

Tuesday, 18th May, 1982

| 10.00 a.m. | Hospital rounds in Jahra Hospital. |

Wednesday, 19th May, 1982

| 10.00 a.m. | Clinical Session, Mubarak Hospital with Dr. M. K. Emara |

Thursday, 20th May, 1982

9.00 a.m.	To visit Farwania Hospital
10.30 a.m.	Panel discussion in Farwania Hospital on Family Doctor Practice in Cardiology
	Chairman: Dr. M. K. Emara
	Members: Dr. D. B. Linder
	Dr. Saad Zaghloul
	Dr. Ashmawi Abdel Wahab

81C—12/0101
Seminar on Academic Education

Objectives:	The visit of Dr. L. T. Cotton, MCh., FRCS, Dean, King's College Hospital, Medical School, University of London.
Place:	Mubarak Al Kabir Hospital, Ahmadi Hospital, Sabah Hospital.
Duration:	7 days from 24th of October 1981 till 30th of October 1981.
Organiser:	Joint Board of Postgraduate Medical Education.
Programme Director:	Prof. F. F. Fenech.
Participants:	Doctors interested in the subject.
Programme:	

24th October, 1981 (Saturday)

9.00 a.m.	Professor F. F. Fenech's Office
	Department of Medicine, Mubarak Al Kabir Hospital
	Visit to Medical School
12.00 noon	Meeting with Dean
	Faculty of Medicine

25th October, 1981 (Sunday)

10.00 a.m.	Meeting with Dr. Na'il Al Naqeeb
	Undersecretary
	Ministry of Public Health

| 12.00 noon | Meeting with Dr. N. Al Kazemi and Dr. E. Ruzyllo Training Division, Ministry of Health Dasmah |

26th October, 1981 (Monday)

| 8.00 a.m. | Undergraduate Teaching Session Department of Surgery Prof. B. Ekloff |
| 1.00 p.m. | Faculty Seminar Topics to be chosen by lecturer |

27th October, 1982 (Tuesday)

| 10.00 a.m. | Visit to Ahmadi Hospital and Kuwait Oil Company Complex. Departure to Ahmadi at 10.00 a.m. and return in late afternoon. Lunch and Lecture at Ahmadi—topic to be chosen by Dr. L. T. Cotton. |

28th October, 1981 (Wednesday)

| 8.00 a.m. | Operating Session Department of Surgery Mubarak Al Kabir Hospital Prof. B. Eklof |

29th October, 1981 (Thursday)

| 8.00 a.m. | Lecture at Sabah Hospital Surgical Department Dr. Sudad Sabri |

81C—1420
Seminar on Gastroenterology

Objectives:	The visit of Prof. Martin Kalser, Miami University. To teach recent advances in the field of gastroenterology.
Place:	Al Sabah Hospital, Department of Medicine, Endoscopy Unit.
Duration:	6 days, 24th April, 1982 till 29th April 1982.
Organiser:	The Training Division in cooperation with the Office of International Medical Education, University of Miami.
Programme Director:	Dr. Basil Al Naqeeb.
Participants:	The course is aimed at gastroenterologists and doctors interested in gastroenterology.

Programme:

Saturday, 24th April, 1982

11.00 a.m.   To meet Prof. A. R. Yousof, Head of the Department of Medicine, Al Sabah Hospital

12.00 noon   Visit to the Endoscopy Unit of the Department of Medicine
Head of the Unit
Dr. Basil Al Naqeeb

Sunday, 25th April, 1982

10.00 a.m.   Hospital rounds with Dr. Basil Al Naqeeb

1.00 p.m.   To meet Prof. A. M. Yousof, Dean of the Medical Faculty

Monday, 26th April, 1982

10.00 a.m.   Clinical Session, Farwania Hospital with Dr. Ashmawi

Tuesday, 26th April, 1982

11.00 a.m.   To meet Dr. Basil Al Naqeeb, Al-Sabah Hospital

12.00 noon   Prof. Martin Kalser, lecture on: Pancreatic Diseases

Wednesday, 28th April, 1982

9.00 a.m.   To meet Prof. F. Fenech, Chairman of Medicine, Mubarak Hospital

10.00 a.m.   Clinical Session, Mubarak Hospital

Thursday, 29th April, 1982

10.30 a.m.   Prof. Martin Kalser, lecture on: Small Intestine Absorption, at Jahra Hospital

81C—1601
The Nephrology Seminars

Objectives: The visit of Dr. Chisholm S. Ogg, B.Sc., MB, ChB, FRCP, MRCS, Renal Physician and Director of Dialysis and Transplant Unit, Guy's Hospital, London.
To teach advances in the field of nephrology.
To give lectures for the MRCP Part I Course and for the MRCP Part II Course.

Place (Venue): Al Sabah Hospital, Ahmadi Hospital, Amiri Hospital, Chest Hospital.

Duration: 10 days, from 27th March till 5th April 1981.

Organiser: Ministry of Public Health.

Programme Director: Prof. F. F. Fenech, Chairman of the Department of Medicine, Al Sabah Hospital.

Participants: The physicians of the above-mentioned hospitals, doctors participating in the MRCP Part I Course, the MRCP Part II Course and under graduates.

Programme:

Saturday, 28th March, 1981

9.00 a.m.	O.P. Clinic, Amiri Hospital (Renal Unit) (Dr. H. Wood)
5.30 p.m.	Lecture (MRCP Part I Course) Glomerulonephritis Lecture Room 105 Faculty of Medicine

Sunday, 29th March, 1981

10.30 a.m.	Visit to Ahmadi Hospital and Kuwait Oil Company Complex (Dr. J. McIntyre and Dr. J. G. Lloyd)

Monday, 30th March, 1981

9.00 a.m.	Grand Round, Amiri Hospital (Kidney Unit)
12.00 noon	Clinical Meeting, Amiri Hospital Topic to be chosen by Dr. Ogg
5.00 p.m.	Renal Medicine Data (MRCP Part II Course) Lecture Room 105 Faculty of Medicine

Tuesday, 31st March, 1981

9.00 a.m.	Visit to Transplant Unit Chest Hospital
12.00 noon	Clinical Meeting The Present State of Dialysis and Transplantation Seminar Room, Department of Medicine, Al Sabah Hospital

Wednesday, 1st April, 1981

9.00 a.m.	Undergraduate Teaching Round Amiri Hospital (Dr. H. Wood)
5.30 p.m.	Lecture (MRCP Part I Course) Acute Renal Failure Lecture Room 105 Faculty of Medicine

Thursday, 2nd April, 1981

10.00 a.m.	Clinical Session (MRCP Part II Course) Amiri Hospital

Saturday, 4th April, 1981

4.30 p.m. Lecture (MRCP Part I Course)
Chronic Renal Failure
Lecture Room 105
Faculty of Medicine

81C—1701
Seminar on Endocrinology

Objectives: The visit of Dr. J. McKenzie, Miami University.
To teach recent advances in the field of Endrocrinology.

Place: Al Adan Hospital, Al Sabah Hospital, Farwania Hospital, Mubarak Hospital.

Duration: 6 days, from 5th June, 1982 till 10th June, 1982.

Organiser: Training Division in cooperation with the Office of International Medical Education, University of Miami.

Programme Director: Dr. A. Maarafi.
Participants: The course is aimed at endocrinologists and doctors interested in endocrinology.

Programme:

Saturday, 5th June, 1982

9.00 a.m. To meet Dr. A. Maarafi, Head of Dept. of Medicine, Al Adan Hospital
10.00 a.m. Hospital rounds with Dr. A. Maarafi

Sunday, 6th June, 1982

9.00 a.m. To meet Prof. A. R. Yousof, Head of Department of Medicine, Al Sabah Hospital
10.00 a.m. Clinical Session, Al Sabah Hospital
12.00 noon Dr. John M. McKenzie, lecture on:
Hyperthyroidism, Grave's Disease

Monday, 7th June, 1982

9.00 a.m. To meet Prof. F. Fenech, Chairman of Medicine, Mubarak Hospital
10.00 a.m. Clinical Session, Mubarak Hospital

Tuesday, 8th June, 1982

10.00 a.m. Clinical Session, Mubarak Hospital

Wednesday, 9th June, 1982

10.00 a.m. Hospital rounds in Jahra Hospital

Thursday, 10th June, 1982

9.00 a.m. Visit to Farwania Hospital

10.30 a.m.   Panel discussion in Farwania Hospital on
                              Family Doctor Practice in Endocrinology
                              Chairman: Dr. A. Maarafi

                              Members: Dr. John McKenzie
                                       Dr. Saad Zaghloul
                                       Dr. Ashmawi Abdel Wahab

81C—1801
Advances in Medicine, Particularly in the Field of Haematology

Objectives: The visit of Professor John Richmond, MD, FRCP
                           Professor of Medicine, University of Sheffield.
                           To teach recent advances in the field of haematology.

Place: Al Sabah Hospital, Ahmadi Hospital, Amiri Hospital,
                           Farwania Hospital, Adan Hospital.

Duration: 14 days—from 6th Feb. 1981 till 20th Feb. 1981.

Organiser: Ministry of Public Health.

Programme Director: Prof. F. F. Fenech, Chairman of the Department of
                           Medicine, Al Sabah Hospital.

Participation: Internists and training doctors in the five hospitals
                           (MRCP Part I Course, MRCP Part II Course), attend-
                           ing lectures, clinical rounds and instruction session.

Programme:

                           7th February, 1981 (Saturday)

10.00 a.m.   Teaching Round Ward 1, Al Sabah
                           (Undergraduates)
5.30 p.m.   Lecture (MRCP Part I Course) Iron Deficiency and
                           Iron Overload
                           Faculty of Medicine

                           8th February, 1981 (Sunday)

10.30 a.m.   Visit to Ahmadi Hospital and Kuwait Oil Company
                           Complex
                           Lecture at Ahmadi—topic to be chosen by Professor
                           Richmond

                           9th February, 1981 (Monday)

9.00 a.m.   Lymphoma Clinic, Radiotherapy Department,
                           Al Sabah Hospital (Dr. Samir Mutawa)
4.00 p.m.   Oral Session (MRCP Part II Course)
                           Department of Medicine, Al Sabah Hospital

10th February, 1981 (Tuesday)

10.30 a.m.   Teach-in Session on Haemolytic Anaemia
                     (Seminar Room)
12.00 noon   Clinical Meeting—Lecture The Spleen

11th February, 1981 (Wednesday)

9.00 a.m.   Visit to Amiri Hospital, Department of Medicine (Dr.
                     Basil Naqeeb and Dr. A. Hafez)
5.30 p.m.   Lecture (MRCP Part I Course) Bleeding Disorders—
                     Clinical and Laboratory Diagnosis
                     Faculty of Medicine

12th February, 1981 (Thursday)

9.00 a.m.   Farwania Hospital
                     Long cases—(MRCP Part II Course)

14th February, 1981 (Saturday)

9.00 a.m.   Visit to Adan Hospital, Medical Department (Dr.
                     Emara)
5.30 p.m.   Lecture (MRCP Part I Course) Polycythaemia and
                     Myeloproliferative Disorders
                     Faculty of Medicine

15th February, 1981 (Sunday)

9.00 a.m.   Visit to Farwania Hospital, Medical Department (Dr.
                     Ashmawi)

16th February, 1981 (Monday)

9.00 a.m.   Lymphoma Clinic, Radiotherapy Department, Al
                     Sabah Hospital (Dr. Samir Mutawa)
11.00 a.m.—1.00 p.m. Seminar on Neurological Complications of Systemic
                     Disease

17th February, 1981 (Tuesday)

10.00 a.m.—11.30 a.m. Teach-in Session Topic to be chosen by Professor Rich-
                     mond
                     C.P.C. A Case of Abdominal Mass in a 24 Year Old
                     Man

18th February, 1981 (Wednesday)

9.00 a.m.   Teaching Round—Ward 12, Al Sabah Hospital
5.30 a.m.   Lecture (MRCP Part I Course) Valvular Heart Disease
                     Faculty of Medicine

19th February, 1981 (Thursday)

9.00 a.m.   Long Cases·(MRCP Part II Course)
                     Ward 2 Medical, Al Sabah Hospital

81C—1802
Haematological Seminar

Objectives:	The visit of Dr. Robert Hume, M.D., F.R.C.P., F.R.C.P.G. Consultant Physician, Southern General Hospital, Glasgow. To teach recent advances in Haematology.
Place:	Al Sabah Hospital, Mubarak Hospital, Ahmadi Hospital, Amiri Hospital.
Duration:	8 days, 6th—13th March, 1982.
Organiser:	Discipline Committee for Medicine and Joint Board of Postgraduate Medical Education.
Programme Director:	Professor F. F. Fenech, Chairman of Medicine, Medical Faculty.
Participants:	Internists and training doctors (MRCP Part I Course, MRCP Part II Course) attending lectures, clinical rounds and instruction session.

Programme:

Saturday, 6th March, 1982

9.00 a.m.	Meeting with Professor F. F. Fenech Department of Medicine, Mubarak Al-Kabeer
5.30 p.m.	M.R.C.P. Part I Course Topic: Macrocytic Anaemia

Sunday, 7th March, 1982

9.00 a.m.	Meeting with Professor A. R. Yousof, Department of Medicine, Sabah Hospital—Teaching Round
12.00 noon	Clinical Meeting

Monday, 8th March, 1982

9.00 a.m.	Visit to Hospital (Dr. A. Lulu)
4.00 p.m.—6.00 p.m.	M.R.C.P. Part II Course, Slides Oral Session with Professor A. M. Yousuf

Tuesday, 9th March, 1982

10.30 a.m.	Visit to Ahmadi Hospital (Dr. J. G. Lloyd) and Kuwait Oil Company Complex Departure to Ahmadi at 10.30 a.m. and return in late afternoon Lunch and Lecture at Ahmadi Topic: to be chosen by lecturer

Wednesday, 10th March, 1982

9.00 a.m.	Teaching Ward Round Mubarak Al-Kabeer Hospital
12.00 noon	Clinical Meeting
4.30 p.m.	M.R.C.P. Part I Course Topic: Polycythemia and Myeloproliferative Disorders

Thursday, 11th March, 1982

10.00 a.m.	M.R.C.P. Part II Course Clinical Session with Pofessor A. M. Yousuf, Chest Hospital

Saturday, 13th March, 1982

10.00 a.m.	Amiri Hospital, Haematological Dept. (Dr. A. Hafez)
5.30 p.m.	M.R.C.P. Part I Course Topic: Investigations and Management of Thrombo-cytopenias

81C—1803
Seminar on Haematology

Objectives:	The visit of Dr. Abdel A. Yunis, Miami University. To teach recent advances in the field of Haematology.
Place:	Mubarak Hospital, Al Sabah Hospital, Al Adan Hospital, Ibn Sina Hospital, Farwania Hospital.
Duration:	6 days, from 22nd May, 1982 till 27th May, 1982.
Organiser:	Training Division in cooperation with the Office of International Medical Education, University of Miami.
Programme Director:	Prof. Ladislav Chrobak.
Participants:	The course is aimed at haematologists and doctors interested in haematology.
Programme:	

Saturday, 22nd May, 1982

9.00 a.m.	To meet Prof. Ladislav Chrobak, Mubarak Al Kabir Hospital
10.00 a.m.	Clinical Session with Prof. Ladislav Chrobak and Dr. Thomas Lipsic

Sunday, 23rd May, 1982

8.00 a.m.	Dr. Adel A. Yunis, lecture on: Bone Marrow Function Mubarak Al Kabir Hospital
10.00 a.m.	Clinical Session with Prof. Ladislav Chrobak and Dr. Thomas Lipsic

Monday, 24th May, 1982

10.00 a.m.   Clinical Session with Dr. Ahmed Hafez Yousof
                               Maternity Hospital

Tuesday, 25th May, 1982

9.00 a.m.   To meet Dr. St. Lopaciuk
                               Ibn Sina Hospital
12.00 noon   Dr. Adel A. Yunis, lecture on:
                               Nutritional Anaemias
                               Al Sabah Hospital

Wednesday, 26th May, 1982

10.00 a.m.   Clinical Session with Dr. A. Snigurovicz, Al Sabah
                               Hospital

Thursday, 27th May, 1982

9.00 a.m.   To visit Farwania Hospital
10.30 a.m.   Panel discussion in Farwania Hospital on Family Doc-
                               tor Practice in Haematology
                               Chairman: Prof. Ladislav Chrobak
Members: Dr. A. A. Yunis
          Dr. Abdul Aziz Haseneen
          Dr. Saad Zaghloul
          Dr. Ashmawi Abdel Wahab
          Dr. Ahmed Faud Khalil

Outline of the Panel Discussion on (X)

1. *Introduction:*
   General characteristics of (X) as a clinical science and recent advances in that field.

2. *Role of Early Diagnosis of Diseases in the Field of (X):*
   Clinical meanings and importance
   Methodological possibilities
   When and how to cooperate with specialists.

3. *Role of Genetic Factors in (X):*
   Study health conditions of family members.

4. *Role of Living Conditions of the Patient:*
   Economic conditions of the family
   Customs of the family
   Other factors.

5. *Practical Possibilities for the Family Medicine Doctor in Diagnosis and Treatment in the (X) Diseases.*

6. *Importance of Follow-up by the Family Medicine Doctor of the Treated Patient.*

7. *Answers of the Members of the Panel Discussion to Questions from the Floor.*
   (X) Pulmonology
       Endocrinology
       Cardiology
       Haematology
       Neurology
       Pediatrics
       Gynaecology and Obstetrics
       Radiology

81C—1901
Seminar on Hyperlipidemia

Objectives:	The visit of Dr. Haruo Nakamura, M.D., Ph.D., Associate Professor, School of Medicine, Jiket University, Department of Internal Medicine, Aoto Hospital, Tokyo, Japan. To teach advances in lipids metabolism.
Place:	Mubarak Al Kabir Hospital, Sabah Hospital, Ahmadi Hospital.
Duration:	20th—27th March, 1982.
Organiser:	Discipline Committee for Medicine.
Programme Director:	Prof. F. F. Fenech.
Participants:	Doctors interested in the subject.

Programme:

20th March, 1982 (Saturday)

9.00 a.m.	Meeting with Prof. F. F. Fenech Department of Medicine Mubarak Al Kabir Hospital
11.30 a.m.	Meeting with Prof. A. R. Yousuf Sabah Hospital

21st March, 1982 (Sunday)

10.00 a.m.	Meeting with Prof. A. R. Yousuf Sabah Hospital
10.30 a.m.	C.C.U.—Sabah Hospital
12.00 noon	Lecture at Sabah Hospital Topic: Hyperlipoproteinaemia

22nd March, 1982 (Monday)

9.00 a.m.	Visit to Lipid Research Lab. Sabah Hospital

23rd March, 1982 (Tuesday)

10.00 a.m.	Visit to Ahmadi Hospital and Kuwait Oil Company Complex. Departure to Ahmadi at 10.00 a.m. and return in late afternoon. Lunch and Lecture at Ahmadi—topic to be chosen by Dr. H. Nakamura.

24th March, 1982 (Wednesday)

9.00 a.m.	Meeting with Prof. F. F. Fenech Department of Medicine Mubarak Al Kabir Hospital
12.00 noon	Clinical Meeting Mubarak Al Kabir Hospital Topic: Hyperlipoproteinaemia

25th March, 1982 (Thursday)

9.00 a.m.	Meeting with Prof. A. R. Yousuf Sabah Hospital
10.00 a.m.	Lipid Research Lab, Sabah Hospital Meeting to be discussed future plan

27th March, 1982 (Saturday)

8.00 a.m.	5th year curriculum course Lecture in Mubarak Al Kabir Hospital Topic: Hyperlipidaemia

81C—2001
Seminar on Rheumatology

Objectives:	The visit of Dr. H. Berry, MA, DM, MRCP., Consultant Physician, Department of Rheumatology, King's College Hospital, Denmark Hill, London, U.K.
Place:	Mubarak Al Kabir, Sabah Hospital.
Duration:	7 days, from 17th April till 24th April, 1982.
Organiser:	Discipline Committee for Medicine.
Programme Director:	Professor F. Fenech, Chairman of Medicine
Participants:	Doctors in various medical disciplines involved in rheumatology.
Programme:	

Saturday, 17th April, 1982

9.00 a.m.	Meeting with Prof. F. F. Fenech Department of Medicine Mubarak Al Kabir Hospital

Sunday, 18th April, 1982

9.30 a.m.
Meeting with Prof. A. R. Yousuf
Department of Medicine
Sabah Hospital
Teaching Round

Monday, 19th April, 1982

9.00 a.m.
Mubarak Out-patient Session
(Dr. M. Sattar, Rheumatologists)

11.00 a.m.— 1.00 p.m.
5th Year Curriculum Course
Multidisciplinary Seminar
Topic: Rheumatoid Arthritis

4.00 p.m.— 6.00 p.m.
MRCP Part II Course
Rheumatology—data and slides

Tuesday, 20th April, 1982

10.30 a.m.
Visit to Ahmadi Hospital
(Dr. J. G. Lloyd)
and Kuwait Oil Company Complex
Departure to Ahmadi at 10.30 a.m. and return in late af-
ternoon
Lunch and Lecture at Ahmadi
Topic: to be chosen by lecturer

Wednesday, 21st April, 1982

9.00 a.m.
Mubarak Al-Kabeer Hospital
Teaching Session in the Wards

12.00 noon
Clinical Meeting—Lecture to be chosen by Lecturer

5.30 p.m.
Lecture (MRCP Part I Course)
Topic: Sero-Negative Arthropathies

Thursday, 22nd April, 1982

9.30 a.m.
M.R.C.P. Part II Course
Mock Clinical Session
with Dr. M. K. Emara

Saturday, 24th April, 1982

9.00 a.m.
Visit to Farwania Hospital
Teaching Session
(Dr. Abdul Wahab Ashmawi)

81C—2301
Transplantation Surgery

Objectives:
The visit of Dr. H. H. Newsome, Professor and Vice
Chairman, Dept. of Surgery, Virginia Commonwealth
University, Virginia, U.S.A., aims:
to exchange opinions and experiences with surgeons
and nephrologists,

to teach advances in the field of transplantation surgery.

Place:	Department of Surgery Al Sabah Hospital Chest Hospital Amirie Hospital Farwania Hospital Adan Hospital Ahmadi Hospital
Duration:	2 weeks, from 3. 1. 1981 till 6. 1. 1981.
Organiser:	Ministry of Public Health.
Programme Director:	Prof. G. M. Abouna Chairman of Surgery Department Al Sabah Hospital
Participation:	Surgeons of the above-mentioned hospitals.
Programme:	

Sunday, 4. 1. 1981

8.30 a.m.	Dept. of Surgery—Renal Transplantation Unit (Prof. G. M. Abouna at Chest Hospital, Transplantation Surgery Outpatient Clinic
10.30 a.m.	Dept. of Surgery, Al Sabah Hospital

Monday, 5. 1. 1981

8.00 a.m.	Operating Theatre, Al Sabah Hospital
11.00 a.m.—12.00 noon	Ward Round—medical students (Ward 14)
4.00 p.m.	Transplant Meeting, Transplant Surgery Unit, Chest Hospital

Tuesday, 6. 1. 1981

7.30 a.m.	Morbidity and Mortality Conference, Lecture Room Ward 14, Al Sabah Hospital
8.30 a.m.	Ward Round (Professorial Unit)
11.00 a.m.—12.00 noon	Professors round, lecture room Dept. of Surgery Ward 14
12.00 noon— 1.00 p.m.	Vascular meeting Lecture Room Ward 14
6.00 p.m.	Special lecture, Nutritional Aspects in Surgery. Allied Health and Nursing Auditorium Al Sabah Hospital

Wednesday, 7. 1. 1981

8.00 a.m.	Al Sabah Hospital, Ward 4 Ward Round (Dr. Mallick and Dr. Abu Naem)
10.00 a.m.	Teaching Round, Medical Students, Ward 4 (Students from Ward 1 and 4)
11.00 a.m.	Renal Transplantation, Chest

Thursday, 8. 1. 1981

8.00 a.m.	Surgical Grand Rounds. Allied Health and Nursing Auditorium Al Sabah Hospital—Fluid and Electrolyte Therapy
10.00 a.m.	Combined Oncology Conference, Dept. of Radiotherapy, Al Sabah Hospital

Saturday, 10. 1. 1981

8.00 a.m.	Amirie Hospital, Dept. Surgery (Dr. J. Oomen and Dr. Al-Sayar)
1.00 p.m.	Amirie Hospital Outpatients

Sunday, 11. 1. 1981

8.00 a.m.	Dept. of Surgery, Farwania Hospital Dr. Abu Jaba

Monday, 12. 1. 1981

8.00 a.m.	Dept. of Surgery, Adan Hospital Dr. Mustafa Abdul Shafi

Tuesday, 13. 1. 1981

8.00 a.m.	Dept. of Surgery, Al Sabah Hospital Ward Round (Professorial Unit)
8.30 a.m.	Visit Ahmadi Hospital

Wednesday, 14. 1. 1981

8.00 a.m.	Transplantation surgery, Chest Hospital (Prof. G. M. Abouna)
12—1.00 p.m.	Tutorial, Residents and Registrars Lecture Room, Ward 14, Dept. of Surgery, Al Sabah Hospital

Thursday, 15. 1. 1981

8.00 a.m.	Surgical Grand Rounds Allied Health and Nursing Auditorium, Al Sabah Hospital: Some Aspects of Thyroid and Para-thyroid Surgery.
10.00 a.m.	Combined Oncology Conference Dept. of Surgery, Ward 14 Al Sabah Hospital

81C—2302
Seminar on Surgery

Objectives:	The visit of Dr. Joseph Timmes, Miami University. To teach recent advances in the field of Surgery.
Place:	Chest Hospital, Mubarak Hospital, Al Sabah Hospital.
Duration:	6 days, 29th May, 1982 till 3rd June, 1982.
Organiser:	Training Division in cooperation with the Office of International Medical Education, University of Miami.
Programme Director:	Dr. Taiseer Abu N'ema.
Participants:	The seminar is aimed at surgeons and all doctors interested in the lecture.

Programme:

Saturday, 29th May, 1982

7.30 a.m.— 1.00 p.m. Visit Chest Hospital
(Dr. Osama Abdul Majid)

Sunday, 30th May, 1982

7.30 a.m.— 1.00 p.m. Visit Chest Hospital
(Dr. Hani Shuhaiber)

Monday, 31st May, 1982

7.30 a.m.— 1.00 p.m. Visit Chest Hospital
(Dr. Osama and Dr. Hani)

Tuesday, 1st June, 1982

7.30 a.m.—11.30 a.m. Visit Chest Hospital
(Dr. Osama and Dr. Hani)
12.00 noon Cardiology / cardiac surgery meeting

Wednesday, 2nd June, 1982

7.30 a.m.— 1.00 p.m. Visit Sabah Hospital
(Dr. Sadad Sabri)

Thursday, 3rd June, 1982

10.00 a.m. Visit Mubarak Hospital
Grand Rounds
12.00 noon Dr. Joseph Timmes, lecture on:
Cardio-thoracic Surgery

81C—2303
Seminar on Surgery

Objectives: The visit of Dr. Abdul Islami, Miami University.
To teach recent advances in the field of Surgery.

Place: Lecture Room, Al Sabah Hospital.

Duration: 6 days, 29th May, 1982 till 3rd June, 1982.

Organiser: Training Division in cooperation with the Office of International Medical Education, University of Miami.

Programme Director: Dr. Taisser Abu N'ema.

Participants: The course is aimed at surgeons and all doctors interested in the lecture.

Programme:

Saturday, 29th May, 1982

9.00 a.m. Visit Dr. Basil Al Naqeeb, Gastroenterology Al Sabah Hospital

Sunday, 30th May, 1982

9.00 a.m. Visit Mubarak Hospital, Department of Surgery—Unit D (Dr. Jacob Oommen).

12.00 noon Morbidity and Mortality conference

Monday, 31st May, 1982

8.00 a.m. Visit Farwania Hospital
(Dr. Abu Jabal)

Tuesday, 1st June, 1982

8.00 a.m. Visit Adan Hospital
(Dr. Cheriyan)

Wednesday, 2nd June, 1982

8.00 a.m. Visit Mubarak Hospital
(Prof. Abouna and Prof. Eklof)

1.30 p.m. Oncology meeting
(Dr. Taiseer Abu N'ema)

Thursday, 3rd June, 1982

9.00 a.m. Visit Al Sabah Hospital
(Dr. Sadad Sabri, Head, Dept. of Surgery)

12.00 noon Dr. Abdul Islami, lecture on:
Gastrointestinal Tract

81C—23/1704
(Seminar, Conference, Lectures, etc.)

Objectives: The visit of Prof. Sten Tiblin
Department of Surgery
Malmo, University of Lund, Sweden.

To teach recent advances in the field of surgery of endocrinology.

Place: Mubarak Al Kabir Hospital, Ahmadi Hospital, Adan Hospital, Farwania Hospital.

Duration: 13 days, from 1st of March 1982 till 13th of March 1982.

Organiser: Joint Board of Postgraduate Medical Education.

Programme Director: Prof. Bo Eklof, Chairman of Surgery, Faculty of Medicine.

Participants: The seminar is aimed at surgeons interested in endocrine surgery.

Programme: POSTGRADUATE LECTURES
28th February, 1982 (Sunday)

Ahmadi: Hypercalcemia: Diagnostic and Therapeutic Challenge

1st March, 1982 (Monday)

12.30 p.m.—1.30 p.m.   Cold Thyroid Nodule
Conference Room, Mubarak

8th March, 1982 (Monday)

12.30 p.m.—1.30 p.m.   Multiple Endocrine Neoplasia
Conference Room, Mubarak

9th March, 1982 (Tuesday)

Adan Hospital
Thyroid Carcinoma

11th March, 1982 (Thursday)

10.00 a.m.   Mubarak Auditorium
Surgical Treatment of Hyperparathyroidism

13th March, 1982 (Saturday)

Farwania Hospital
Breast Carcinoma

15th March, 1982 (Monday)

12.30 p.m.—1.30 p.m.   Hypertension due to Endocrine Causes
Conference Room, Mubarak

22nd March, 1982 (Monday)

12.30 p.m.—1.30 p.m.   Diagnostic and Surgical Pitfalls in Endocrine Surgery
Conference Room, Mubarak

25th March, 1982 (Thursday)

10.00 a.m.   Hypercalcemia: Diagnostic and Therapeutic Challenge

81C—2401
Cardiosurgical Seminar

Objectives: The visit of Professor Gordon K. Danielson.
                       To discuss and practice open heart surgery.

Place: Chest Hospital.

Duration: 7 days, 13th Feb.—19th Feb. 1982.

Organiser: Joint Board of Postgraduate Medical Education.

Programme Director: Dr. Hani J. Shuhaiber, Consultant Cardiac Surgeon,
                       Chest Diseases Hospital.

Participants: Surgeons and cardiologists interested in heart diseases.

Programme:

Saturday, 13th February, 1982

8.00 a.m.   Open Heart Surgery at the Chest Hospital with Dr.
                       Hani Shuhaiber

Sunday, 14th February, 1982

8.00 a.m.   Open Heart Surgery at the Chest Hospital with Dr.
                       Hani Shuhaiber
12.00 noon   Dr. Gordon K. Danielson lecture on,
                       Advances in the Treatment of Congenital Heart
                       Diseases
                       Lecture room in Mubarak Hospital

Monday, 15th February, 1982

8.00 a.m.   Open Heart Surgery at the Chest Hospital with Dr.
                       Hani Shuhaiber

Tuesday, 16th February, 1982

8.00 a.m.   Open Heart Surgery at the Chest Hospital with Dr.
                       Hani Shuhaiber

Wednesday, 17th February, 1982

8.00 a.m.   Out patient session with cardiac surgical follow-up
11.00 a.m.   Cardiac meeting in the Chest Hospital

Thursday, 18th February, 1982

10.15 a.m.   Dr. Gordon K. Danielson lecture on,
                       Advances in the Treatment of Acquired Heart Disease
                       Lecture room in Mubarak Hospital

81C—2402
Seminar on Cardiac Surgery

Objectives:

The visit of Dr. Terence English
Consultant Cardio Thoracic Surgeon
Pappworth Hospital.
To teach the advances in heart surgery.

Place:

Chest Hospital.

Duration:

10 days, from 14th of March 1982 till 23rd of March 1982.

Organiser:

Joint Board of Postgraduate Medical Education.

Programme Director:

Dr. Hani J. Shuhaiber
Consultant Cardiac Surgeon
Chest Disease Hospital.

Participants:

Surgeons interested in Cardiac Surgery.

Programme:

13th March, 1982 (Saturday)

A.M.

Arrival at the airport to be received by Dr. Hani J. Shuhaiber

14th March, 1982 (Sunday)

A.M.

Open Heart Surgery at the Chest Hospital with Dr. Hani J. Shuhaiber

15th March, 1982 (Monday)

A.M.

Open Heart Surgery at the Chest Hospital with Dr. Hani J. Shuhaiber

P.M.

Lecture on: The Roll of Surgery in Ischaemic Heart Diseases will be given in the Chest Disease Hospital, Ground Floor, Lecture Room at 6 p.m.

16th March, 1982 (Tuesday)

A.M.

Open Heart Surgery at the Chest Hospital with Dr. Hani J. Shuhaiber

P.M.

Lecture on: The Management of Cardio Thoracic Trauma will be given in Mubarak Hospital, main Auditorium at 6 p.m.

A.M.

Out patient session with cardiac surgical follow-up

P.M.

Attending cardiac meeting in the Chest Hospital

18th March, 1982 (Thursday)

A.M.

Lecture on: The Present Status of Cardiac Transplantation will be given in Mubarak Hospital, Main Auditorium at 10 a.m.

P.M.

Visit to the Ministry of Health

20th March, 1982 (Saturday)

A.M.   Open Heart Surgery at the Chest Hospital with Dr. Hani J. Shuhaiber

21st March, 1982 (Sunday)

A.M.   Open Heart Surgery at the Chest Hospital with Dr. Hani J. Shuhaiber
P.M.   Lecture in the Cardiac Department Seminar

22nd March, 1982 (Monday)

A.M.   Open Heart Surgery at the Chest Hospital with Dr. Hani J. Shuhaiber

81C—2403
Seminar on Cardiac Surgery

Objectives: The visit of Dr. Donald Ross from National Heart Hospital.

Place: Chest Hospital.

Duration: 5 days, 3rd April—7th April, 1982.

Organiser: Discipline Committee for Surgery.

Programme Director: Dr. Hani J. Shuhaiber, Consultant Cardiac Surgeon, Chest Diseases Hospital.

Participants: Cardiac Surgeons.

Programme:

Saturday, 3rd April, 1982

Open Heart Surgery at the Chest Hospital with Dr. Hani J. Shuhaiber

Sunday, 4th April, 1982

Open Heart Surgery at the Chest Hospital with Dr. Hani J. Shuhaiber

6.30 p.m.   Lecture on: The Present Position and Indications for Surgery in Heart Diseases
                        (Chest Hospital, Ground Floor, Lecture Room)

Monday, 5th April, 1982

Open Heart Surgery at the Chest Hospital with Dr. Hani J. Shuhaiber

Tuesday, 6th April, 1982

Open Heart Surgery at the Chest Hospital with Dr. Hani J. Shuhaiber

6.30 p.m.	Lecture on: Coronary Artery Surgery in Heart Diseases (Mubarak Hospital, Main Auditorium)

Wednesday, 7th April, 1982

8.00 a.m.—11.00 a.m.	Out Patient Session with cardiac surgical follow-up and visit to the Ministry of Health Attending Cardiac Meeting in the Chest Hospital

81C—2404
Seminar of Vascular Surgery

Objectives: The visit of Professor Robert Kistner
University of Hawaii, Honolulu, USA.

Place: Department of Surgery
Mubarak Hospital.

Duration: 10 days, 24th April—3rd May, 1982.

Organiser: Joint Board of Postgraduate Medical Education.

Programme Director: Prof. Bo Eklof.

Participants: Surgeons and all doctors interested.

Programme:

Sunday, 25th April 1982

7.30 a.m.	Mubarak Hospital—Mortality and Morbidity Conference
8.30 a.m.	Vascular clinic
1.30 p.m.	Oncology Conference

Monday, 26th April 1982

8.00 a.m.	Mubarak Hospital—X-Ray Conference Unit B.
9.00 a.m.	Ward Rounds
4—6 p.m.	Symposium on Venous Reconstructive Surgery, Main Auditorium Panel: Dr. Kistner, Dr. Eklof, Dr. Mathew, Dr. Zyke, Dr. Taiseer, Dr. Thulesius

Tuesday, 27th April 1982

9.30 a.m.	Visit KOC Hospital, Ahmadi Lecture: Surgical Approach to Chronic Venous Disease

Wednesday, 28th April 1982

8.00 a.m.	Mubarak Hospital, Operating Session

Thursday, 29th April 1982

8.00 a.m.	Ward Rounds
10.00 a.m.	Grand Round Present Status of Below-Knee Artery Reconstruction (Prof. Kistner)

Saturday, 1st May, 1982

8.00 a.m.   Mubarak Hospital, Operating Session

Sunday, 2nd May, 1982

8.00 a.m.   Meet Prof. G. Abouna and the Transplant Department
1.00 p.m.   Meet the Dean of the Faculty of Medicine

Monday, 3rd May, 1982

8.00 a.m.   Mubarak Hospital—Unit A, Outpatient Clinic
2—4 p.m.   Problem Cases in Venous Surgery—discussion in lec-
                             ture room of consultant area

81C—23/1401
Surgery of the Alimentary System

Objectives: To teach recent advances in the field of surgery of the
                       alimentary system.

Place: Sheraton Hotel.

Duration: 5 days, 1st February—5th February, 1982.

Organiser: Discipline Committee of Surgery, and Area Executive
                       Committee for Continuing Medical Education of the
                       Joint Board.

Programme Director: Professor George M. Abouna, Department of Surgery,
                       Mubarak Al Kabeer Hospital.

Guest lecturers: Dr. Thomas Demeester, Professor of Surgery, Universi-
                       ty of Chicago Medical School, U.S.A.
                       Dr. J. M. Greep, Prof. of Surgery and Dean, Faculty of
                       Medicine, University of Limberg, Maastricht, Holland.
                       Dr. David Johnston, Prof. of Surgery, University of
                       Leeds, England.
                       Dr. George Johanston, Consultant Surgeon, Royal Vic-
                       toria Hospital, Belfast, Northern Ireland.
                       Dr. Nils G. Kock, Professor of Surgery, University of
                       Gotenborg, Sweden.
                       Dr. A. R. Moosa, Professor of Surgery, University of
                       Chicago Medical School, Chicago, U.S.A.
                       Dr. Marshal Orloff, Professor and Chairman, Dept. of
                       Surgery, University of California, U.S.A.
                       Dr. Atef Sallam, Professor of Surgery, Emory, Universi-
                       ty, Atlanta, Georgia, U.S.A.
                       Dr. James Thompson, Prof. and Chairman, Department
                       of Surgery, University of Texas Medical Branch,
                       Galveston, U.S.A.
                       Dr. J. G. Turcotte, Prof. and Chairman, Department of
                       Surgery, University of Michigan, Ann Arbor, U.S.A.

Dr. Timothy S. Harrison, Professor of Surgery and Physiology, The Milton S. Hershey Medical Center, Pennsylvania State University, U.S.A.

Local lecturers: Dr. George M. Abouna, Professor of Surgery, Kuwait University and Head, Organ Transplant Service, Mubarak Hospital.

Na'il Al-Naqeeb, Undersecretary, Ministry of Public Health, Surgeon, Mubarak Hospital.

Dr. Basil Al Naqeeb, Chief, Gastroenterology Dept., Al Sabah Hospital.

Dr. Husam Baissouni, Chief of Radiology Dept., Al Sabah Hospital.

Dr. Abdulla Hehbehani, Senior Surgical Registrar, Mubarak Al Kabeer Hospital.

Dr. M. S. Adnani, Dept. of Pathology, Kuwait University.

Dr. Majeed Alwan, Surgeon, Al Sabah Hospital.

Dr. Ahmad Abu-Jabal, Chief of Surgery, Farwania Hospital.

Dr. Joseph Cheriyan, Chief of Surgery, Adan Hospital.

Dr. Letchka Vassiliva, Dept. of Gastroenterology, Al Sabah Hospital.

Dr. A. Lindgren, Dept. of Pathology, Kuwait University.

Dr. Largs G. Lindberg, Professor of Pathology, Kuwait University.

Dr. Samir Mutawah, Radiotherapist, Dept. of Radiotherapy, Al Sabah Hospital.

Dr. Kumar Mahajian, Associate Professor of Surgery, Kuwait University.

Dr. J. S. Jacob, Dept. of Gastroenterology, Al Sabah Hospital.

Dr. Taiseer Aby Naema, Assistant Prof. of Surgery, Kuwait University.

Dr. Yousof Omar, Chief of Radiotherapy Dept., Al Sabah Hospital.

Dr. Jacob Oomen, Surgeon, Mubarak Al Kabeer Hospital.

Dr. Sadad Sabri, Chief of Surgery, Al Sabah Hospital, Kuwait.

Participants: The course is aimed at surgeons and doctors interested in gastroenterology.

Programme:

Monday, 1st February, 1982

ESOPHAGUS—I

Chairmen: Dr. Na'il Al Naqeeb
            Prof. Tom DeMeester

10.00 a.m.—10.30 a.m.   Current Methods of Investigation of Esophageal Disease
(Tom DeMeester)

10.30 a.m. — 11.00 a.m.	Carcinoma of the Esophagus—Techniques and Results of Surgical Therapy (Tom DeMeester)
11.00 a.m. — 11.30 a.m.	Carcinoma of the Esophagus—The Role of Radiotherapy in Treatment—Kuwait experience
11.30 a.m. — 11.50 a.m.	*PANEL DISCUSSION* (Dr. Na'il Al Naqeeb, Moderator) (Dr. T. DeMeester, Dr. Yousof Omar)

ESOPHAGUS—II
Chairmen: Dr. DeMeester, Dr. J. Oomen

11.50 a.m. — 12.10 p.m.	Reflux Esophagitis, Medical Management (Basil Al-Naqeeb and J. S. Jacob)
12.10 p.m. — 12.30 p.m.	Reflux Esophagitis, Surgical Management (Tom DeMeester)
12.30 p.m. — 1.00 p.m.	*PANEL DISCUSSION* Dr. Jacob Oomen (Moderator) Dr. T. DeMeester, Dr. Basil Al-Naqeeb
1.00 p.m. — 2.30 p.m.	LUNCH (BALL ROOM B)

STOMACH AND DUODENUM—I

Chairmen: Dr. Basil Al-Naqeeb
Dr. Husam Baissouni

2.40 p.m. — 2.50 p.m.	Gastro-Intestinal Manifestations of Some Endocrine Disorders (Dr. Timothy S. Harrison)
2.50 p.m. — 3.10 p.m.	The Role of Ultrasound in Diagnosis of Disease of the Alimentary System (Letchka Vassiliva and Basil Al-Naqeeb)
3.10 p.m. — 3.30 p.m.	The Role of Aspiration Cytology in the Diagnosis of Diseases of the Alimentary System (A. Lindgren and Lars G. Lindberg)
3.30 p.m. — 4.00 p.m.	*PANEL DISCUSSION* Dr. Basil Al-Naqeeb (Moderator) Dr. T. S. Harrison, Dr. L. Vassiliva, Dr. A. Lindgren, Dr. H. Baissouni
4.00 p.m. — 4.30 p.m.	BREAK
4.30 p.m. — 6.00 p.m.	Motion Picture and Videotape Presentation
8.00 p.m.	Reception and Dinner (The Grand Ball Room, Sheraton Hotel)

Tuesday, 2nd February, 1982

STOMACH AND DUODENUM—II

Chairmen: Prof. J. M. Greep
Dr. Ahmed Abp Jabal

8.00 a.m.— 8.30 a.m.	Gastro-Intestinal Hormones (James Thompson)
8.30 a.m.— 9.00 a.m.	Current Treatment of Chronic Gastric Ulcer (David Johnston)
9.00 a.m.— 9.30 a.m.	Highly Selective Vagotomy for Duodenal Ulcer— Long-term results (David Johnston)
9.30 a.m.—10.00 a.m.	Critical Evaluation of the Operation for Duodenal Ulcer (James Thompson)
10.00 a.m.—10.30 a.m.	*PANEL DISCUSSION* Dr. J. M. Greep (Moderator) Dr. James Thompson Dr. David Johnston, Dr. Abu Jabal
10.30 a.m.—11.00 a.m.	COFFEE BREAK

STOMACH AND DUODENUM—III
Chairmen: Dr. Timothy Harrison,
               Dr. Joseph Cheriyan

11.00 a.m.—11.30 a.m.	The Perforated and Stenosed Duodenal Ulcer (David Johnston)
11.30 a.m.—12.00 noon	The Zollinger Ellison Syndrome (James Thompson)
12.00 noon—12.30 p.m.	*PANEL DISCUSSION* Dr. T. Harrison (Moderator), Dr. David Johnston, Dr. James Thompson, Dr. Joseph Cheriyan
12.30 p.m.— 2.00 p.m.	LUNCH BREAK (BALL ROOM—B)

LIVER—I

Chairmen: Dr. Yousof Omar, Dr. Sadad Sabri

2.00 p.m.— 2.20 p.m.	Primary Hepato-Cellular Carcinoma in Kuwait—Histo- pathological Appraisal (M. S. Al-Adnani)
2.20 p.m.— 2.40 p.m.	The Surgical Treatment Liver—The Local Experience of Hydatid Disease of the Liver (G. M. Abouna, Majeed Alwan)
2.40 p.m.— 3.00 p.m.	Management of Primary and Metastatic Tumours (J. G. Turcotte)
3.00 p.m.— 3.20 p.m.	*PANEL DISCUSSION* Dr. M. S. Al-Adnani (Moderator) Dr. Majeed Alwan Dr. J. G. Turcotte Dr. Marshall Orloff

LIVER—II
Chairman: Dr. Marshall Orloff

3.20 p.m.— 3.40 p.m.	Strategies in Management of Hepatic Trauma (J. G. Turcotte)
3.40 p.m.— 4.00 p.m.	Hemobelia (James Thompson)
4.00 p.m.— 4.30 p.m.	*PANEL DISCUSSION* Dr. Marshall Orloff (Moderator) Dr. J. G. Turcotte Dr. James Thompson Dr. J. M. Greep
4.30 p.m.— 5.00 p.m.	COFFEE BREAK
5.00 p.m.— 6.00 p.m.	Motion Picture and Video Tape Presentation

Wednesday, 3rd February, 1982

PORTAL HYPERTENSION—I

Chairman: Dr. J. G. Turcotte

8.00 a.m.— 8.20 a.m.	Radiological Evaluation of Patients with Portal Hypertension (Husam Baissouni)
8.20 a.m.— 8.50 a.m.	Hemodynamic Evaluation and Selection of Patients for Total or Selective Shunting Operations (Atef Sallam)
8.50 a.m.— 9.10 a.m.	Esophageal Transaction Using Circular Stapling Gun (George Johnston)
9.10 a.m.— 9.30 a.m.	Early Experience of Surgical Treatment of Portal Hypertension (G. M. Abouna, A. Menkarios, Basil Al-Naqeeb, Omer Al Farouk, H. Yousof, H. Baissouni)
9.30 a.m.—10.00 a.m.	*PANEL DISCUSSION* Dr. J. G. Turcotte (Moderator) Dr. Atef Salam Dr. G. Johnston Dr. G. M. Abouna Dr. H. Baissouni
10.00 a.m.—10.30 a.m.	COFFEE BREAK

PORTAL HYPERTENSION—I

Chairman: Dr. Atef Salam

10.30 a.m.—11.00 a.m.	Techniques and results of Meso-Caval Shunt (J. G. Turcotte)
11.00 a.m.—11.30 a.m.	Techniques and results of Porto-Caval Shunt (Marshall Orloff)

11.30 a.m.—12.00 noon	Techniques and Results of Distal Spleno-Renal Shunt (Atef Salam)
12.00 a.m.—12.30 p.m.	*PANEL DISCUSSION* Dr. Atef Salam (Moderator) Dr. J. G. Turcotte Dr. Marshall Orloff
12.30 a.m.— 2.00 p.m.	LUNCH BREAK

SPECIAL SESSION
G. M. Abouna (Moderator)

2.00 p.m.— 2.15 p.m.	Upper G.I. Haemorrhage in Kuwait (Basil Al Naqeeb)
2.15 p.m.— 2.30 p.m.	Bleeding Esophageal Varices (Marshall Orloff)
2.30 p.m.— 3.00 p.m.	*PANEL DISCUSSION* Dr. Basil Al Naqeeb (Moderator) Dr. Marshall Orloff, Dr. Atef Salam Dr. J. Turcotte, Dr. G. Johnston

PANCREAS AND BILIARY SYSTEM—I
Chairman: Dr. A. R. Roosa
Dr. Taiseer Abu Naema

3.00 p.m.— 3.30 p.m.	Acute Cholecystitis (Orloff)
3.30 p.m.— 4.00 p.m.	Pancreatic Resection for Chronic Pancreatitis (J. G. Turcotte)
4.00 p.m.— 4.30 p.m.	PANEL DISCUSSION Dr. Moosa (Moderator), Dr. J. Turcotte, Dr. J. Greep
4.30 p.m.— 5.00 p.m.	COFFEE BREAK
5.00 p.m.— 6.00 p.m.	Motion Picture Presentation

Thursday, 4th February, 1982

PANCREAS AND BILIARY SYSTEM — II
Chairmen: Dr. George Johnston
Dr. Abdulla Behbehani

8.00 a.m.— 8.20 a.m.	Pancreatic Cancer—How can we achieve early diagnosis (A. R. Moosa)
8.20 a.m.— 8.50 a.m.	Diagnosis and Management of Endocrine Tumours of Pancreas (Dr. James Thompson)

8.50 a.m.— 9.10 a.m.	Total Pancreatectomy—when and how (A. R. Moosa)

PANEL DISCUSSION

9.10 a.m.— 9.30 a.m.	Panel discussion Dr. J. G. Turcotte (Moderator) Dr. J. M. Greep, Dr. A. R. Moosa Dr. Timothy Harrison

PANCREAS AND THE BILIARY SYSTEM—III

Chairmen: Prof. James Thompson
Dr. Basil Al-Naqeeb

9.30 a.m.— 9.50 a.m.	Investigation and Management of Jaundice (George Johnston)
9.50 a.m.—10.10 a.m.	Management of Retained Stones in the Bile Ducts (J. M. Greep)
10.10 a.m.—10.30 a.m.	Endoprosthesis for Internal and External Biliary Drainage (Greep)
10.30 a.m.—10.50 a.m.	*PANEL DISCUSSION* Prof. J. Thompson (Moderator), Dr. Marshall Orloff, Dr. George Johnston, Dr. J. M. Greep, Dr. Basil Al-Naqeeb

INTESTINE—I

Chairmen: Dr. Nils G. Kock
Dr. Samir Motawa

11.20 a.m.—11.40 a.m.	The Obstructed Colon (A. R. Moosa)
11.40 a.m.—12.00 noon	Surgical Management of Inflammatory Bowel Disease (Nils Kock)
12.00 noon—12.20 p.m.	Intestinal Lymphoma in Kuwait (Yousof Omar, Basil Al-Naqeeb, Abdulla Behbehani, Samir Motawa, M. Barakat)
12.20 p.m.—12.40 p.m.	Conventional Intestinal Stomas and Indications (Nils G. Kock)

INTESTINE—I (Cont'd)

12.40 p.m.— 1.00 p.m.	Nils Kock (Moderator), Basil Al-Naqeeb A. R. Moosa, S. Motawa
1.00 p.m.— 2.30 p.m.	*LUNCH BREAK* (BALL ROOM—B)

INTESTINE—II
Chairmen: Dr. David Johnston
Dr. Kumar Mahajan

2.30 p.m.— 3.00 p.m.	Preservation of the Ileocecal Valve Ulcerative Colitis (David Johnston)
3.00 p.m.— 3.30 p.m.	Continent Stomas—Progress Report (Nils G. Kock)
3.30 p.m.— 4.00 p.m.	Carcinoma of the Recto-Sigmoid treated with Stapling Gun (David Johnston)

PANEL DISCUSSION

4.00 p.m.— 4.30 p.m.	Dr. David Johnston (Moderator) Dr. Basil Al Naqeeb, Dr. Nils G. Kock Dr. George Johnston, Dr. A. R. Moosa
4.30 p.m.— 4.45 p.m.	SUMMING UP (Prof. G. Abouna)
4.45 p.m.	COFFEE AND CLOSE

81C—2601
Urinary Calculi

Objectives: To teach recent advances in the field of pathological mechanisms and clinical pictures of urinary calculi.

Place: Auditorium—Mubarak Al-Kabeer Hospital.

Duration: One day, 15th February, 1982.

Organiser: Discipline Committee of Surgery and Area Executive Committee for Continuing Medical Education of the Joint Board.

Programme Director: Dr. Holmquist, Professor of Urology Department of Surgery.

Participants: All surgeons and physicians interested in urology and nephrology.

Programme:

Monday, 15th February, 1982

1.00 p.m.
Introduction
(Prof. Holmquist)
Renal Mechanism of Calculus Formation
(Prof. O. Thulesius)
Renal Tubular Acidosis as a Cause of Calculi Formation
(Prof. Johnny)
Hyperparathyroidism
(Dr. Shridhar)
Stone Formation in Bilharziasis
(Dr. Pawar)

2.30 p.m.
Suggestions on a Mutual Investigation Programme of Patients with Stone Disease
(Prof. Holmquist)

Prophylactic Treatment with Thiazides and its Physio-
logical Background
(Prof. Thulesius)
Surgical Treatment
(Dr. Shridhar)
Electrohydraulic Treatment of Bladder-Stones
(Prof. Holmquist)
Final Remarks
(Prof. Holmquist)

All the papers will last 10—15 minutes and will be followed by a discussion.

Evaluation of the Course on Urinary Calculi

The meeting dealing with urinary calculi was held with local teachers and aimed at giving a modern and up-to-date aspect of urinary calculi. After an introduction Professor Thulesius gave the physiological aspects of stone formation of different kinds such as cystinurea, uric acid stones, hyperocalat, ideopathic hypercalcuria and so on. After that Professor Johnny presented the problems with some tubular defects, mainly tubular acidosis. Tubular acidosis might be the background of stone formation especially in young people. Dr. Shridar talked about hyperparathyroidism and Dr. Pawar about stone formation in Bilharzia where the stones are formed in the ureter, which is a very unusual site of stone formation. After a brief discussion document for a mutual investigation programme was presented, it was mentioned that we are planning to start a joint clinic in cooperation with Professor Johnny and the nephrology department to which patients with complicated stones might be referred. Thereafter prophylactic treatment was discussed regarding cystinurea and uric acid stones. Prof. Thulesius described the mechanism behind the prophylactic Thiazid treatment. This treatment has been used, for example, in Sweden for two or three years in complicated cases, and this prophylactic treatment has reduced the frequency from 1 stone yearly to 0.01 stone yearly. This treatment is very promising and will be started here in Kuwait and controlled and followed up by the joint outpatient clinic just mentioned. Finally, surgical treatment was discussed, especially the more difficult part of it viz. Staghom Calculi. The future in this field will probably be a percutaneous nephrostomy combined with ultrasound destroying of the stone through this pathway. The last paper dealt with the Electrohydraulic treatment of bladder-stones, and the new appliance which has now come to Mubarak Hospital was demonstrated.

As a whole the meeting was very much appreciated, but the real target group viz. the junior staff, was absent with a few exemptions. Most of the audience consisted of Senior Registrars and Consultants. Therefore, one has to find new forms in order to also attract the junior staff. Probably this is partly a question of time. The next Postgraduate Course on Urology will probably be held in the evening.

In the evening we had an appreciated social programme with sauna, refreshments and dinner, hosted and sponsored by the Wolf Company.

81C—2602
Distal Ureteric Structures in Bilharzia

Objectives: To teach the advances in urology.

Place: S A S Hotel.

Duration:	Afternoon meeting on May 31st, 1982.
Organiser:	Dr. Joseph Cheriyan Adan Hospital Dr. Bo Holmquist Mubarak Hospital
Coordinator:	Dr. Abu Jabal Farwania Hospital
Participants:	Surgeons, registrars and all doctors interested.
Programme:	

Monday, 31st May, 1982

5.00 p.m.	Introduction Dr. Cheriyan—10 minutes Investigation and Indication of Surgery Dr. Salman Shukhry, Sabah Hospital—10 minutes Urodynamic studies Dr. Pawar, Mubarak Hospital—10 minutes
	Surgical Technique The Adan Model Dr. Malikowsky—5 minutes The Sabah Model Dr. Salman Shukhry—5 minutes The Farwania Model Dr. Ghazali—5 minutes The Mubarak Model Dr. Holmquist—5 minutes
	Follow-up The Adan Model Dr. Malikowsky—5 minutes The Sabah Model Dr. Salman Shukhry—5 minutes The Farwania Model Dr. Ghazali—5 minutes The Mubarak Model Dr. Holmquist—5 minutes
6.30 p.m.	Discussion
Social Programme	Sponsor—Park Davis
7.00 p.m.—8.30 p.m.	Refreshments
8.30 p.m.	Dinner, SAS Hotel

81C—27/2801
Course in Surgery of the Hand

Objectives:	To provide instruction in the basic principles of hand surgery. It is designed for interested surgical consult-

ants and senior registrars. A basis in reconstructive surgery either orthopaedic or plastic surgery is desirable.

Place: Dept. of Orthopaedics, Sulaibhikat, Hospital and possibly also the Faculty of Medicine.

Duration: 2 weeks, from Nov. 7th—19th, 1981.

Organisers: Prof. J. I. P. James M.S., F.R.C.S., F.R.A.C.S.,
Dr. Kamal Helmi, Hand Surgeon, and
Dr. M. Sherieff (Ophthalmology)

Programme Director: Prof. J. I. P. James M.S., F.R.C.S.

Participation: Consultants, senior registrars and registrars from Kuwait and from the neighbouring countries.
The full course is restricted to 10 participants, as much of the instruction is given in outpatient clinics and at operative sessions. The lectures will be open to a wider audience.
Applications should be sent to Professor J. I. P. James, The Orthopaedic Hospital, Sulaibikhat, P. O. Box. 4079, Kuwait, by September 1st, 1981.

Programme: *Lectures:*
Mr. Guy Pulvertaft, F.R.C.S., Emeritus Consultant, Hand Surgeon: Derby
Mr. D. W. Lamb, F.R.C.S. (E), Orthopaedic Surgeon: Edinburgh
Mr. N. Barton, F.R.C.S., Orthopaedic Surgeon: Nottingham.
Mr. Hugh Brown, T.D., O.H.S., F.R.C.S. Plastic Surgeon: Newcastle.
Professor J. I. P. James M.S., F.R.C.S., F.R.A.C.S. (Hon): Kuwait
Dr. Kamal Helmi, F.R.C.S., Hand Surgeon: Kuwait

November 7th—12th
November 14th—19th

Saturday	7th	8.00 a.m.	Outpatient clinic Dr. Helmi and visitors
Sunday	8th	8.00 a.m.	Operating session
Monday	9th	8.00 a.m.	Outpatient clinic
Tuesday	10th	8.00 a.m.	Operating session
Wednesday	11th	8.00 a.m.	Operating session
Thursday	12th	8.00 a.m.	Clinical conference

LECTURE AND AUDIO-VISUAL PROGRAMME (PROVISIONAL)

4.00 p.m.—6.00 p.m.

| Nov. 7th | Introduction: Injuries of the Hand | Prof. J. I. P. James |
| | Functional Anatomy of the Hand. Film. | Mr. G. Pulvertaft |

Nov. 8th	The Wounded Hand: Examination and Assessment	Mr. G. Pulvertaft
	Primary Treatment	Mr. N. Barton
Nov. 9th	Skin Loss and Replacement	Mr. H. Brown
	Tendon Injury and Repair	Mr. G. Pulvertaft
Nov. 10th	Fractures of the Metacarpals and Phalanges	Mr. N. Barton
	Peripheral Nerve Injuries	Prof. J. I. P. James
Nov. 11th	Reconstruction of Paralytic and Post Traumatic Problems	Mr. D. W. Lamb
	Volkman's Ischaemic Contracture	Prof. J. I. P. James
Nov. 14th	Congenital Deformities of the Hand	Mr. D. W. Lamb
	Burns of the Hand	Mr. H. Brown
Nov. 15th	Amputations	Mr. N. Barton
	Microsurgery in the Hand	Dr. Kamal Helmi
Nov. 16th	Rheumatoid Arthritis	Mr. N. Barton
	Nerve Compression Syndromes	Mr. D. W. Lamb
Nov. 17th	The Infected Hand	Mr. D. W. Lamb
	After Care. The Stiff Hand	Mr. G. Pulvertaft
Nov. 18th	QUESTIONS AND ANSWERS	

81C—2901
Paediatric Surgery

Objectives:	The visit of Professor Nobuhiko Komi, M.D. Professor of Surgery, School of Medicine, University of Tokushima, Japan. To teach recent advances in the field of Paediatric Surgery.
Place:	Ibn Sina Hospital, Mubarak Hospital, Sabah Hospital, Farwania Hospital, Adan Hospital.
Duration:	14 days, from 25th November—10th December 1981.
Organiser:	Discipline Committee for Surgery of the Joint Board for Postgraduate Education.
Programme Director:	Dr. Kazue, Ibn Sina Hospital.
Participants:	Surgeons of the above-mentioned hospitals and training doctors in the five hospitals attending lectures, clinical rounds and instruction sessions.
Programme:	

25th November, 1981 (Wednesday)

9.00 a.m.	Visit Mubarak Hospital (Prof. Abouna)
10.30 a.m.	Visit Ibn Sina Hospital (Dr. Mahmoud El Bedr)

26th November, 1981 (Thursday)

8.00 a.m.   Sabah Hospital Surgical Grand Round
Congenital Biliary Malformations
(Dr. S. Sabri and Dr. R. Mallick)

28th November, 1981 (Saturday)

8.30 a.m.   Visit Farwania Hospital—Department of Surgery (Dr.
Abu Jabal)
Lecture: Biliary Obstruction

29th November, 1981 (Sunday)

8.00 a.m.   Ibn Sina Hospital, Outpatient Dept.
(Dr. Kazue)

30th November, 1981 (Monday)

11.00 a.m.   Dept. of Paediatrics—Mubarak Hospital
(Prof. Paul Agius)
Lecture: Malrotations of the Intestine

1st December, 1981 (Tuesday)

8.00 a.m.   Ibn Sina Hospital—Paediatric Surgery Department:
Grand Rounds, Journal Club and Ward Rounds.

2nd December, 1981 (Wednesday)

Operating Theatre, Ibn Sina Hospital
(Dr. Kazue)

3rd December, 1981 (Thursday)

11.00 a.m.   Mubarak Al Kabeer Hospital—Surgical Grand Rounds
(Prof. Abouna and Prof. Eklof)
Title "Experimental Studies on the Congenital Malfor-
mations using Fetal Surgery"

5th December, 1981 (Saturday)

8.00 a.m.   Ibn Sina Hospital (Dr. Issa and Dr. Bedr)

6th December, 1981 (Sunday)

8.00 a.m.   Outpatient Department; Ibn Sina Hospital
(Dr. Kazue and Dr. Issa)

7th December, 1981 (Monday)

12.00 noon   Farwania Hospital (Dept. of Paediatrics)
(Dr. Ahmed Kamal)
Lecture: Surgical Emergencies in Children

8th December, 1981 (Tuesday)

7.50 a.m.   Adan Hospital, Dept. of Surgery and Paediatrics
(Dr. Cherian and Dr. Fernando)
Lecture: Congenital Biliary Malformations

9th December, 1981 (Wednesday)

8.00 a.m.   Operating Theatre, Ibn Sina Hospital
                             (Dr. Kazue)

10th December, 1981 (Thursday)

11.00 a.m.   Department of Paediatrics, Al Sabah Hospital
                             (Dr. Abdulla Rashid)
                             Lecture: Surgical Emergencies in Neonates

81C—2902
Seminar on Paediatric Surgery

Objectives: The visit of Dr. John Scott F.R.C.S.
                             Consultant Pediatric Surgeon
                             Newcastle Upon Tyne, England.
                             To teach the advances in Paed. Surgery.

Place: Nursing Institute, Sabah Hospital
                             Ibn Sina Hospital
                             Mubarak Hospital
                             Farwania Hospital.

Duration: 14 days, 20th April—3rd May, 1982.

Organiser: Discipline Committee for Surgery of the Joint Postgrad-
                             uate Board.

Programme Director: Professor George M. Abouna.

Participants: Surgeons and all doctors interested.

Programme:

Tuesday, 20th April 1982

8.00 a.m.   Journal club, Ibn Sina Hospital
9.30 a.m.   Grand Rounds, Ward 1, 2 and 3
12.00 noon   Lecture on Abnormalities of Ureters, Bladder and
                             Urethra
                             Nursing Institute, Sabah Hospital

Wednesday, 21st April 1982

8.00 a.m.   Outpatient clinic, Ibn Sina Hospital
11.00 a.m.   Operation theatre, Ibn Sina Hospital

Thursday, 22nd April 1982

10.00 a.m.   Seminar on Urinary Incontinence and Enuresis
                             Nursing Institute, Sabah Hospital

Saturday, 24th April 1982

8.00 a.m.   Outpatients, Ibn Sina Hospital
11.00 a.m.   Operation theatre

6.00 p.m.	Postgraduate lecture Management of Malformations of Gastrointestinal Tract Mubarak Al Kabir Hospital

Sunday, 25th April 1982

8.00 a.m.	Paediatric Dept. Mubarak Hospital (Dr. Hassan Abdul Majeed)

Monday, 26th April 1982

8.00 a.m.	Outpatient clinic Ibn Sina Hospital
11.00 a.m.	Operation theatre

Tuesday, 27th April 1982

8.00 a.m.	Journal Club Ibn Sina Hospital
9.30 a.m.	Grand Rounds Ward 1, 2 and 3
12.00 noon	Lecture on Neonatal Surgical Intensive Care Nursing Institute, Sabah Hosp.

Wednesday, 28th April 1982

8.00 a.m.	Outpatient clinic Ibn Sina Hospital
11.00 a.m.	Operation theatre

Thursday, 29th April 1982

10.00 a.m.	Lecture on Investigation and Management of Sex Chromosome Mosaic and Delayed Puberty Nursing Institute, Sabah Hospital

Saturday, 1st May 1982

8.00 a.m.	Visit Dept. of Surgery and Paediatrics Farwania Hospital (Dr. Abu Jabal)
11.00 a.m.	Operation theatre Ibn Sina Hospital

Sunday, 2nd May 1982

8.00 a.m.	Outpatient clinic Ibn Sina Hospital

Monday, 3rd May 1982

8.00 a.m.	Dept. of Paediatrics Mubarak Hospital (Dr. Hassan Abdul Majeed)

81C—3301
Seminar on Paediatrics

Objectives: The visit of Prof. Akram M. Tamer, Miami University. To teach recent advances in the field of Paediatrics.

Place: Al-Sabah Hospital, Maternity Hospital, Farwania Hospital, Al-Adan Hospital.

Duration: 6 days, from 8th May—13th May 1982.

Organiser: Training Division in cooperation with the Office of International Medical Education, University of Miami.

Programme Director: Dr. Promod Mullick.

Participants: The course is aimed at paediatricians and doctors interested in paediatrics.

Programme:

Saturday, 8th May, 1982

8.30 a.m.—11.30 a.m.   Ward Round in Sabah Hospital of Wards 2 and 9
12.00 noon—1.00 p.m.   Lecture Survey of Recent Advances in Paediatrics
Sabah Hospital, O.P.D. Lecture Room

Sunday, 9th May, 1982

8.30 a.m.—11.30 a.m.   Maternity Hospital—Neonatal Ward Rounds
12.00 noon—1.00 p.m.   Lecture The High Risk Neonate
Lecture Theatre—Maternity

Monday, 10th May, 1982

8.30 a.m.—10.30 a.m.   Case presentation and discussion with D.C.M. candidates
Ward—1, Al-Sabah Hospital
10.30 a.m.—11.30 a.m.   Lecture I Childhood Allergy
O.P.D. Lecture Room, Al-Sabah Hospital
12.00 noon—1.00 p.m.   Lecture II Childhood Allergy
O.P.D. Lecture Room, Al-Sabah Hospital

Tuesday, 11th May, 1982

9.00 a.m.—11.30 a.m.   Ward Rounds with Consultants, Staff, and Postgraduates in Al-Jahra Hospital
12.00 noon—1.00 p.m.   Dr. Akram M. Tamer, Lecture on:
Antibiotic Prescribing in Childhood
Jahra Hospital

Wednesday, 12th May, 1982

9.00 a.m.—11.30 a.m.   Ward Round with Consultants, Staff and Postgraduates at Adan Hospital
12.00 a.m.—1.00 p.m.   Lecture: Sudden Infant Death Syndrome
Al-Adan Hospital

Thursday, 13th May, 1982

8.30 a.m.—10.00 a.m.	Ward Rounds with Consultants, Staff and Postgraduates at Farwania Hospital
10.30 a.m.	Panel Discussion in Farwania Hospital on: Family Doctor Practice in Paediatrics Chairman: Dr. Promod Mullick Members: Dr. Akram M. Tamer Dr. Saad Zaghloul Dr. Ashmawi Abdel Wahab Dr. Ahmed Fuad Khalil

81C—33/1403
Course in Paediatric Gastro-Enterology

Objectives: The visit of Dr. J. T. Harries, Reader in Paediatrics and Hon. Consultant Physician, Institute of Child Health, The Hospital for Sick Children, Great Ormond Street, London, aims:
To exchange views and experiences in Gastro-Enterology with Paediatricians and Postgraduate Doctors in Kuwait.
To teach advances in the field of Gastro-Enterology.
To discuss research programmes.

Place: Department of Paediatrics
Al-Sabah Hospital
Mubarak Hospital
Farwania Hospital
Adan Hospital
Jahra Hospital.

Duration: 2 weeks, from 5. 2. 1982 to 18. 2. 1982.

Organiser: Ministry of Public Health.

Programme Director: Prof. Abdulla A. A. Al-Rashied, Chairman of Paediatric Department, Al-Sabah Hospital.

Participation: The paediatricians and postgraduates of the above-mentioned hospitals.

Programme:

Saturday, 6th February, 1982

9.00 a.m.	Dept. of Paediatrics, Al-Sabah Hospital
12.00 noon—1.00 p.m.	Lecture: Modern Trends in Gastro-Enterology Paed. Lecture Room O.P.D., Al-Sabah Hospital

Sunday, 7th February, 1982

8.30 a.m.—11.00 a.m.	Ward Round in Ward 2, 3 and 4 with the Consultants and Resident Staff Al-Sabah Hospital

5.00 p.m.   Special Lecture: Allied Health and Nursing
Auditorium, Al-Sabah Hospital

Monday, 8th February, 1982

8.30 a.m.—11.00 a.m.   Ward Round in Ward 5, 6 and 8 with Consultants and
Resident Staff, Al-Sabah Hospital

12.00 noon—1.00 p.m.   Lecture: Infective Diarrhoea and Vomiting
Paed. Lecture Room O.P.D., Al-Sabah Hospital

5.00 p.m.   Lecture: Small Intestinal Enteropathies
                             Allied Health and Nursing
Auditorium, Al-Sabah Hospital

Tuesday, 9th February 1982

8.30 a.m.   Round in the Neo-Natology Unit,
Maternity Hospital, with the Consultants and the Paediatric Staff

12.00 noon—1.00 p.m.   Lecture: Development of Structure and Functions of
the G.I.T.

5.00 p.m.   Exocrine Pancreatic Function in Premature and
Full-Term Neonates
Allied Health and Nursing Auditorium
Al-Sabah Hospital

Wednesday, 10th February, 1982

8.30 a.m.—10.30 a.m.   Mubarak Hospital, Paediatric Dept.
Ward Round with Consultants and Resident Staff

11.00 a.m.—1.00 p.m.   Research Meeting with Consultant
Mubarak Hospital

5.00 p.m.   Panel Discussion
Persistent Neonatal Jaundice
Allied Health and Nursing Auditorium
Al-Sabah Hospital

Thursday, 11th February, 1982

8.30 a.m.—10.30 a.m.   Undergraduate Teaching Ward Round
Mubarak Hospital

11.30 a.m.—1.00 p.m.   Lecture: Selective Inborn Errors of Absorption
Lecture Room, Paediatric Dept.
Al-Sabah Hospital

Saturday, 13th February, 1982

8.30 a.m.—11.00 a.m.   Ward Rounds with Consultants and Residents
Adan Hospital

12.00 noon—1.00 p.m.   Research meeting
Consultants
Adan Hospital

5.00 p.m.   Lecture: Inborn Errors of Hepatic Metabolism
Allied Health and Nursing Auditorium
Al-Sabah Hospital

Sunday, 14th February, 1982

8.30 a.m.—11.30 a.m.	Ward Rounds Farwania Hospital
12.00 noon—1.00 p.m.	Research Meeting Consultant Farwania Hospital
5.00 p.m.	Seminar: Active Chronic Hepatitis Allied Health and Nursing Auditorium Al-Sabah Hospital

Monday, 15th February, 1982

8.30 a.m.—11.00 a.m.	Ward Rounds with Consultants and Resident Staff Jahra Hospital
12.00 noon—1.00 p.m.	Case Discussion and Research Discussion Jahra Hospital
6.00 p.m.	Lecture: Gastro-Intestinal Immunology Allied Health and Nursing Auditorium Al-Sabah Hospital

Tuesday, 16th February, 1982

8.30 a.m.—11.30 a.m.	Discussion Regarding Research Programme and Presentation of Patients of Clinical Interest Al-Sabah Hospital
12.00 noon—1.00 p.m.	Lecture: Cow's Milk Protein Allergy Lecture Room O.P.D. Al-Sabah Hospital

Wednesday, 17th February, 1982

8.30 a.m.—10.30 a.m.	Tutorial for D.C.H. candidates Al-Sabah Hospital
11.30 a.m.—1.00 p.m.	Clinico—Pathological Conference Al-Sabah Hospital Lecture Room
5.00 p.m.	Seminar on Investigatory Techniques Allied Health and Nursing Auditorium Al-Sabah Hospital

Thursday, 18th February, 1982

10.00 a.m.	Seminar on I. V. Alimentation Lecture Room, Al-Sabah Hospital
11.00 a.m.	Symposium on Protracted Diarrhoea Al-Sabah Hospital

81C—33/1402
Recent Advances and Current Paediatric Gastro-Enterology

Objectives:	The visit of Dr. Adrian C. Douwes, Paediatrics Gastro-Enterologist, Children's Department, Free University Hospital, Amsterdam, Netherlands aims:

To review the recent advances and current practice in paediatric gastroenterology.
To exchange views and experiences in gastroenterology with paediatricians and postgraduates.
To discuss research programmes.

Place: Department of Paediatrics
                        Al-Sabah Hospital
                        Mubarak Hospital
                        Farwania Hospital
                        Adan Hospital
                        Jahra Hospital.

Duration: 2 weeks, from 5. 2. 1982—19. 2. 1982

Organiser: Ministry of Public Health.

Programme Director: Prof. Abdulla A. A. Al-Rashied, Chairman, Paediatric Department, Al-Sabah Hospital.

Participants: Paediatricians and postgraduates of the above-mentioned hospitals.

Programme:

Saturday, 6th February, 1982

10.00 a.m.   Dept. of Paediatrics, Al-Sabah Hospital
 5.00 p.m.   Special Lecture—Allied Health and Nursing Auditorium, Al-Sabah Hospital

Sunday, 7th February, 1982

8.30 a.m.—10.30 a.m.   Mubarak Hospital, Paediatric Department
                        Ward Round with Consultants and Resident Staff
12.00 noon—1.00 p.m.   Lecture: Gastrointestinal Physiology
                        Lecture room O.P.D.
                        Al-Sabah Hospital

Monday, 8th February, 1982

8.30 a.m.—11.00 a.m.   Undergraduate Teaching Round
                        Mubarak Hospital
11.30 a.m.—1.00 p.m.   Discussion Regarding Research with Consultants
                        Mubarak Hospital
3.30 p.m.—4.00 p.m.   Lecture: Protein—Losing Enteropathies
                        Allied Health and Nursing Auditorium
                        Al-Sabah Hospital

Tuesday, 9th February, 1982

9.00 a.m.—12.00 noon   Ward Round in Ward 2, 3 and 4 with the Consultants
                        Residents Staff
                        Al-Sabah Hospital
3.30 p.m.—4.30 p.m.   Diarrhoeal Problems and Management in the Neonate
                        Allied Health and Nursing Auditorium
                        Al-Sabah Hospital

Wednesday, 10th February, 1982

8.30 a.m. — 11.30 a.m.	Ward Round in Ward 5, 6 and 8 with Consultants and Resident Staff Al-Sabah Hospital
12.00 noon — 1.00 p.m.	Lecture: Intestinal Malabsorption in Infancy and Childhood Lecture Room O.P.D. Al-Sabah Hospital
5.00 p.m.	Panel Discussion Persistent Neonatal Jaundice Allied Health and Nursing Auditorium Al-Sabah Hospital

Thursday, 11th February 1982

8.30 a.m. — 11.30 a.m.	Round in the Neo-Natology Unit Maternity Hospital, Al-Sabah Hospital with Consultants and Paediatric Staff

Saturday, 13th February, 1982

8.30 a.m. — 11.00 a.m.	Ward Round with Consultants and Resident Staff Farwania Hospital
12.00 noon — 1.00 p.m.	Lecture: Gastrointestinal Allergy Lecture Room O.P.D. Al-Sabah Hospital

Sunday, 14th February, 1982

8.30 a.m. — 11.30 a.m.	Ward Rounds, Adan Hospital
12.00 noon — 1.00 p.m.	Research Meeting with Consultants and Adan Hospital
5.00 p.m.	Seminar — Active Chronic Hepatitis Allied Health and Nursing Auditorium Al-Sabah Hospital

Monday, 15th February, 1982

8.30 a.m. — 11.00 a.m.	Tutorial for D.C.H. Candidates Al-Sabah Hospital
11.30 a.m. — 1.00 p.m.	Panel Discussion on Microbiology and Chemotherapy of the G.I.T. in Acute Infantile Gastroenteritis Al-Sabah Hospital Lecture Room
4.30 p.m. — 5.30 p.m.	Lecture: Gastrointestinal Hormones Allied Health and Nursing Auditorium Al-Sabah Hospital

Tuesday, 16th February, 1982

8.30 a.m. — 11.30 a.m.	Ward Rounds with Consultants and Paediatric Staff Jahra Hospital
12.00 noon — 1.00 p.m.	Discussion Regarding Research with Consultants Jahra Hospital

4.00 p.m.	Symposium on Pancreatic Disease in Infancy and Childhood Allied Health and Nursing Auditorium Al-Sabah Hospital

Wednesday, 17th February, 1982

8.30 a.m. — 11.00 a.m.	Clinical Discussion on Hepatobiliary Disease in Children Al-Sabah Hospital

Thursday, 18th February, 1982

8.30 a.m. — 9.30 a.m.	Discussion Regarding Research Programme Al-Sabah Hospital
10.00 a.m. — 12.00 noon	Seminar on I.V. Alimentation Lecture Room O.P.D. Al-Sabah Hospital
3.30 p.m. — 4.30 p.m.	Special Lecture Allied Health and Nursing Auditorium Al-Sabah Hospital

81C—3701
Intensive Course in Gynaecology and Obstetrics

Objectives:	To update the knowledge of doctors working in the Gynaecology and Obstetrics discipline. To increase the proficiency of said doctors in better understanding and tackling problems related to gynaecological and obstetrical diseases. To help candidates wishing to sit for the M.R.C.O.G. Part II.
Place:	Lecture Room and Wards in the Maternity Hospital, Kuwait.
Duration:	14 days, from 20th March, 1982—1st April, 1982.
Organiser:	Discipline Committee for Gynaecology and Obstetrics of the Joint Board of Postgraduate Medical Education.
Programme Director:	Dr. Aly El-Tanir.
Participants:	All interested doctors working in Gynaecology and Obstetrics.
Visiting Lecturers:	From U.K., Professor J. Pinkerton, Professor M. Macnaughton, Dr. Henry, Mr. Arthur Williams, Dr. F. Loeffler, Professor Philip Myerscough.
Programme:	

Saturday, 20th March, 1982

10.00 a.m. — 1.00 p.m.	Prof Pinkerton Prof. Macnaughton Dr. Henry

2.30 p.m.— 3.30 p.m.   Prof. Pinkerton, lecture on:
                           Urinary Tract Infections in Obstetrics and Gynaecology
3.30 p.m.— 4.30 p.m.   Prof. Macnaughton, lecture on:
                           Premature Labour
5.00 p.m.— 6.00 p.m.   Dr. Henry, lecture on:
                           Carcinoma in Situs of the Cervix and its Management

Sunday, 21st March, 1982

10.00 a.m.— 1.00 p.m.   Prof. Pinkerton
                           Prof. Macnaughton
                           Dr. Henry
2.30 p.m.— 3.30 p.m.   Prof. Macnaughton, lecture on:
                           Maternal and Perinatal Mortality
3.30 p.m.— 4.30 p.m.   Dr. Henry, lecture on:
                           Placental Dysfunction and the Small-for-Dates Baby
5.00 p.m.— 6.00 p.m.   Prof. Pinkerton, lecture on:
                           Onset of Labour

Monday, 22nd March, 1982

10.00 a.m.— 1.00 p.m.   Prof. Pinkerton
                           Prof. Macnaughton
                           Dr. Henry
2.30 p.m.— 3.30 p.m.   Dr. Henry, lecture on:
                           Family Planning
3.30 p.m.— 4.30 p.m.   Prof. Pinkerton, lecture on:
                           The Normal and Abnormal Puerperium
5.00 p.m.— 6.00 p.m.   Prof. Macnaughton, lecture on:
                           Anaemia in Pregnancy

Tuesday, 23rd March, 1982

10.00 a.m.— 1.00 p.m.   Prof. Pinkerton
                           Prof. Macnaughton
                           Dr. Henry
2.30 p.m.— 3.30 p.m.   Prof. Pinkerton, lecture on:
                           The Modern Management of Placenta Praevia
3.30 p.m.— 4.30 p.m.   Prof. Macnaughton, lecture on:
                           Hormones in Obstetrics and Gynaecology
5.00 p.m.— 6.00 p.m.   Dr. Henry, lecture on:
                           Obstetric Trauma and Ruptured Uterus

Wednesday, 24th March, 1982

10.00 a.m.— 1.00 p.m.   Prof. Pinkerton
                           Prof. Macnaughton
                           Dr. Henry
2.30 p.m.— 3.30 p.m.   Prof. Macnaughton, lecture on:
                           Hormones in Obstetrics and Gynaecology
3.30 p.m.— 4.30 p.m.   Dr. Henry, lecture on:
                           Caesarean Section
5.00 p.m.— 6.00 p.m.   Prof. Pinkerton, lecture on:
                           Diseases of the Vulva

Thursday, 25th March, 1982

10.00 a.m.— 1.00 p.m.	Prof. Pinkerton Prof. Macnaughton Dr. Henry
2.30 p.m.— 3.30 p.m.	Dr. Henry, lecture on: Unstable Life
3.30 p.m.— 4.30 p.m.	Prof. Pinkerton, lecture on: The Acute Abdomen in Pregnancy
5.00 p.m.— 6.00 p.m.	Prof. Macnaughton, lecture on: Carcinoma of the Cervix

81C—3702
Seminar on Obstetrics and Gynaecology

Objectives:
The visit of Dr. Allen McLeod, Miami University.
To teach recent advances in the field of Obstetrics and Gynaecology.

Place:
Maternity Hospital, Mubarak Hospital, Farwania Hospital, Jahra Hospital.

Duration:
6 days, from 26th June, 1982—1st July, 1982.

Organiser:
Training Division in cooperation with the Office of International Medical Education, University of Miami.

Programme Director:
Dr. Ahmad Nabil Mustafa.

Participants:
The seminar is aimed at gynaecologists.

Programme:

Saturday, 26th June, 1982

9.00 a.m.—10.00 a.m. 10.00 a.m.	To meet Dr. Hassan Hathout, Head, Maternity Hospital Ward rounds with consultants, staff and postgraduates at Maternity Hospital

Sunday, 27th June, 1982

10.00 a.m.	Ward rounds with consultants, staff and postgraduates at Maternity Hospital
12.00 noon	Dr. Allen McLeod, lecture on: Perinatology

Monday, 28th June, 1982

10.00 a.m.	Hospital rounds in Jahra Hospital with Dr. Sahim Yassin

Tuesday, 29th June, 1982

10.00 a.m.	Hospital rounds in Al-Adan Hospital with Dr. Samir Mustafa Kamel

Wednesday, 30th June, 1982

10.00 a.m.   Hospital rounds in Mubarak Hospital

Thursday, 1st July, 1982

9.00 a.m.   To visit Farwania Hospital
10.30 a.m.   Panel discussion in Farwania Hospital on
Family Doctor Practice in Obstetrics and Gynaecology
Chairman: Dr. A. N. Mustafa
Members: Dr. Allen McLeod
             Dr. Saad Zaghloul
             Dr. Hani Mahmoud Auda

81C—4301
Family Medicine Practice

Objectives: The Joint Board, according to the instructions of the Ministry of Public Health, Kuwait, has formed a Discipline Committee for Family Medicine. This important decision means that the National Health Care System of Kuwait is going to be modernised in the field of outpatient care and in general practice.
To formulate in that respect the objectives and requirements in different fields of medicine.
To discuss this problem with foreign visitors.
To discuss with doctors from outpatient clinics and health centers principles of family medicine practice in different fields of medicine.

Place: Farwania Hospital.

Duration: Once a week on Thursday, from 6th May—15th July, 1982.

Organiser: Training Division in Collaboration with Discipline Committee for Family Medicine of the Joint Board of Postgraduate Education.

Programme Director: Dr. Saad Zaghloul, Director, Farwania Hospital.

Participants: Doctors from Health Centers and Outpatient Clinics.

Programme: see below *Outline of the Panel Discussion.*

Thursday, 29th April, 1982

6.00 p.m.   Panel discussion in Farwania Hospital on Family Doctor Practice in Respiratory Diseases
Chairmen: Dr. Ellul-Micallef and
               Dr. Shaaban
Members: Dr. Sami I. Said
             Dr. Saad Zaghloul
             Dr. Ashmawi Abdel Wahab

Thursday, 13th May, 1982

10.30 a.m.   Panel discussion in Farwania Hospital on
                              Family Doctor Practice in Paediatrics
                              Chairman: Dr. Promoda Mullick
                              Members: Dr. Akram M. Tamer
                                        Dr. Saad Zaghloul
                                        Dr. Ashmawi Abdel Wahab
                                        Dr. Ahmed Fuad Khalil

Wednesday, 19th May, 1982

10.30 a.m.   Panel discussion in Farwania Hospital on
                              Family Doctor Practice in Cardiology
                              Chairman: Dr. M. K. Emara
                              Members: Dr. D. B. Linder
                                        Dr. Saad Zaghloul
                                        Dr. Ashmawi Abdel Wahab

Thursday, 27th May, 1982

10.30 a.m.   Panel discussion in Farwania Hospital on
                              Family Doctor Practice in Haematology
                              Chairman: Prof. Ladislav Chrobak
                              Members: Dr. A. A. Yunis
                                        Dr. Abdul Aziz Hasaneen
                                        Dr. Saad Zaghloul
                                        Dr. Ashmawi Abdel Wahab
                                        Dr. Ahmed Faud Khalil

Thursday, 10th June, 1982

10.30 a.m.   Panel discussion in Farwania Hospital on
                              Family Doctor Practice in Endocrinology
                              Chairman: Dr. A. Maarafi
                              Members: Dr. John McKenzie
                                        Dr. Saad Zaghloul
                                        Dr. Ashmawi Abdel Wahab
                                        Dr. Ahmed Faud Khalil

Thursday, 17th June, 1982

10.30 a.m.   Panel discussion in Farwania Hospital on
                              Family Doctor Practice in Neurology
                              Chairman: Dr. R. A. Shakir
                              Members: Dr. Nobel David
                                        Dr. Saad Zaghloul
                                        Dr. Ashmawi Abdel Wahab
                                        Dr. Farouk Al Kayzi, from Ibn Sina Hospi-
                                        tal

Thursday, 24th June, 1982

10.30 a.m.   Panel discussion in Farwania Hospital on
                              Family Doctor Practice with Radiology

Chairman: Dr. M. D. Al Tamami
Members: Dr. E. Russell
Dr. Saad Zaghloul
Dr. M. Shafeeq

Thursday, 1st July, 1982

10.30 a.m.

Panel discussion in Farwania Hospital on
Family Doctor Practice in Obstetrics and Gynaecology
Chairman: Dr. A. N. Mustafa
Members: Dr. Allen McLeod
Dr. Saad Zaghloul
Dr. Hani Mahmoud Auda

Thursday, 15th July, 1982

8.30 p.m.

Panel discussion in Farwania Hospital on
Family Doctor Practice in Psychiatry and Behavioural
Sciences
Chairman: Dr. Mohamed El-Islam
Members: Dr. Burton Goldstein
Dr. Hussein Darwish
Dr. Saad Zaghloul

Outline of the Panel Discussion on (X)
(see page 210)

1. *Introduction:*
   General characteristics of (X) as a clinical science and recent advances in that field

2. *Role of Early Diagnosis of Disease in the Field of (X):*
   Clinical meanings and importance
   Methodological possibilities
   When and how to cooperate with specialists

3. *Role of Genetic Factors in (X):*
   Study health conditions of family members

4. *Role of Living Conditions of the Patient:*
   Economic conditions of the family
   Customs of the family
   Other factors

5. *Practical Possibilities for the Family Medicine Doctor in Diagnosis and Treatment in (X) Diseases.*

6. *Importance of Follow-up by the Family Medicine Doctor of the Treated Patient.*

7. *Answers of the Members of the Panel Discussion to the Questions from the Floor.*

(X) Pulmonology
Endocrinology
Cardiology
Haematology
Neurology

Paediatrics
Gynaecology and Obstetrics
Radiology
Psychiatry and Behavioural Sciences

81C—4401
Two Months Refresher Course
for Primary Health Centre Doctors

Objectives:	To instruct and discuss common medical problems in general practice. To assist the doctors of Primary Health Centers in dealing with their everyday professional problems.
Methods:	To enable all doctors to take part in this training each lecture of the course will be repeated, and accordingly doctors in each Health Centre will be divided into 2 groups: A and B.

General Organisation of the Course

7.20	An attendance list has to be signed by each doctor taking part in the course.
7.30—10.00	Lectures in Al-Sabah Hospital.
10.00—11.00	Time to enable doctors to return to their Health Centres.
11.00—13.30	Practical activities of doctors' normal in-service work. At that time doctors may expect a tutor's visit with whom he may discuss his professional problems.
Place:	The training will be performed in Al-Sabah Hospital, Conference Room in the Old Institute of Nursing, on Saturdays.
Duration:	2 months, from April 4th, 1981—May 30th, 1981, for doctors belonging to group A on

4th of April
11th of April
18th of April
25th of April
2nd of May
9th of May
16th of May
23rd of May
30th of May.

Organiser:	Discipline Committee for Community Medicine.
Programme Director:	Dr. Sami Mattar, Director of the Department of External Medical Services.
Participants:	Doctors belonging to Group A.

Programme:

4th of April, 1981

7.30—8.15	Organisation and Functions of Medical Health Districts
8.20—9.05	Early Diagnosis of Tuberculosis
9.10—9.55	Chronic Respiratory Failure

11th of April 1981

7.30—8.15	Assessment and Management of Common Paediatric Emergencies
8.20—9.05	Treatment of Burns
9.10—9.55	Early Diagnosis of Cancer

18th of April, 1981

7.30—8.15	Early Diagnosis of Cancer
8.20—9.05	Heart Failure Management
9.10—9.55	Coronary Care

25th of April, 1981

7.30—8.15	Examination of the Eye, External Eye Diseases
8.20—9.05	Peptic Ulcer
9.10—9.55	Acute Abdomen

2nd of May, 1981

7.30—8.15	Chronic Hepatitis
8.20—9.05	Disease of Gall Bladder and Pancreas
9.10—9.55	Interpretation of Liver Function Tests

81C—54/9601
Ultra-Sound in Ophthalmology

Objectives: The visit of Dr. Vernon Smith F.R.C.S., Consultant Ophthalmic Surgeon from Birmingham Eye Hospital. To teach the advances in ophthalmology.

Place: Al-Sabah Hospital, Eye Department and Conference Room of Ibn Sina Hospital.

Duration: 12 days, 4th July, 1981—16th July, 1981.

Organiser: Joint Board of Postgraduate Medical Education.

Programme Director: Dr. S. M. M. Sheriff, M.B., F.R.C.S., D.O. (Lond.). Head of Eye Department.

Participants: Ophthalmologists.

Programme:

Saturday, 4th July, 1981

8.00 a.m.—1.00 p.m.	Ophthalmic Clinic and Discussion of Cases

Sunday, 5th July, 1981

8.00 a.m.—1.00 p.m.   Surgical Operations

Monday, 6th July, 1981

8.00 a.m.—1.00 p.m.   Clinical Demonstration—Ultra Sonography

Tuesday, 7th July, 1981

8.00 a.m.—1.00 p.m.   Surgical Operations

Wednesday, 8th July, 1981

8.00 a.m.—1.00 p.m.   Ophthalmic Clinic and Discussion of Cases

Thursday, 9th July, 1981

                        Clinical Meeting and Lectures
8.30 a.m.   Dr. Vernon Smith, lecture on
                        Basic Principals of Ultra-Sound
12.30 p.m.   Dr. Vernon Smith, lecture on
                        Diagnostic Ultra-Sound in Ophthalmology

Saturday, 11th July, 1981

8.00 a.m.—1.00 p.m.   Ophthalmic clinic and discussion of cases

Sunday, 12th July, 1981

6.30 p.m.   Dr. Vernon Smith, lecture on
                        Orbital surgery

Monday, 13th July, 1981

8.00 a.m.—1.00 p.m.   Clinical demonstration—Ultra Sonography

Tuesday, 14th July, 1981

8.00 a.m.—1.00 p.m.   Surgical operations

Wednesday, 15th July, 1981

8.00 a.m.—1.00 p.m.   Ophthalmic clinic and discussion of cases

Thursday, 16th July, 1981

8.30 a.m.   Dr. Vernon Smith, lecture on
                        Exenteration
12.30 p.m.   Dr. Vernon Smith, lecture on
                        Orbital trauma

81C—5402
Retinopathy

Objectives: The visit of Mr. J. D. Scott, F.R.C.S., Director of Retina
                        Service, Adenbrooks Hospital, Cambridge, U.K.
                        To discuss the clinical problems of retinopathy.

Place:	The Ophthalmic Department, Ibn Sina Hospital.
Duration:	9 days, from 12th October, 1981—20th October, 1981.
Organiser:	Joint Board of Postgraduate Medical Education.
Programme Director:	Dr. S. M. M. Sheriff, M.B., F.R.C.S., D.O. (Lond.), Chairman of the Eye Department.
Participants:	Ophthalmologists and all doctors interested are invited to attend.
Programme:	

Monday, 12th October, 1981

7.30 a.m.—10.00 a.m.	Clinic
10.30 a.m.— 1.30 p.m.	Clinic

Tuesday, 13th October, 1981

7.30 a.m.—10.00 a.m.	Operating
10.30 a.m.— 1.30 p.m.	Operating

Wednesday, 14th October, 1981

7.30 a.m.—10.00 a.m.	Clinic
10.30 a.m.— 1.00 p.m.	Operating

Thursday, 15th October, 1981

7.30 a.m.—10.00 a.m.	Clinical demonstration
12.00 noon	Mr. John Scott's lecture on Use of Silicone Fluid in Retinal Surgery

Saturday, 17th October, 1981

7.30 a.m.—10.00 a.m.	Clinic
10.30 a.m.— 1.30 p.m.	Operating
6.30 p.m.	Mr. John Scott's lecture on Management of Diabetic Retinopathy

Sunday, 18th October, 1981

7.30 a.m.—10.00 a.m.	Clinic
10.30 a.m.— 1.30 p.m.	Operating

Monday, 19th October, 1981

7.30 a.m.—10.00 a.m.	Clinic
10.30 a.m.— 1.30 p.m.	Operating
6.30 p.m.	Mr. John Scott's lecture on Prophylaxis of Retinal Detachment

Tuesday, 20th October, 1981

7.30 a.m.—10.00 a.m.	Clinic
10.30 a.m.— 1.30 p.m.	Operating

81C—5403
Seminar on Ophthalmology

Objectives: The visit of Dr. W. M. Haining, F.R.C.S., Ophthalmic
                       Consultant.
                       To teach the advances in ophthalmology.

Place: Ophthalmic Department, Ibn Sina Hospital.

Duration: 10 days, 2nd November, 1981—14th November, 1981.

Organiser: Joint Board of Postgraduate Medical Education.

Programme Director: Dr. S. M. M. Sheriff, M.B., F.R.C.S., D.O. (Lond.),
                       Head of Eye Department.

Participants: Ophthalmologists and all interested doctors.

Programme:

                       Monday, 2nd November, 1981

6.00 p.m.—7.30 p.m.   Video Funduscopy and Fluroscopy
                       Lecture, Dr. Haining

                       Thursday, 5th November, 1981

12.00 p.m.—1.00 p.m.   Lens Implantation
                       Lecture, Dr. Haining

                       Monday, 9th November, 1981

6.00 p.m.—7.30 p.m.   Ocular Manifestations in Systemic Disease
                       Lecture, Dr. Haining

                       Thursday, 12th November, 1981

12.00 noon—1.00 p.m.   Photocoagulation
                       Lecture, Dr. Haining

81C—5404
Clinical Seminar on Ophthalmology

Objectives: The visit of Dr. Harvey Lincoff, M.D., Ophthalmic Sur-
                       geon, Retina Service, New York Hospital, and Cornell
                       School of Medicine.
                       To teach recent advances in the field of Ophthalmology.
                       To exchange experiences in clinical work.

Place: Ibn Sina Hospital.

Duration: 10 days, from 19th April, 1982—29th April, 1982.

Organiser: Discipline Committee for Surgery, Joint Board of Post-
                       graduate Education.

Programme Director: Dr. S. M. M. Sheriff, M.B., F.R.C.S., D.O. (Lond.),
                       Chairman of the Eye Department.

Participants: All Ophthalmologists in Kuwait.

Programme:

Monday, 19th April, 1982

7.30 a.m.—10.00 a.m.   Eye Clinic—to see cases and to hold clinical discussions

10.00 a.m.—1.30 p.m.   Eye Clinic—to see cases and to hold clinical discussions

6.00 p.m.   Lecture: the topic will be given later

Tuesday, 20th April, 1982

7.30 a.m.—10.00 a.m.   Eye Clinic—to see cases and to hold clinical discussions

10.00 a.m.—1.30 p.m.   Operations
6.00 p.m.   Lecture: the topic will be given later

Wednesday, 21st April, 1982

7.30 a.m.—10.00 a.m.   Eye Clinic—to see cases and to hold clinical discussions

10.00 a.m.—1.30 p.m.   Operations
6.00 p.m.   Lecture: the topic will be given later

Thursday, 22nd April, 1982

7.30 a.m.—9.30 a.m.   Referred cases from other departments
10.00 a.m.—12.00 noon   Clinical Meeting
12.00 noon—1.00 p.m.   Lecture: the topic will be given later

Saturday, 24th April, 1982

7.30 a.m.—10.00 a.m.   Eye Clinic—to see cases and to hold clinical discussions

10.00 a.m.—1.30 p.m.   Operations
6.00 p.m.   Lecture: the topic will be given later

Sunday, 25th April, 1982

7.30 a.m.—10.00 a.m.   Eye Clinic—to see cases and to hold clinical discussions

10.00 a.m.—1.30 p.m.   Operations
6.00 p.m.   Lecture: the topic will be given later

Monday, 26th April, 1982

7.30 a.m.—10.00 a.m.   Eye Clinic—to see cases and to hold clinical discussions

10.00 a.m.— 1.30 p.m.   Operations
6.00 p.m.   Lecture: the topic will be given later

Tuesday, 27th April, 1982

7.30 a.m.—10.00 a.m.   Eye Clinic—to see cases and to hold clinical discussions

| 10.00 a.m.—1.30 p.m. | Operations |
| 6.00 p.m. | Lecture: the topic will be given later |

Wednesday, 28th April, 1982

7.30 a.m.—10.00 a.m.	Eye Clinic—to see cases and to hold clinical discussion
10.00 a.m.—1.30 p.m.	Operations
6.00 p.m.	Lecture: the topic will be given later

Thursday, 29th April, 1982

7.30 a.m.—9.30 a.m.	Referred cases from other departments
10.00 a.m.—12.00 noon	Clinical Meeting
12.00 noon—1.00 p.m.	Lecture: the topic will be given later

81C—5405
Clinical Seminar on Ophthalmology

Objectives:	The visit of Dr. Jeff Davies, Consultant Ophthalmic Surgeon, Eye Department, Kings College Hospital, London, U.K.
	To teach recent advances in the field of Ophthalmology. To exchance experiences in clinical work.
Place:	Ibn Sina Hospital, Eye Clinic.
Duration:	12 days, from 8th May, 1982—20th May, 1982.
Organiser:	Discipline Committee for Surgery, Joint Board of Postgraduate Education.
Programme Director:	Dr. S. M. M. Sheriff, M.B., F.R.C.S., D.O. (Lond.), Chairman of the Eye Department.
Programme:	

Saturday, 8th May, 1982

7.30 a.m.—10.00 a.m.	Eye Clinic—to see cases and to hold clinical discussions
10.00 a.m.—1.30 p.m.	Eye Clinic—to see cases and to hold clinical discussions
6.00 p.m.	Lecture: the topic will be given later

Sunday, 9th May, 1982

7.30 a.m.—10.00 a.m.	Eye Clinic—to see cases and to hold clinical discussions
10.00 a.m.—1.30 p.m.	Operations
6.00 p.m.	Lecture: the topic will be given later

Monday, 10th May, 1982

| 7.30 a.m.—10.00 a.m. | Eye Clinic—to see cases and to hold clinical discussions |

10.00 a.m.—1.30 p.m.	Operations
6.00 p.m.	Lecture: the topic will be given later

Tuesday, 11th May, 1982

7.30 a.m.—10.00 a.m.	Eye Clinic—to see cases and to hold clinical discussions
10.00 a.m.—1.30 p.m.	Operations
6.00 p.m.	Lecture: the topic will be given later

Wednesday, 12th May, 1982

7.30 a.m.—10.00 a.m.	Eye Clinic—to see cases and to hold clinical discussions
10.00 a.m.—1.00 p.m.	Operations
6.00 p.m.	Lecture: the topic will be given later

Thursday, 13th May, 1982

7.30 a.m.—9.30 a.m.	Referred cases from other departments
10.00 a.m.—12.00 noon	Clinical Meeting
12.00 noon—1.00 p.m.	Lecture: the topic will be given later

Saturday, 15th May, 1982

7.30 a.m.—10.00 a.m.	Eye Clinic—to see cases and to hold clinical discussions
10.00 a.m.—1.30 p.m.	Operations
6.00 p.m.	Lecture: the topic will be given later

Sunday, 16th May, 1982

7.30 a.m.—10.00 a.m.	Eye Clinic—to see cases and to hold clinical discussions
10.00 a.m.—1.30 p.m.	Operations
6.00 p.m.	Lecture: the topic will be given later

Monday, 17th May, 1982

7.30 a.m.—10.00 a.m.	Eye Clinic—to see cases and to hold clinical discussions
10.00 a.m.—1.30 p.m.	Operations
6.00 p.m.	Lecture: the topic will be given later

Tuesday, 18th May, 1982

7.30 a.m.—10.00 a.m.	Eye Clinic—to see cases and to hold clinical discussions
10.00 a.m.—1.30 p.m.	Operations
6.00 p.m.	Lecture: the topic will be given later

Wednesday, 19th May, 1982

7.30 a.m.—10.00 a.m.	Eye Clinic—to see cases and to hold clinical discussions
10.00 a.m.—1.30 p.m.	Operations
6.00 p.m.	Lecture: the topic will be given later

Thursday, 20th May, 1982

7.30 a.m.—9.30 a.m.	Referred cases from other departments
10.00 a.m.—12.00 noon	Clinical meetings
12.00 noon—1.00 p.m.	Lecture: the topic will be given later

81C—5601
Seminar on Dermatology

Objectives: The visit of Prof. Henry Menn from Miami University.

Place: Department of Dermatology, Sabah Hospital.

Duration: 3 days from Saturday the 18th of April, 1981, to Monday the 20th of April, 1981.

Organiser: Training Division in collaboration with D.C.F.M.

Programme Director: Dr. M. M. Selim, M.D.

Participants: Consultants and registrars in dermatology, Physicians preparing for Part I, M.R.C.P.

Programme: Round table discussion,
clinical consultations.
2 lectures, one on cutaneous manifestations of systemic diseases and the other on chemosurgery of cutaneous cancer.
Round table discussions covering plans for Kuwait Dermatology Center, the situation of post-graduate education in dermatology, Kuwait and fields where further future cooperation could be established.

81C—56/7902
Medical Mycology

Objectives: The visit of Professor Paul H. Jacobs, Stanford University.
To train participants in diagnosis and management of dermatophytosis.

Place: Kuwait University, Medical Faculty, Lecture Room No. 106, MDL No. 1.

Duration: 5 days, from 9th January, 1982—12th January, 1982.

Organiser: Discipline Committee for Medicine.

Programme Director: Dr. M. M. Selim, M.D.
Dr. Karol Kleibl, M.D., Ph.D., Co-Director.

Participants: Dermatologists, Microbiologists, Pathologists, Paediatricians, Internists, General Practitioners, Medical Students, Selected Technicians.

Programme:

Friday, 8th January, 1982

Arrival and preparation of material for the course

Saturday, 9th January, 1982

Morning
5.00 p.m.—8.00 p.m.

Preparation of material for the course
Introduction to medical mycology:
classification, epidemiology, diagnostic tests, therapeutic considerations, new trends and immunological methods in medical mycology, self-assessment

Sunday, 10th January, 1982

5.00 p.m.—8.00 p.m.

Superficial dermatophyte infections.
Yeast-like organisms.
Practical demonstrations. Self-assessment.

Monday, 11th January, 1982

5.00 p.m.—8.00 p.m.

The problem of T. versicolor in tropical areas. Tinea nigra. Sub-cutaneous infections: sporotrichosis, chromoblastomycosis. Practical demonstrations. Self-assessment

Tuesday, 12th January, 1982

5.00 p.m.—8.00 p.m.

The systemic mycosis:
Coccidiodomycosis, Histoplasmosis, North and South American Blastomycosis, Cryptococcosis, Mycetomas, Actinomycosis, Nocardiosis, Self-assessment.
Round table discussion

N.B.

1. The practical sessions with the assistance of Mrs. Jacobs will be conducted with 100 slides of histopathological material demonstrating the morphology and special staining characteristics and direct preparations from fungal colonies.
2. A handout will be prepared by Prof. Jacobs for duplication.

81C—5603
Seminar on Dermatology

Objectives:

The visit of Professor Malcolm Greaves.
To participate in continuing medical education, postgraduate teaching in dermatology and advice regarding current research and patient care.

Place: Department of Dermatology, Al-Sabah Hospital.

Duration: 6 days, from 6th February, 1982—11th February, 1982.

Organiser: Discipline Committee for Medicine.

Programme Director: Dr. M. M. Selim, M.D.

Participants: Residents and Registrars in Dermatology, Interested Physicians, Medical Students.

Programme:

Saturday, 6th February 1982

8.00 a.m.—12.00 noon   Outpatient
(for consultation)
Khaldeyah Skin Clinic

5.00 p.m.— 6.00 p.m.   Lecture: What is New in Dermatology
(for dermatologists)
Khaldeyah Skin Clinic

Sunday, 7th February, 1982

8.00 a.m.—12.00 noon   Outpatient
(for consultation)
Khaldeyah Skin Clinic

5.00 p.m.— 6.00 p.m.   Lecture: The Skin and Disorders of Metabolism
(dermatologists and interested physicians)
Khaldeyah Skin Clinic

Monday, 8th February, 1982

8.00 a.m.—12.00 noon   Outpatient
(for consultation)
Amiri State Hospital, Skin Outpatients

Tuesday, 9th February, 1982

8.00 a.m.—12.00 noon   Round table discussion about research and cutaneous medicine
(for consultants)
Light Therapy Unit (Khawla)

5.00 p.m.— 6.00 p.m.   Lecture: Skin Markers of Endocrine Diseases
(dermatologists and interested physicians)
Khaldeyah Skin Clinic

Wednesday, 10th February, 1982

8.00 a.m.—12.00 noon   Outpatient
(for consultation)
Amiri State Hospital, Skin Outpatients

5.00 p.m.— 6.00 p.m.   Lecture: Rational Basis in Antihistamine Therapy
(dermatologists and interested physicians)
Khaldeyah Skin Clinic

Thursday, 11th February, 1982

8.00 a.m.—12.00 noon   Grand round
(dermatologists)
Light Therapy Unit (Khawla)

81C—5901
The Neurology Seminars

Objectives:	The visit of Dr. I. T. Draper, M.D., F.R.C.P., Consultant Neurologist, Southern General Hospital, Glasgow. To teach advances in neurology.
Place (Venue):	Al-Sabah Hospital, Ibn Sina Hospital, Farwania Hospital, Faculty of Medicine, Lecture Room 105.
Duration:	9 days, 14th—22nd March, 1981.
Organiser:	Ministry of Public Health.
Programme Director:	Prof. F. Fenech, Chairman of Medicine, Al-Sabah Hospital.
Participants:	The physicians of the above-mentioned hospitals, the neurologists and doctors participating in M.R.C.P. Part I Course, in M.R.C.P. Part II Course.

Programme:

Saturday, 14th March, 1981

11.00 a.m.	Neuro-Radiology Meeting, Radiology Department, Al-Sabah Hospital
5.30 p.m.	Lecture (M.R.C.P. Part I Course) Multiple Sclerosis Lecture Room 105, Faculty of Medicine

Sunday, 15th March, 1981

9.00 a.m.	Visit to Farwania Hospital (Dr. Ashmawi) Lecture Topic to be decided by Dr. Draper Teaching Ward Round

Monday, 16th March, 1981

9.00 a.m.	Postgraduate Teaching Round, Ward 2, Al-Sabah (Dr. Shakir)
11.30 a.m.	Visit to Ibn Sina Hospital (Dr. R. Shakir)
5.00 p.m.	Neurology Slide Show (M.R.C.P. Part II Course), Lecture Room 105, Faculty of Medicine

Tuesday, 17th March, 1981

9.30 a.m.	Outpatient Clinic, Al-Sabah Hospital (Dr. R. Shakir)
12.00 noon	Clinical Meeting, Seminar Room, Al-Sabah Hospital

Wednesday, 18th March, 1981

9.30 a.m.	Undergraduate Teaching Ward Round, Ward 2, Al-Sabah Hospital (Dr. Ghasan)

5.30 p.m.	Lecture (M.R.C.P. Part I Course) Extrapyramidal Syndrome Lecture Room 105, Faculty of Medicine

Thursday, 19th March, 1981

10.00 a.m.	Clinical Session (M.R.C.P. Part II Course) Ward 3, Al-Sabah Hospital

Saturday, 21st March, 1981

9.30 a.m.	Undergraduate Teaching Ward Round Ward 5, Al-Sabah Hospital (Dr. Karnik)
12.30 p.m.	Lunch at Faculty Club
5.30 p.m.	Lecture (M.R.C.P. Part I Course) Muscle Disorders and Myasthenia Lecture Room 105 Faculty of Medicine

81C—5902
Neurological Seminar

Objectives:	The Visit of Dr. J. P. Ballantyne, Consultant Neurologist, Southern General Hospital, Glasgow, Scotland. To teach recent advances in neurology.
Place:	Ibn Sina Hospital, Mubarak Al-Kabir Hospital, Ahmadi Hospital, Adan Hospital.
Duration:	8 days, from 20th—27th March, 1982.
Organiser:	Joint Board for Postgraduate Medical Education.
Programme Director:	Prof. F. F. Fenech, Chairman of the Department of Medicine, Al-Sabah Hospital and Dr. R. A. Shakir, Head of the Neurology Unit.
Participants:	Neurologists and internists, training doctors (M.R.C.P. Part I Course, M.R.C.P. Part II Course) attending lectures, clinical rounds and instruction sessions.
Programme:	

20th March, 1982 (Saturday)

9.00 a.m.	Meeting with Dr. R. A. Shakir Ibn Sina Hospital Grand Round and X-Ray meeting
5.30 p.m.	Lecture (M.R.C.P. Part I Course) Topic: Demyelinating Disease

21st March, 1982 (Sunday)

9.00 a.m.	Meeting with Professor F. F. Fenech Department of Medicine

Mubarak Al-Kabir Hospital
Teaching Ward Round

22nd March, 1982 (Monday)

9.00 a.m.	Outpatient Session Ibn Sina Hospital
5.00 a.m.—6.00 p.m.	M.R.C.P. Part II Course Neurology—Slides

23rd March, 1982 (Tuesday)

10.30 a.m.	Visit to Ahmadi Hospital (Dr. J. G. Lloyd) and Kuwait Oil Company Complex Lunch and Lecture at Ahmadi— Topic to be chosen by lecturer.

24th March, 1982 (Wednesday)

9.00 a.m.	Mubarak Al-Kabir Hospital Teaching Ward Round
12.00 noon	Clinical Meeting
5.30 p.m.	Lecture, M.R.C.P. Part I Course Topic: Neuromuscular Disorders

25th March, 1982 (Thursday)

10.00 a.m.	M.R.C.P. Part II Course Mock Clinical Session Adan Hospital (Dr. M. K. Emara)

27th March, 1982 (Saturday)

9.00 a.m.	Ibn Sina Hospital Grand Round and X-Ray Meeting
4.30 a.m.—5.30 p.m.	M.R.C.P. Part I Course Topic: Extrapyramidal Syndromes

81C—5903
Seminar on Neurology

Objectives:	The visit of Dr. Nobel David, Miami University. To teach recent advances in the field of neurology.
Place:	Al-Sabah Hospital, Ibn Sina Hospital, Jahra Hospital, Farwania Hospital, Al-Adan Hospital.
Duration:	6 days, from 12th June, 1982—17th June, 1982.
Organiser:	Training Division in cooperation with the Office of International Medical Education, University of Miami.
Programme Director:	Dr. R. A. Shakir.
Participants:	The course is aimed at neurologists and doctors interested in neurology.

Programme:

12th June, 1982 (Saturday)

8.30 a.m.	Ibn Sina Hospital Ward 4 Ward Round
10.30 a.m.	X-Ray Meeting

13th June, 1982 (Sunday)

8.30 a.m.	Ibn Sina Hospital Ward 4 Students' Clinical Teaching

14th June, 1982 (Monday)

8.30 a.m.	Adan Hospital Dr. Amin Marafio

15th June, 1982 (Tuesday)

8.30 a.m.	Ibn Sina Hospital Ward 4 Clinical Case Presentation

16th June, 1982 (Wednesday)

10.30 a.m.	Mubarak Al-Kabir Hospital Dr. R. Shakir
12.00 noon	Clinical Meeting Medicine Department Mubarak Al-Kabir Hospital

17th June, 1982 (Thursday)

9.00 a.m.	To visit Farwania Hospital
10.00 a.m.	Panel discussion in Farwania Hospital on Family Doctor Practice in Neurology Chairman: Dr. R. A. Shakir Members: Dr. Nobel David Dr. Saad Zaghloul Dr. Ashmawi Abdel Wahab Dr. Farouk Al Kayzi, from Ibn Sina Hospital

81C—6101
Seminar on Psychiatry

Objectives:	The visit of Burton J. Goldstein, Miami University. To teach recent advances in the field of psychiatry and the behavioural sciences.
Place:	Lecture Room, Al-Sabah Hospital.

Duration:	6 days, from 1st May, 1982—6th May, 1982.
Organiser:	Training Division in cooperation with the Office of International Medical Education, University of Miami.
Programme Director:	Prof. M. F. El-Islam, F.R.C.P., F.R.C. Psych.
Participants:	The course is aimed at psychiatrists and doctors interested in psychiatry and the behavioural sciences.
Programme:	

Saturday, 1st May, 1982

9.00 a.m.—12.00 noon   Clinical Teaching (Inpatients)

Sunday, 2nd May, 1982

9.00 a.m.—11.00 a.m.   Clinical Teaching (Outpatients)
11.00 a.m.—12.00 noon   Dr. Burton J. Goldstein, M.D.,
lecture on: Psychopharmacology

Monday, 3rd May, 1982

9.00 a.m.—12.00 noon   Clinical Teaching (Inpatients)

Tuesday, 4th May, 1982

9.00 a.m.—12.00 noon   Clinical Teaching (Outpatients)

Wednesday, 5th May, 1982

9.00 a.m.—12.00 noon   Clinical Teaching (Inpatients)

Thursday, 6th May, 1982

9.00 a.m.—10.00 a.m.   Lecture 2
10.00 a.m.—11.00 a.m.   Open Discussion

Remark: Clinical Teaching includes bedside teaching, ward rounds, case conferences and individual case consultations.

81C—6301
Radiological Seminar

Objectives:	The visit of Professor Uno Erickson, Head of the Department of Diagnostic Radiology, Uppsala University. To discuss the organisational conditions for Kuwait X-Ray departments. To get advice on principles and facilities for the postgraduate teaching of Kuwait radiologists.
Place (Venue):	Mubarak Hospital, Sabha Hospital, Chest Hospital, Ibn Sina Hospital, Adan Hospital, Farwania Hospital and Al-Jahra Hospital.
Duration:	7 days, from 13th January, 1982 till 19th January, 1982.

Organiser:	Discipline Committee for Radiology.
Programme Director:	Prof. Dr. Leo Steinhart.
Participants:	Radiologists, selected technicians.
Programme:	

Wednesday, 13th January, 1982

Arrival and preparation of material for the seminar

Thursday, 14th January, 1982

9.00 a.m.— 2.00 p.m.	Visit to the Chest Hospital (Cardiology) Mubarak Hospital
8.00 p.m.	Social arrangement Dinner in Marriot Hotel

Friday, 15th January, 1982

Social programme arranged by the Public Relation Office of the Ministry of Public Health

Saturday, 16th January, 1982

8.00 a.m.— 2.00 p.m.	Visit to Mubarak Hospital or Chest Hospital

Sunday, 17th January, 1982

8.00 a.m.— 2.00 p.m.	Visit to Sabah Hospital and Ibn Sina Hospital

Monday, 18th January, 1982

8.00 a.m.— 2.00 p.m.	Visit to Adan Hospital and Farwania Hospital

Tuesday, 19th January, 1982

8.00 a.m.— 2.00 p.m.	Visit to Jahra Hospital
6.00 p.m.	Meeting in Mubarak: to discuss the ideas and proposals of Prof. Erickson

81C—63/3302
Seminar on Paediatric Radiology

Objectives:	The visit of Dr. Richard Heller Professor of Paediatric Radiology Director Paediatric Radiology Vanderbilt University, Nashville, Tennessee, U.S.A. To teach recent advances in paediatrics radiology.
Place:	Auditorium Al-Mubarak Hospital.
Duration:	2nd March, 1982—10th March, 1982.
Organiser:	Discipline Committee for Radiology.
Programme Director:	Dr. M. A. Rudwan.

Participants:	Radiologists, all doctors are cordially invited. Professor Hellar will be available for consultations in the Radiology Dept., Ibn Sina Hospital. Visits to other hospitals have been arranged.

Programme:

2nd March, 1982 (Tuesday)

5.30 p.m.   Paediatric Radiology in Music City
U.S.A. (Nashville, Tennessee), and an evaluation of the newborn with an abdominal mass

3rd March, 1982 (Wednesday)

5.30 p.m.   Hirschsprung's Disease

6th March, 1982 (Saturday)

. 5.30 p.m.   Wilm's Tumour and the newborn with respiratory distress

7th March, 1982 (Sunday)

5.30 p.m.   Paediatric fractures and the battered child

8th March, 1982 (Monday)

5.30 p.m.   Fundamentals of Paediatric G.I. Radiology

9th March, 1982 (Tuesday)

5.30 p.m.   Paediatric Pulmonary Disease

10th March, 1982 (Wednesday)

5.30 p.m.   Paediatric radiology quiz and review

81C—6303
Seminar on Radiology

Objectives:	The visit of Dr. Russel, Miami University. To teach recent advances in the field of radiology.
Place:	Al-Adan Hospital, Mubarak Hospital, Sabah Hospital, Jahra Hospital, Farwania Hospital.
Duration:	6 days, from 19th June, 1982—24th June, 1982.
Organiser:	Training Division in cooperation with the Office of International Medical Education, University of Miami.
Programme Director:	Dr. Mohi Al Din Al Tamani.
Participants:	The course is aimed at radiologists and doctors interested in clinical radiology.

Programme:

Saturday, 19th June, 1982

9.00 a.m.	To meet Dr. Mohi Al Din Al Tamani
	Head, Radiology Dept., Al-Adan Hospital
10.00 a.m.	Clinical Session with Dr. Al Tamani

Sunday, 20th June, 1982

8.30 a.m.	To meet Prof. Leo Steinhart, Chairman
	Radiology, Mubarak Hospital
9.00 a.m.	Clinical Session with Prof. Leo Steinhart
12.00 noon	Dr. Edward Russell, lecture on:
	Special Procedures Radiologist
	(angiographers)
	Lecture Room, Mubarak Hospital

Monday, 21st June, 1982

9.00 a.m.	Clinical Session with
	Dr. Hosam Bassioni—Medical Building
	Dr. M. Radwan—Ibn Sina Hospital
12.00 noon	Dr. Edward Russell, lecture on:
	Surgical Radiology
	Sabah Hospital

Tuesday, 22nd June, 1982

10.00 a.m.	Clinical Session with
	Dr. Mohammed Zahran, Jahra Hospital

Wednesday, 23rd June, 1982

10.00 a.m.	Clinical Session with
	Dr. Mohammed Shafeeq, Farwania Hospital

Thursday, 24th June, 1982

9.00 a.m.	To visit Farwania Hospital
10.30 a.m.	Panel discussion in Farwania Hospital on
	Family Doctor Practice with Radiology
	Chairman: Dr. M. D. Al Tamani
	Members: Dr. E. Russell
	Dr. Saad Zaghloul
	Dr. M. Shafeeq

81C—67/1201
Overview of Nuclear Medicine

Objectives: The visit of Dr. M. N. Maisey, M.D., F.R.C.P., Director, Department of Nuclear Medicine, Guy's Hospital, London.
To teach advances in the field of Nuclear Medicine.
To give lectures for the M.R.C.P. Part I Course and the M.R.C.P. Part II Course.

Place (Venue):	Al-Sabah Hospital, Ahmadi Hospital, Mubarak Medical School and Al-Adan Hospital.
Duration:	One week from 21st—27th March, 1981.
Organiser:	Ministry of Public Health.
Programme Director:	Prof. F. F. Fenech, Chairman of the Department of Medicine, Al-Sabah Hospital.
Participants:	The physicians of the above-mentioned hospitals, doctors participating in the M.R.C.P. Part I Course, the M.R.C.P. Part II Course and undergraduates.

Programme:

Saturday, 21st March, 1981

10.00 a.m.	Visit to Radiotherapy Department (Dr. Yusuf Omar) Al-Sabah Hospital
5.30 p.m.	Lecture (M.R.C.P. Part I Course) Thyroid Disease—Diagnostic and Management Aspects Lecture Room 105 Faculty of Medicine

Sunday, 22nd March, 1981

10.30 a.m.	Visit to Ahmadi Hospital and Kuwait Oil Company Complex Lunch and Lecture at Ahmadi— topic to be chosen by Dr. Maisey

Monday, 23rd March, 1981

11.00 a.m.	Visit to Mubarak Medical School with Professor Fenech and Mr. Ronald Johnson (Meet in Mr. Johnson's Office, Faculty of Medicine)
1.00 p.m.	Cardiac Meeting (Chest Hospital) Cardiac Imaging (Professor A. M. Yousof)
5.00 p.m.	M.R.C.P. Part II Neuroendocrinology Data Lecture Room 105 Faculty of Medicine

Tuesday, 24th March, 1981

12.00 noon	Clinical Meeting Overview of Nuclear Medicine Seminar Room, Department of Medicine Al-Sabah Hospital

Wednesday, 25th March, 1981

9.00 a.m.	Nuclear Medicine Department Radiotherapy Department, Al-Sabah

5.30 p.m.   Lecture (M.R.C.P. Part I Course)
                               Role of Nuclear Medicine
                               Lecture Room 105
                               Faculty of Medicine

                               Thursday, 26th March, 1981

10.00 a.m.   Mock Clinicals (M.R.C.P. Part II Course)
                               Adan Hospital

81C—67/6502
Nuclear Medicine and its Clinical Application

Objectives: To deliver a series of lectures to inform members of the
                              medical profession of the capabilities and limitations of
                              nuclear medicine in clinical practice, and to make them
                              aware of the availability of some investigative proce-
                              dures and their correct application.

Place: Lecture Room
                              Radiotherapy and Radioisotope Department, Sabah
                              Hospital.

Duration: 3 months, from 19th December, 1981 to 12th March,
                              1982.

Organiser: Radiotherapy and Radioisotope Department with
                              cooperation of Discipline Committee for Medicine.

Programme   Director: Dr. Y. T. Omar, Head of Radiotherapy Dept.
                              Sabah Hospital.

Lecturer: Prof. Dr. Hussein Abdel Daiem

Participants: All interested members of the medical profession in dif-
                              ferent medical and surgical specialities.

Programme: A series of lectures on nuclear medicine and its clinical
                              application according to the following programme:

                              Sunday, 19th December, 1981

12.00 noon—1.00 p.m.   Bone Scanning I
                              Pharmaceuticals and Clinical Applications

                              Sunday, 26th December, 1982

12.00 noon—1.00 p.m.   Bone Scanning II
                              Role in Orthopaedic Problems

                              Sunday, 2nd January, 1982

12.00 noon—1.00 p.m.   Tumour Seeking Agents

Sunday, 9th January, 1982

12.00 noon—1.00 p.m.   Gallium Imaging
                              Relation with CT Scanning

Sunday, 16th January, 1982

12.00 noon—1.00 p.m.   Deep Venous Thrombosis

Sunday, 30th January, 1982

12.00 noon—1.00 p.m.   Pulmonary Perfusion and Ventilation

Sunday, 5th February, 1982

12.00 noon—1.00 p.m.   Myocardial Imaging

Sunday, 12th February, 1982

12.00 noon—1.00 p.m.   Brain Flow and Scanning
                              Post and Present Status

Sunday, 5th March, 1982

12.00 noon—1.00 p.m.   Evaluation of Renal Flow

Sunday, 12th March, 1982

12.00 noon—1.00 p.m.   Blood Pool Studies

81C—65/0903
Cancer Education and Control

Objectives: To survey the recent advances in the field of oncology.
                           To explore the problems of cancer education and con-
                           trol.

Place: Mubarak Hospital Auditorium.

Duration: 5 days, from 23rd till 27th January 1982.

Organiser: Discipline Committee for Medicine and Department of
                           Radiotherapy, Sabah Hospital.

Programme Director: Dr. Y. T. Omar with cooperation of Dr. J. Brousil, Dr.
                           R. Morrison, and Dr. M. S. Motawi.

Guest Lecturers: Dr. T. B. Brewin, Deputy Director
                           Institute of Radiotherapy and Oncology
                           Western Infirmary, Glasgow, U.K.

                           Dr. Z. Dienstbier
                           Director, Institute of Biophysics and Nuclear Medi-
                           cine, Charles University, Prague, Czechoslovakia

                           Dr. M. G. Hanna
                           Director, Frederick Cancer Research
                           Centre, Maryland
                           U.S.A.

Dr. G. O'Conor
Director, International Affairs
National Cancer Institute
Bethesda, Maryland, U.S.A.

Dr. L. Price
Consultant Medical Oncologist
Institute of Cancer Research, London

Dr. Vang
Chairman, Department of Surgery
Central Hospital, Eskjo, Sweden

Dr. U. Veronesi, President, U.I.C.C.
Director, Institute Nazionale per lo
Studio e la Cura dei Tumori, Milan, Italy

Local Lecturers: Dr. G. M. Abouna
Professor of Surgery and Head
of Transplant Unit, Medical School

Dr. S. M. Ali
Chairman, Department of Pathology
Sabah Hospital

Dr. M. Y. Ali
Chairman and Professor of Pathology
Medical School

Dr. J. Brousil
Consultant, Nuclear Medicine
Dept. of Radiotherapy, Sabah Hospital

Dr. B. Eklof
Chairman and Professor of Surgery
Medical School

Dr. N. El-Naqeeb
Undersecretary
Ministry of Public Health

Dr. F. F. Fenech
Chairman and Professor of Medicine
Medical School

Dr. H. Hathout
Chairman and Professor of Gynaecology
Medical School

Dr. J. Mayza
Consultant Oncological Surgeon
Mubarak Hospital

Dr. R. Morrison
Consultat Radiotherapist
Dept. of Radiotherapy
Sabah Hospital

Dr. M. S. Motawi
Consultant Radiotherapist
Dept. of Radiotherapy
Sabah Hospital

Dr. Y. T. Omar
Chairman, Department of Radiotherapy
Sabah Hospital

Prof. E. Ruzyllo
Head of Training Division
Dept. of Public Health and Planning

Dr. L. Steinhart
Chairman and Professor of Radiology
Medical School

Dr. A. M. Yousof
Dean. Medical School
Kuwait University

Participants: It is addressed to various medical disciplines involved in oncology and to anyone who may be interested in the proposed programme.

Programme:

Saturday, 23rd January, 1982

4.00 p.m.   Dr. L. A. Price
Tumour Growth Kinetics and its Effect on Therapy and Prognosis

4.30 p.m.   Dr. U. Veronesi
Presentation of Thyroid Carcinoma
Dr. H. Hathout
Cancer Cervix in Kuwait
Dr. Na'il Al Naqeeb
Personal Experience with Head and Neck Cancer

6.00 p.m.   *Panel:*
Multidisciplinary Management in Cancer
Moderator:
Dr. U. Veronesi
Discussents:
Dr. M. G. Hanna
Dr. M. S. Motawi
Dr. L. A. Price
Dr. U. Veronesi

Sunday, 24th January, 1982

4.00 p.m.   Dr. U. Veronesi
Melanoma
Dr. M. G. Hanna
Status of Immunotherapy in Cancer Management

5.00 p.m.   Dr. L. A. Price
Increasing Potential for Curability of Head and Neck Tumours
Dr. R. Morrison
Combination of CT and RT in Squamous Cell Carcinoma of Head and Neck

6.00 p.m.   *Panel:*
                             Cancer Undergraduate Education
                             Moderator:
                             Dr. B. Eklof
                             Discussents:
                             Dr. G. M. Abouna
                             Dr. T. B. Brewin
                             Dr. Z. Dienstbier
                             Dr. U. Veronesi

                             Monday, 25th January, 1982

4.00 p.m.   Dr. T. B. Brewin
                             Comparing Response Rates and Assessment of Results
4.30 p.m.   Dr. M. S. Motawi
                             Childhood Hodgkin's Disease
                             Dr. U. Veronesi
                             Breast Cancer
                             Dr. O'Conor
                             International Collaboration in Cancer
6.00 p.m.   *Panel:*
                             Cancer Post-Graduate Education
                             Moderator:
                             Dr. A. M. Yousof
                             Discussants:
                             Dr. Morrison
                             Dr. Na'il Al Naqeeb
                             Dr. L. A. Price
                             Prof. E. Ruzyllo
                             Dr. A. R. Yousof

                             Tuesday, 26th January, 1982

4.00 p.m.   Dr. G. O'Conor
                             Development of Cancer Programme
4.30 p.m.   Dr. Y. T. Omar
                             Cancer Registry
                             Dr. A. Modtjabai
                             WHO and Cancer Control
                             Dr. L. Lindberg
                             Cytology in Cancer Control
6.00 p.m.   *Panel:*
                             Cancer Centre Organisation
                             Moderator:
                             Dr. Na'il Al Naqeeb
                             Discussents:
                             Dr. J. Mayza
                             Dr. R. Morrison
                             Dr. G. O'Conor
                             Dr. Y. T. Omar
                             Dr. U. Veronesi

Wednesday, 27th January, 1982

4.00 p.m.	Dr. Z. Dienstbier Role of Nuclear Medicine in Cancer Management with Particular Reference to Hodgkin's Disease
4.30 p.m.	Dr. M. G. Hanna Active Specific Immunotherapy in Colorectal Cancer Dr. J. Brousil Computer Contribution to the Enhancement of Reliability of Nuclear Medicine Examinations in Oncology
6.00 p.m.	*Panel:* Cost Benefit Analysis *Moderator:* Dr. Y. T. Omar *Discussants:* Dr. M. Y. Ali Dr. T. B. Brewin Dr. L. Steinhart Dr. Johannes Vang

81C—6901
Advances in Anaesthesia and Intensive Care

Objectives:	The visit of Professor Jordanov, Professor of Anaesthesia and I.C.U., and Chairman of Postgraduate Education Board, Sofia, Bulgaria. To see and discuss the advances in Anaesthesia and I.C.U., in Kuwait especially in the New Hospitals. Interchange of ideas with the senior consultants and members of the Standing Committee for Anaesthesia on Post-Graduate Training and continuing medical education.
Place:	Al-Sabah Hospital Maternity, Chest Diseases, Suliebekhat, Gahra, Adan, Farwania, Ibn Sina and Mubarak Hospitals.
Duration:	31 days from 17th of February till 20th March 1981.
Organiser:	Ministry of Public Health.
Programme Director:	Dr. Mohamed M. Motaweh, Chairman, Department of Anaesthesia, Sabah, Chest Diseases and Infectious Diseases Hospitals.
Participants:	All anaesthetists in the above-mentioned hospitals.
Programme:	

18th February, 1981 (Wednesday)

11.00 a.m.	Department of Anaesthesia Dr. M. M. Motaweh, Sabah Hospital

19th February, 1981 (Thursday)

9.00 a.m.—11 a.m.   Meeting
Dr. M. M. Motaweh, Sabah Hospital

20th February, 1981 (Friday)

Weekly Holiday

21st February, 1981 (Saturday)

9.00 a.m.— 1.00 p.m.   Visit to Theatres
Dr. A. M. Obeid Discussion: Organisation and equipment of the Department of Anaesthesia, Ibn Sina Hospital

22nd February, 1981 (Sunday)

9.00 a.m.— 1.00 p.m.   Visit to I.C.U., Dr. A. M. Obeid
Visit round the Hospital
Discussion: Anaesthesia for Ophthalmic Surgery—
Anaesthesia for Outpatients and Day Cases Ibn Sina
Hospital

23rd February, 1981 (Monday)

9.00 a.m.— 1.00 p.m.   Visit to Faculty of Medicine
Kuwait University

24th February, 1981 (Tuesday)

Meeting with Undersecretary
Health Ministry

28th February, 1981 (Saturday)

9.00 a.m.— 1.00 p.m.   Operating List, Dr. Khairy Nagib
Farwania Hospital

1st March, 1981 (Sunday)

9.00 a.m.— 1.00 p.m.   Dr. Khairy Nagib, I.C.U.
Scientific Meeting: Recent Developments of New Mus-
cle Relaxant Drugs. Basic Characteristics in Animal
Experiments and Clinical Practice, Farwania Hospital

2nd March, 1981 (Monday)

9.00 a.m.— 1.00 p.m.   Scientific Meeting, El-Gahra Hospital

3rd March, 1981 (Tuesday)

9.00 a.m.— 1.00 p.m.   Operation Theatre, Neurosurgery
Sabah Hospital

4th March, 1981 (Wednesday)

9.00 a.m.— 1.00 p.m.   Dr. Khairy Nagib, Operating List
Discussion:
Organisation and Equipment of Department of Anaesthesia.
Anaesthesia for Outpatients and Day Cases
Farwania Hospital

5th March, 1981 (Thursday)

9.00 a.m.—10.00 a.m.   Dr. Khairy Nagib, Lecture Scientific Meeting
Recent Advances in Treatment of Chest Injuries
Farwania Hospital

7th March, 1981 (Saturday)

9.00 a.m.— 1.00 p.m.   Orthopaedic Surgery, Dr. Omran Quader
Discussion: Anaesthesia for Ophthalmic Surgery Suliebekhat Hospital

8th March, 1981 (Sunday)

9.00 a.m.— 1.00 p.m.   Ophthalmic Surgery, Dr. Omran Quader
Suliebekhat Hospital

9th March, 1981 (Monday)

9.00 a.m.— 1.00 p.m.   Dr. Mayan Yacoub
Visit round the Theatres and I.C.U.
Mubarak Hospital

10th March, 1981 (Tuesday)

9.00 a.m.— 1.00 p.m.   Operation List Dr. A. G. El-Gohary
Discussion: Organisation and Equipment of Department of Anaesthesia
Adan Hospital

11th March, 1981 (Wednesday)

9.00 a.m.— 1.00 p.m.   Visit to I.C.U., Dr. A. G. El-Gohary
Discussion: Long Term Respiratory Care
Main Problems and Their Management
Adan Hospital

12th March, 1981 (Thursday)

9.00 a.m.— 1.00 p.m.   Scientific Meeting, Dr. A. G. El-Gohary
Recent Advances in Treatment of Chest Injuries
Adan Hospital

14th March, 1981 (Saturday)

9.00 a.m.— 1.00 p.m.   Dr. M. M. Motaweh
Operation Theatre
Discussion: Anaesthesia for Outpatients and Day Cases
Sabah Hospital

15th March, 1981 (Sunday)

9.00 a.m.— 1.00 p.m.	Dr. M. M. Motaweh Open Cardiac Surgery, Session Visit to I.C.U., Chest Disease Hospital

16th March, 1981 (Monday)

9.00 a.m.—11.00 a.m.	Operation List, Dr. A. S. Okasha Maternity Hospital
11.00 a.m.— 1.00 p.m.	Visit to the Ministry of Health

17th March, 1981 (Tuesday)

9.00 a.m.—11.00 a.m.	I.C.U.—Discussion, Dr. A. S. Okasha Respiratory Insufficiency and Failure Maternity Hospital
11.00 a.m.— 1.00 p.m.	Neurosurgical Theatre Dr. M. M. Motawah, Sabah Hospital

18th March, 1981 (Wednesday)

9.00 a.m.— 1.00 p.m.	Dr. H. A. F. Yousef Scientific Meeting: Long Term Respiratory Care, Main Problems and Their Management Modern Trends in Anaesthetic Techniques Organisation and Equipment of the Department of Anaesthesia Gahara Hospital

19th March, 1981 (Thursday)

8.00 a.m.— 9.00 a.m.	Scientific Meeting Recent Trends in I.C.U. Centralisation Dr. M. M. Motaweh, Sabah Hospital
9.30 a.m.—10.30 a.m.	Post-Graduate Training and Teaching in Anaesthesia, Dr. M. M. Motaweh Sabah Hospital

81C—69/24/4502
Recent Advances in Open Heart Surgery, Anaesthesia and Intensive Care

Objectives:	The visit of Dr. John Simpson, FFARCS., Senior Consultant, Anaesthetist, National Heart Hospital, London, U.K. To teach the advances in Anaesthesia in the Field of Open Cardiac Surgery, stressing Paediatric Open Cardiac Surgery. Anaesthesia—Interchange of Ideas about Speciality Training Staff Members from Kuwait in the Field of Paediatric Open Cardiac Surgery Anaesthesia and Intensive Care.

Place:	Al Sabah Hospital, Chest Diseases, Adan, Farwania, Ibn Sina, Mubarak Hospitals.	
Duration:	11 days, from 10th April till 20th April 1981.	
Organiser:	Discipline Committee for Anaesthesiology.	
Programme Director:	Dr. Mohamed M. Motaweh, Chairman, Dept. of Anaesthesia, Sabah, Chest Diseases and Infectious Diseases Hospitals.	
Participants:	All Anaesthetists in Kuwait.	

Programme:

Saturday, 11th April 1981

9.00 a.m.— 2.00 p.m.	Open Cardiac Surgery Anaesthesia, Surgical Session	Chest Diseases Hospital
6.00 p.m.— 7.30 p.m.	*Lecture:* Treatment of Severe Hypoxcaemia	Chest Diseases Hospital Lecture Room

Sunday, 12th April, 1981

8.00 a.m.— 1.00 p.m.	Closed Cardiac Surgery Anaesthesia session	Chest Disease Hospital
5.30 p.m.	Attendance at Opening Ceremony of the 6th Kuwait Medical Association Congress	Hilton Hotel

Monday, 13th April, 1981

8.00 a.m.— 1.00 p.m.	Rounds, Operation Sessions	Sabah Hospital
6.45 p.m.— 8.15 p.m.	Pannel Discussion for Postgraduate Training and Teaching	Hilton Hotel

Tuesday, 14th April, 1981

8.00 a.m.— 1.00 p.m.	Rounds, Operation Theatres Intensive Care Unit and Emergenca Area, accompanied by Dr. Khairy Nageeb	Farwania Hospital
6.00 p.m.— 7.30 p.m.	*Lecture:* Support for the Failing Heart	Chest Disease Hospital Lecture Room

Wednesday, 15th April, 1981

8.00 p. m.—12.00 noon	Round in Pre-Natural Unit Dr. Daverjan Visiting of Emergency Service Dept. Mr. Abdul Reda Abbas	Maternity Hospital Emergency Service Dept.

| 12.30 p.m. | Meeting with the Undersecretary of the Ministry of Public Health, accompanied by Dr. Mohamed M. Motaweh and Dr. Hani Shoubaier | Ministry of Public Health |

Thursday, 16th April, 1981

	Scientific Meetings	Al Sabah Hospital
9.00 a.m. — 10.15 a.m.	*Lecture:* Anaesthesia for Children and Cardiac Surgery	Chest Diseases Hospital Lecture Room
10.00 a.m. — 11.30 a.m.	*Lecture:* Post-Operative Problems in Children	Chest Disease Hospital Lecture Room
12.00 noon	*Meeting:* With His Excellency, The Minister of Public Health accompanied with Dr. Mohamed M. Motaweh and Dr. Hani Shoubaier	Ministry of Health

Saturday, 18th April, 1981

| 7.30 a.m. — 2.00 p.m. | Thoracic Surgery Session and Anaesthesia at Operation Theatre | Chest Diseases Hospital |

Sunday, 19th April, 1981

9.00 a.m. — 11.30 a.m.	Round in Mubarak Hospital Dr. Mian Mohamed Yacoub	Mubarak Hospital
12.00 noon — 1.30 p.m.	Round in Adan Hospital Intensive Care Unit Dr. Ahmed Galal Al-Gohari	Adan Hospital
6.00 p.m. — 7.30 p.m.	*Lecture:* Brain Damage	Chest Diseases Hospital Lecture Room

81C—6903
Initiation of Primary F.F.A.R.C.S. Course in Kuwait

Objectives:	The visit of Prof. M. D. Vickers, Professor of Anaesthetics Welsh National School of Medicine, Cardiff. To teach recent advances in postoperative analgesia. To teach how to conduct clinical trials. To discuss the organisation of the Primary F.F.A. Course in Kuwait.
Place:	All hospitals in Kuwait.
Duration:	15 days from 25th April to 6th May 1981.
Organiser:	Ministry of Public Health.
Programme Director:	Dr. Mohamed M. Motaweh, Chairman, Department of Anaesthesia.
Participants:	All anaesthetists in Kuwait.

Programme:

25th April, 1981 (Saturday)

8.30 a.m.— 1.00 p.m.   Operation List, Chest Operation
Chest Diseases Hospital
6.00 p.m.— 7.30 p.m.   Tutorial: Design of Clinical Trials
Chest Diseases Hospital, Lecture Room

26th April, 1981 (Sunday)

8.00 a.m.— 1.30 p.m.   Open Cardiac Surgery Session
Chest Diseases Hospital

27th April, 1981 (Monday)

8.30 a.m.— 1.00 p.m.   Operations List and I.C.U.
Maternity Hospital
6.00 p.m.— 7.30 p.m.   Tutorial: Organisation of Clinical Trials
Chest Diseases Hospital
Lecture Room

28th April, 1981 (Tuesday)

8.30 a.m.— 1.00 p.m.   Operation Lists
Sulibekhat Hospital

29th April, 1981 (Wednesday)

8.30 a.m.— 1.00 p.m.   Operation Lists and I.C.U.
Adan Hospital
6.00 p.m.— 7.30 p.m.   Lecture: Trends in Monitoring of Patients
Chest Diseases Hospital
Lecture Room

30th April, 1981 (Thursday)

9.00 a.m.—10.30 a.m.   Scientific Meeting of Sabah Hospital
Chest Diseases Hospital, Lecture Room
Tutorial: Analysis of Research Results

2nd May, 1981 (Saturday)

8.30 a.m.—12.30 noon   Visit to Ibn Sina Hospital
Ibn Sina Hospital
6.00 p.m.— 7.30 p.m.   Lecture: New Methods of Postoperative Analgesia
Chest Diseases Hospital
Lecture Room

3rd May, 1981 (Sunday)

8.30 a.m.— 1.00 p.m.   Operation Lists and I.C.U.
Mubarak Hospital

4th May, 1981 (Monday)

8.30 a.m.— 1.00 p.m.	Operation Lists and I.C.U. Farwania Hospital
6.00 p.m.— 7.30 p.m.	Lecture: Occupational Hazards of Theatre Staff Chest Diseases Hospital Lecture Room

5th May, 1981 (Tuesday)

8.30 a.m.—12.30 noon	Operation Lists Jahra Hospital

6th May, 1981 (Wednesday)

9.00 a.m.—12.20 noon	Operation Lists Sabah Hospital
6.00 p.m.— 7.30 p.m.	Lecture: Developments in Medicine Relevant to Anaesthesia Chest Diseases Hospital Lecture Room

81C—69/30/4504
Advances in Neurosurgical Anaesthesia and Intensive Care

Objectives:	The visit of Dr. William Fitch, Senior Lecturer, Royal Infirmary, University of Glasgow, Scotland. To teach recent advances in the field of Neurosurgical Anaesthesia and Intensive Care. Orientation tutorials regarding Primary F.F.A. Examination.
Place:	Al-Sabah Hospital, Chest Diseases Hospital, Ibn Sina Hospital, Farwania, Mubarak Hospital and Al-Adan Hospital.
Duration:	17 days, from 18th October to 3rd November 1981.
Organiser:	Discipline Committee for Anaesthesiology and Intensive Care.
Programme Director:	Dr. Mohamed M. Motaweh, Chairman, Anaesthesia Dept. of Sabah, Chest and Infectious Diseases Hospital.
Participants:	All anaesthetists in Kuwait.
Programme:	

Monday, 19th October, 1981

9.00 a.m.	Visit to Open Cardiac Surgery Session in Chest Diseases Hospital	Chest Diseases Hospital

Tuesday, 20th October, 1981

8.30 a.m.	Neurosurgical List	Ibn Sina Hospital
5.30 p.m.	Lecture: Pre-operative Assessment of Fitness for Anaesthesia Discussion of Risk Factors before Anaesthesia and Surgery	Chest Diseases Hospital

Wednesday, 21st October, 1981

8.30 a.m.	Neurosurgical List	Ibn Sina Hospital

Thursday, 22nd October, 1981

Tutorial Physiology — Chest Diseases Hospital

8.30 a.m.	A. Physiology of the Autonomic Nervous System
9.45 a.m.	B. The Control of Respiration

Saturday, 24th October, 1981

8.30 a.m.	Neuro-Radiology Meeting	Ibn Sina Hospital
5.30 p.m.	Lecture: Respiratory Abnormalities in Patients with a Head Injury Possible Aetiology and Clinical Implications	Chest Diseases Hospital

Sunday, 25th October, 1981

8.30 a.m.	Neurosurgical List	Ibn Sina Hospital

Monday, 26th October, 1981

8.30 a.m.	Round, Operation Surgical List and Intensive Care Unit	Farwania Hospital
5.30 p.m.	Lecture: The Diagnosis and Management of Smoke Damage to the Lungs. Discussion of Aspects Complicating Major Burns	Chest Diseases Hospital

Tuesday, 27th October, 1981

8.30 a.m.	Neurosurgical List	Ibn Sina Hospital
5.30 p.m.	Tutorial: Pharmacology of the Autonomic Nervous System	Chest Diseases Hospital Lecture Room

Wednesday, 28th October, 1981

8.30 a.m.	Neurosurgical List	Ibn Sina Hospital

Saturday, 31st October, 1981

8.30 a.m.	Surgical Operation Lists and Intensive Care	Al Adan Hospital
5.30 p.m.	Tutorials: Clinical Measurement of Blood Flow through the Organs and Tissues	Chest Diseases Hospital Lecture Room

Sunday, 1st November, 1981

8.30 a.m.	Surgical List and Intensive Care	Mubarak Hospital

Monday, 2nd November, 1981

8.30 a.m.	Operation Lists and Intensive Care	Sabah Hospital
11.00 a.m.	Meeting with the Undersecretary of the Ministry of Public Health	Health Ministry

81C—69/3705
Epidural Analgesia for Labour

Objectives:	The visit of Professor Philip R. Bromage Professor and Chairman, Department of Anaesthesiology, Health Sciences Center University of Colorado, Denver, U.S.A. To demonstrate Epidural Analgesia for Labour. Recent Advances in Acute and Chronic Pain Relief.
Place:	Maternity, Chest Diseases, Ibn Sena, Farwania, Adan and Mubarak Hospitals.
Duration:	14 days from the 6th to the 18th of November, 1981.
Organiser:	Ministry of Public Health, Discipline Committee for Anaesthesiology and Intensive Care.
Programme Director:	Dr. Mohamed M. Motaweh, Chairman, Anaesthesia Department, Sabah, Chest Diseases and Infectious Diseases Hospitals.
Participants:	All Anaesthetists in Kuwait.
Programme:	

Saturday, 7th November, 1981

9.00 a.m.	Round of Open Cardiac Surgery Operation	Chest Diseases Hospital

Sunday, 8th November, 1981

9.00 a.m.	Demonstration, Epidural Analgesia for Labour	Maternity Hospital
5.30 p.m.	Lecture: Subarachnoid-Epidural Anaesthesia Mechanism of Action	Chest Diseases Hospital Lecture Room

Monday, 9th November, 1981

9.00 a.m.	Demonstration Epidural Analgesia for Labour	Maternity Hospital

Tuesday, 10th November, 1981

9.00 a.m.	Pain Relief Demonstration of Intractable Carcinoma by Block	Deep X-Ray Therapy Sabah Hospital
11.00 a.m.	Demonstration, Epid. Analgesia for Labour	Maternity Hospital
5.30 p.m.	Lecture: Subarachnoid Epidural Anaesthesia, Physiological Outcome	Chest Diseases Hospital Lecture Room

Wednesday, 11th November, 1981

9.00 a.m.	Demonstration, Epidural Analgesia for Labour	Maternity Hospital

Thursday, 12th November, 1981

	Sabah Hospital Scientific Meeting	Chest Diseases Hospital Lecture Room
8.30 a.m.	1. Tutorial: Local Anaesthesia, Pharmacology and Anatomy	
9.45 a.m.	2. Pain Mechanisms and Control	

Saturday, 14th November, 1981

9.00 a.m.	Demonstrations, Epidural Analgesia for Surgery	Farwania Hospital
5.30 p.m.	1. Lecture: Obstetrical Anaesthesia, General Principles	Chest Diseases Hospital
6.45 p.m.	2. Regional Anaesthesia for Obstetrics	Chest Diseases Hospital Lecture Room

Sunday, 15th November, 1981

8.30 a.m.	Attendance of a Session of Infection Control Conference	Meridian Hotel

Monday, 16th November, 1981

9.00 a.m.	Demonstration of Pain Relief in Advanced Malignancy Session of Surgical Lists	Mubarak hospital
6.00 p.m.	Lecture: Management of Acute and Chronic Pain	I.C.S. Meeting Sheraton Hotel

Tuesday, 17th November, 1981

9.00 a.m.	Demonstration Epidural Analgesia for Labour	Maternity Hospital
1.00 p.m.	Round in Intensive Care Unit	Adan Hospital

Wednesday, 18th November, 1981

9.00 a.m.	Demonstration Epidural Analgesia in Labour	Maternity Hospital
5.30 p.m.	Lecture: Intra Spinal Narcotics	Chest Diseases Hospital Lecture Room

81C—69/4506
Seminar in Anaesthesia and Intensive Care

Objectives: The visit of Professor Jordan Jordanov, Professor of Anaesthesia and I.C.U. and Vice President of Bulgarian Medical Academy, Sofia, Bulgaria, is intended to:
1. Enable him to see and discuss the advances in Anaesthesia and I.C.U. especially in the new hospitals.
2. Promote the interchange of ideas with the senior consultants and the chairman of the Discipline Committee for Anaesthesiology and Intensive Care on postgraduate training and continuing medical education.
3. Enable him to participate as a member of the delegation of the Peoples Republic of Bulgaria for the Medical Bulgarian-Kuwaiti Week from 27th of February to 3rd March 1982.

Place: Al Sabah Hospital, Old Nursing Institute, Chest Diseases, Al Adan, Jahra, Farwania, Ibn Sina and Mubarak Hospital.

Duration: 31 days from 12th of February to 14th of March, 1982.

Programme Director: Dr. Mohamed M. Motaweh, Chairman, Dept. of Anaesthesia, Sabah, Chest Diseases and Infectious Diseases Hospitals.

Participants: All anaesthetists and doctors from all over Kuwait.

Programme:

Saturday, 13th February, 1982

9.00 a.m.—1.30 p.m.   Visit to Theatre and I.C.U. Ibn Sina Hospital

Sunday, 14th February, 1982

9.00 a.m.—1.30 p.m.   Visit to Theatre and I.C.U. Ibn Sina Hospital

Monday, 15th February, 1982

9.00 a.m.—1.30 p.m.   Visit to Theatre and I.C.U. Ibn Sina Hospital

Tuesday, 16th February, 1982

9.00 a.m.—1.30 p.m.   Visit to Theatre and I.C.U.
                             Ibn Sina Hospital

Wednesday, 17th February, 1982

9.00 a.m.—1.30 p.m.   Visit to Theatre and I.C.U.
                             Ibn Sina Hospital

Thursday, 18th February, 1982

9.00 a.m.—1.30 p.m.   Visit to Theatre and I.C.U.
                             Ibn Sina Hospital

Saturday, 20th February, 1982

9.00 a.m.—1.30 p.m.   Visit to Theatre and I.C.U.
                             Ibn Sina Hospital

Sunday, 21st February, 1982

9.00 a.m.—1.30 p.m.   Visit to Theatre and I.C.U.
                             Ibn Sina Hospital

Monday, 22nd February, 1982

9.00 a.m.—1.30 p.m.   Visit to Theatre and I.C.U.
                             Ibn Sina Hospital

Tuesday, 23rd February, 1982

9.00 a.m.—1.30 p.m.   Visit to Theatre and I.C.U.
                             Ibn Sina Hospital

Wednesday, 24th February, 1982

9.00 a.m.—1.30 p.m.   Visit to Theatre and I.C.U.
                             Ibn Sina Hospital

Saturday, 27th February, 1982

9.00 a.m.—1.30 p.m.   Visit to Theatre and I.C.U.
                             Ibn Sina Hospital
5.00 p.m.   Lecture: Health Care System and Health Services in
                             Bulgaria
                             Old Nursing Institute, Sabah

Sunday, 28th February, 1982

9.00 a.m.—1.30 p.m.   Visit to Theatre and I.C.U.
                             Ibn Sina Hospital
5.00 p.m.   Lecture: Recent Development in Health Manpower
                             Old Nursing Institute, Sabah

Monday, 1st March, 1982

9.00 a.m.—1.30 p.m.   Visit to Theatre and I.C.U.
                             Ibn Sina Hospital

5.00 p.m.   Lecture: Recent Advances in Intensive
                                 Care—Achievements Problems, Further Perspectives
                                 Old Nursing Institute, Sabah

Tuesday, 2nd March, 1982

9.00 a.m.— 1.30 p.m.   Visit to Theatre and I.C.U.
                                 Jahra Hospital

Wednesday, 3rd March, 1982

9.00 a.m.— 1.30 p.m.   Visit to Theatre and I.C.U.
                                 Jahra Hospital
5.00 p.m.   Round table discussion: Acute respiratory failure
                                 Old Nursing Institute, Sabah

Thursday, 4th March, 1982

10.00 a.m.—11.00 a.m.   Lecture: Modern Aspects of Treatment of Patients with
                                 Head Injuries
                                 Jahra Hospital

Saturday, 6th March, 1982

9.00 a.m.— 1.30 p.m.   Visit to Theatre and I.C.U.
                                 Mubarak Hospital

Sunday, 7th March, 1982

9.00 a.m.— 1.30 p.m.   Visit to Theatre and I.C.U.
                                 Mubarak Hospital

Monday, 8th March, 1982

9.00 a.m.— 1.30 p.m.   Visit to Theatre and I.C.U.
                                 Mubarak Hospital

Tuesday, 9th March, 1982

10.00 a.m.—11.00 a.m.   Lecture: Main Topics of Studies and Training of
                                 Undergraduate Students in Anaesthesia, Resuscitation
                                 and Intensive Care
                                 Mubarak Hospital

Wednesday, 10th March, 1982

9.00 a.m.— 1.30 p.m.   Visit to Theatre and I.C.U.
                                 Al Adan Hospital
12.00 noon   Lecture: Continuing Education for the Health
                                 Professions
                                 (Training Division)

Thursday, 11th March, 1982

9.00 a.m.— 1.30 p.m.   Visit to Theatre and I.C.U.
                                 Orthopaedic Hospital

Saturday, 13th March, 1982

10.00 a.m.—11.00 a.m.   Lecture: Specific Requirements for Treatment of
                         Patients in Intensive Care Units

Sunday, 14th March, 1982

9.00 a.m.— 1.30 p.m.   Visit to Theatre and I.C.U.
                         Chest Hospital

81C—6907
Recent Advances in Anaesthesia

Objectives: The visit of Prof. M. D. Vickers, Prof. of Anaesthetics,
                       Welsh National School of Medicine.
                       The Recent Advances in Anaesthesia and Intensive
                       Care.
                       Negotiations for the Second Primary FFARCS., Course
                       in Kuwait.

Place: All Hospitals in Kuwait.

Duration: 12 days from the 18th March to 30th of March 1982.

Programme Director: Dr. Mohamed M. Motaweh, Chairman of Department
                       of Anaesthesia.

Participants: All anaesthetists in Kuwait.

Programme:

Saturday, 20th March 1982

8.30 a.m.— 1.00 p.m.   OCS Session
                         Chest Diseases Hospital

Sunday, 21st March, 1982

8.00 a.m.— 1.30 p.m.   Neurosurgical Lists
                         Ibn Sina Hospital

Monday, 22nd April, 1982

8.30 a.m.— 1.00 p.m.   Operations Lists and I.C.U.
                         Farwania Hospital
6.00 p.m.— 7.00 p.m.   Lecture:
                         Prediction and Prophylaxis of Pulmonary
                         Complications
                         Chest Diseases Hospital, Lecture Room

Tuesday, 23rd March, 1982

8.30 a.m.— 1.00 noon   Operation Lists and I.C.U.
                         Chest Diseases Hospital

Wednesday, 24th March, 1982

8.30 a.m.— 1.00 noon   Operation Lists and I.C.U.
                          Mubarak Hospital

Thursday, 25th March, 1982

9.00 a.m.—10.30 a.m.   Lecture: Respiratory Effects of Some New Analgesics
                          Chest Diseases Hospital
                          Lecture Room

Friday, 26th March, 1982

                          Weekly Holiday

Saturday, 27th March, 1982

8.30 a.m.— 1.00 noon   Operation Lists and I.C.U.
                          Maternity Hospital
6.00 p.m.— 7.00 p.m.   Lecture: A Logical Approach to Neonatal Asphyxia:
                          The Cardiff Inflating Valve
                          Chest Diseases Hospital
                          Lecture Room

Sunday, 28th March, 1982

                          Visit to Ministry of Public Health, Kuwait City

Monday, 29th March, 1982

8.30 a.m.—12.30 noon   Operation Lists and I.C.U.
                          Al Jahra Hospital
6.00 p.m.— 7.00 p.m.   Lecture and Tutorial: The Important Role of the
                          Anaesthetist's Services
                          Chest Diseases Hospital
                          Lecture Room

81C—71/1801
Haematology and Blood Banking

Objectives: To train key technologists in laboratory services.
                         To provide the preliminary training for Kuwaiti medi-
                         cal graduates.

Place: The Adan Hospital Laboratory.

Duration: 3 months, from 7th March, 1981 to 28th May, 1982.

Organiser: The Training Committee for Laboratory Medicine.

Programme Director: Dr. Y. Watanabe, Manager, Laboratory
                         Superintendance, Ministry of Public Health.

Coordinator: Dr. Thomas Lipsic, Consultant Haematologist.

Participants: Kuwaiti with a university diploma and graduates from
                         the Faculty of Science, Kuwait University will have
                         first priority. Applications from personnel outside the
                         above categories can also be accepted.

All applicants should be evaluated before their acceptance. The expected numbers of trainees are approximately 20 to 30.

Programme:

Clinical Haematology

Introduction
  Division, classification, theory, methods etc.
Haemopoiesis
  Cell division, type of multiplication, regulation, DNK, RNK, genetics, kinetics
  Bone marrow
  Regulation, control, production
  Methods, tests: puncture, biopsy, trepano-biopsy, morphology, staining, dynamic
  tests, ERP-study, radioisotope studies
Cytology and Cell Strucutre
  Erythrocyte—RBC
  Development, maturation
  Morphology, Pathology
  Methods, tests, studies
Platelets—Thrombocytes
  Cytology-morphology
  Maturation, utilisation, breakdown
  Function, distribution
  Methods
Coagulation System
  Definition, classification
  Plasma factors, platelets, vessels
  Physiology
  Pathology
  Methods
Parasites in blood
  Classification
  Morphology
  Methods
Haematological Problems in this Region

Blood Banking

Introduction
  History, theory, methods, importance etc.
Antigenic Properties of RBC
  ABO / H / blood group system
  MN Ss blood group system
  D / Rh system / CDE
  P, L, Kell, Fy, Lu, Le and other blood group systems
  Importance of blood groups
  Haemolytic disease of newborn
  Forensic medicine
Antigenic Properties of Platelets
  PL-antigens
  Importance of PL antigens and their relations to HLA
Serum "Blood" Groups

Blood Transfusion Service
  Importance
  Organisation
  Donation
  Blood derivatives, fractions, isolation, preservation, storage
  Technique of the bleeding
  Used materials
  Indication and contraindication of BT, kinds of BT
  Post-transfusional reactions and complications, risk of BT
  Techniques and required documentation in BT

Haemoglobin
  Chemistry, features, nature
  Formation, metabolism, catabolism etc.
  Function, malfunction: dissociation curve, binding of oxygen etc.
  Pathology of Hb / F, A2, C, D, E, etc.
  Methods-Haemoglobinometry, electrophoresis of Hb, spectrometry, fingerprints
  etc.

Iron
  Chemistry, properties, reactions
  Function and content appearance
  Forms, occurrence
  Absorption
  Metabolism
  Methods: staining, biochemistry: absorption, ions, radioisotopic methods
  Pathology

Anaemia
  Definition, classification and toxonomy
  Pathological aspects
  Deficiency anaemia: iron, B12, B8 etc.
  Aplastic-hypoplastic anaemia: primary and secondary
  Haemolytic anaemia: extra and intracorpuscular types, inborn, acquired
  Posthaemorrhagic anaemia
  Methods

Leucocytes—WBC
  Morphology, classification and toxonomy
  Physiology and others
  Maturation, utilisation, breakdown, distribution
  Pathophysiology-pathology
  Methods

Leukemia
  Definition, classification and toxonomy
  Pathological aspects
  Methods

RES-reticuloendothelial system
  Definition, distribution
  Function etc.
  Methods

81C—71/0102
The Histopathology Course

Objectives:	To train key technologists in laboratory services. To provide the preliminary training for Kuwaiti medical graduates.
Place (Venue):	The Histopathology Laboratory, Sabah.
Duration:	10 months, from 15th March, 1981 to 15th January, 1982.
Organiser:	The Training Committee for Laboratory Medicine.
Programme Director:	Dr. Y. Watanabe, Manager, Laboratory Superintendance, Ministry of Public Health.
Coordinator:	Dr. S. M. Ali, Consultant Histopathologist.
Participants:	Kuwaiti with a university diploma and graduates from the Faculty of Science, Kuwait University will have first priority. Applications from personnel outside the above categories can also be accepted. All applicants should be evaluated before their acceptance. The expected numbers of trainees are approximately 20 to 30.

Programme:

Introduction
  The cell
  Methods to examine tissues and cells
The Microscope
  The compound microscope
  The fluorescent microscope
  The dark field microscope
  The polarising microscope
  The phase contrast microscope
  The interference microscope
  The electron microscope
Fixation
Processing
Section Cutting
Adhesions of Sections to Slide
Staining
  Theory of staining
  Preparation of stains
  Basic staining and mounting procedures
  Routine staining
  DNA and RNA
  Special staining including microorganism techniques
Histochemistry
  Carbohydrate
  Lipids
  Amyloid
  Calcium
  Pigments
  Enzymes

Frozen Sections
Museum Mounting
Cytological and Chromosome Techniques
  Preparation of smears
  Fixation
  Staining
  Screening
Recording and Filing
Quality Control

81C—71/08/7903
The Microbiology and Parasitology Course

Objectives:	To train key technologists in laboratory services. To provide the preliminary training for Kuwaiti Medical Graduates.
Place (Venue):	Clinical Microbiology Adan Hospital Laboratory. The Virology Laboratories in the Public Health Laboratory.
Duration:	9 months, from 20th March, 1981 to 15th December, 1981
Organiser:	The Training Committee for Laboratory Medicine.
Programme Director:	Dr. Y. Watanabe, Manager, Laboratory Superintendance, Ministry of Public Health
Coordinator:	Dr. P. R. Hira, Consultant, Parasitologist Dr. Benjamin F. Watson, Consultant Microbiologist Dr. Widad Al-Nakib, Head, Public Health Laboratory (Virologist).
Participants:	Kuwaiti with a university diploma and graduates from the Faculty of Science, Kuwait University, will have first priority. Applications from personnel outside the above categories can be accepted. All applicants should be evaluated before their acceptance. The expected numbers of trainees are approximately 20 to 30.

Programme:

Clinical Bacteriology
Bacterial Physiology and Physiochemistry
  Structure and classification of bacteria
  Biosynthesis
  Bacterial nutrition and growth
  Sterilisation and disinfection
Microbial Genetics
  Genetic transfer
  Molecular aspects of genetics
  Genetic regulation
  Bacterial variation and population dynamics
  Chemotherapeutic actions and genetic implications

Basic Bacteriological Methods
  Basic techniques in bacteriological examinations
  Specimen collection
  Isolation
  Identification
  Serological diagnosis
  Records
  Reports
  Quality control
Bacterial Diseases and Clinical Microbiology
  General principles
  Bacteremia and sepsis
  Central nervous system infections
  Enteric infection—Gastrointestinal infections
  Generalised infection with rash
  Mycobacterial infections
  Respiratory infections
  Tissue infections (localized)
  Urinary tract infections
  Veneral diseases—sexually transmitted diseases

Clinical Virology

Viral Physiology and Other Properties; Bacteriophages
  Structure and classification of viruses
  Replication viruses and interferons
Viral Genetics
  Mutagens, phenotype and genotype
  Genetic interactions and non-genetic interactions
Basic Virological Methods
  Basic techniques in virological examinations
  Specimen collection
  Isolation
  Identification
  Serological diagnosis
  Animal models
  Records
  Reports
  Quality control
Viral Diseases and Clinical Virology
  General principles
  Others (to be decided later)
Rickettsial Infections
  Physiology and classification
  Rickettsioses

Clinical Parasitology

Routine Diagnostic Methods in Clinical Parasitology
  Stool specimens
  Urine specimens, including urine routine
  Blood specimens
Discussions, Seminars Whenever Appropriate

81C—71/0104
Medical Biochemistry

Objectives:	To train key technologists in laboratory services.
Place:	The Adan Hospital Laboratory.
Duration:	7 months from 4th April, 1981 to 30th Sept, 1981.
Organiser:	The Training Committee for Laboratory Medicine.
Programme Director:	Dr. Y. Watanabe, Manager, Laboratory Superintendance, Ministry of Public Health.
Coordinator:	Dr. Barbara Malkiewicz-Wasowicz, Consultant Biochemist.
Participants:	Kuwaiti with a university diploma and graduates from the Faculty of Science, Kuwait University, will have first priority. Applications from personnel without the above categories can also be accepted. All applicants should be evaluated before their acceptance. The expected number of trainees is approximately 20 to 30.

Programme:

Clinical Biochemistry
General Introduction
  Role of clinical biochemistry laboratory
  Daily routine work
  Recording and data processing
  Communication and cooperation between laboratory and users of the services
  Various constraints
Statistics Related to Clinical Biochemistry
  General methods to determine normal ranges—reference values
  Reference values characterizing a single subject
  Intra-individual variations in healthy persons
  Routine laboratory statistics
Accuracy and Precision in Clinical Chemistry
Sources of Variation in Laboratory Measurements
  Preparation of patients for the laboratory investigation
  Collection of specimens
  Storage of the specimens
Quality Control in Clinical Chemistry
  Control of accuracy
  Control of precision
  Internal and external quality control
General Rules for Standardization of Pre-Analytical and Analytical Procedures
Principles of Instrumentation in Clinical Chemistry Laboratory
General Principles for Assessing a New Analytical Method for Routine Use
Water and Electrolytes
  Normal contents of body components
  Water balance—sodium and chloride balance
  Clinical disorders of water and electrolytes

Acid-Base Balance
  Maintenance of normal blood PH
  Compensatory mechanism
  Clinical disorders
Carbohydrate
  Blood glucose
  Diabetes
Lipids
  Classification—metabolism
  Triglyceride, phospholipids, cholosterol, HDL cholesterol
  Plasma lipoproteins
  Activity of lipoprotein lipase
  Hyperlipidaemias
Nitrogenous Compounds
  Metabolism
  Nitrogen balance
  Non-protein nitrogen
  Urea, azotaemia, uric acid, ammonia
  Creatine and creatinine
  Aminoacids
Plasma Proteins
  Metabolism
  Serum proteins: normal and abnormal
  Diseases and plasma proteins
  Electrophoretic patterns
Iron and Other Trace Metals
The Endocrine Glands (a general outline)
  Pituitary
  Thyroid
  Adrenal
  Gonadotrophics: esterogen and progestron
The Liver
  Plasma protein and flocculation tests
  Plasma enzyme: cholinesterases, alkaline phosphatase, transaminases, -gamma-GT
  Detoxication and excretion: bromsulphthalein test
  'Liver function tests'
The kidneys
  Urine formation—clearance in renal function tests
  Proteinuria
  Diseases and biochemical changes of urine
The heart
  Biochemical diagnosis of heart diseases
  Enzyme profiling in diagnosis of myocardial infarction
  Significance of enzyme estimation for monitoring and clinical prognosis
The gastrointestinal tract
  Gastric function tests
  Pancreas tests
  Gastrointestinal disorders and biochemical tests
Nervous System
  Biochemistry in nervous and mental diseases
Biochemical Abnormalities in General
  The steady state and its alteration

Inborn errors; metabolism and normal range
Haemoglobinopathies
Porphylins
Introduction to Toxicology

81C—7105
The Integral Course

Objectives:	To train key technologists in laboratory services, Ministry of Public Health, who can stay long, and
	To provide the preliminary training for Kuwaiti medical graduates.
Place (Venue):	The Adan Hospital Laboratory.
Duration:	4 months from 4th April, 1981 to 16th July, 1981.
Organiser:	The Training Committee for Laboratory Medicine.
Programme Director:	Dr. Y. Watanabe, Manager, Laboratory Superintendance, Ministry of Public Health.
Coordinators:	Dr. Barbara Malkiewicz-Wasowicz Consultat Biochemist
	Dr. Thomas Lipsic, Consultant Haematologist
	Dr. P. R. Hira, Consultant Parasitologist
	Dr. S. M. Ali, Consultant Histopathologist
	Dr. Benjamin F. Watson, Consultant Microbiologist
	Dr. Widad Al-Nakib, Head, Public Health Laboratory (Virologist)
	Mr. Soliman Marzook, Duty Manager, Laboratory Superintendance
Participants:	Kuwaiti with a university diploma and graduates from the Faculty of Science, Kuwait University, will have first priority. Applications from personnel outside the above categories can also be accepted. All applicants should be evaluated before their acceptance. The expected number of trainees is approximately 20 to 30.

Programme:

I. Organisation of Clinical Laboratories—General Information
   Record system
   Inventory system
   Supply system
   General safety precautions
   Data processing system
   Communication and cooperation within the laboratory and between wards and the laboratory, including collection of specimens
II. Clinical Laboratory Statistics
   Basic statistical methods useful in laboratory medicine
   The application of statistical data in laboratory medicine
III. Outline of Quality Control
IV. Instrumentations and Maintainance
   Optical instruments
   Spectrophotometers

Other routine instruments
Counters
  V. Reagents and Their Quality
Reagents suitable for laboratory tests
Long-life and short-life reagents
 VI. Basic Immunology
Immune response
Antigen-antibody reactions
Antibody formation and molecular aspects of antibodies
Complement
Hypersensitivity
Mammalian isoantigens, including blood group substances and transplanta-
tion antigen
Commonly used sero-immunological techniques in the clinical medicine
Future prospects of immunology in connection with laboratory medicine
VII. Computer Application
Introduction to computer hardware
Introduction to computer software
Application of computer science in laboratory medicine
VIII. Library and its Utilisation
Medical library and its systems
Methods of paper surveys
Audiovisual systems

81C—75/7301
Use and Abuse of Antibiotics

Objectives: Refresher course to update the knowledge of Pharmacists of the Pharmacy Division about antibiotics, their
use and abuse, and how to avoid their misuse and
abuse.

Place: The auditorium of the new Mubarak Hospital.

Duration: 6 days, from 14. 2. 1981 till 20. 2. 1981.

Organiser: Dr. Riad Alami, Head of the Pharmacy Division, in
cooperation and coordination with the Kuwait Pharma-
ceutical Society (President: Dr. Abdulla Al-Khars,
Medical School, Kuwait University).

Programme Director: Dr. Riad Alami, Chief Pharmacist.

Participants: The 200 pharmacists of the Pharmacy Division.
Pharmacists belonging to other divisions or centers
such as the control lab., medical stores, manufacturing
plant, and the new hospitals, are all welcome to attend
too.

Programme: *Lectures*

Prof. P. Wilkinson, University of Connecticut, Storrs,
Conn., U.S.A.
Prof. T. Foster, University of Kentucky Medical
Center, Lexington, Kentucky, U.S.A.
Dr. Shahabuddin, Kuwait.

February 14, 1981 (Saturday)

5.00 p.m.   Prof. Wilkinson
                                 Overview of Antibiotics

February 15, 1981 (Sunday)

5.00 p.m.   Prof. Wilkinson
                                 Basic Pharmacokinetic Principles

February 16, 1981 (Monday)

5.00 p.m.   Prof. Foster
                                 Practical Application of Pharmacokinetics for
                                 Antibiotics Therapy

February 17, 1981 (Tuesday)

5.00 p.m.   Prof. Foster
                                 1—A Case Presentation of Aminoglycosides
                                 2—Therapeutic Monitoring for Appropriate Antibiotic
                                 Therapy

February 18, 1981 (Wednesday)

5.00 p.m.   Dr. Shahabuddin
                                 1—Cephalosporins—Overview
                                 2—Cephalosporins, Therapy Monitoring
                                 Consideration

81C—7801
Infection Control

Objectives: To exchange information on infection with Kuwait's
                                 nurses and doctors.
                                 To discuss with Mrs. Julie Carner, Infection Control
                                 Nurse, Centre for Disease Control, Atlanta, U.S.A.,
                                 advances in the field of infection control.

Place (Venue):   All hospitals in Kuwait.

Duration: 14th to 27th February, 1981.

Organiser: The Committee for Infection Control.

Programme Director: Dr. Sadad Sabri

Participants: Infection Control Nursing Officers
                                 Infection Control Teams
                                 Infection Control Trainees
                                 General Nurses and Doctors

Programme:

February 15, 1981 (Sunday)

8.00—10.00 a.m.	Chest Diseases Hospital
	Visit
10.30—12 noon	Psychiatric Hospital
	Seminar
12.30— 1.30 p.m.	Psychiatric Hospital
	Visit

February 16, 1981 (Monday)

8.00—10.00 a.m.	Farwania Hospital
	Visit
10.00—10.30 a.m.	Break
10.30—12 noon	Lecture Room
	Seminar
12.30— 1.30 p.m.	Farwania Hospital
	Visit

February 17, 1981 (Tuesday)

7.30— 8.30 a.m.	Maternity Hospital, Lecture Room
	Discussion on Infection Control
8.30—10.00 a.m.	Maternity Hospital
	Visit
10.00—10.30 a.m.	Break
10.30—12 noon	Wards, Lab. etc.
	Visit
12.00— 1.30 p.m.	Lecture Room
	Seminar

February 18, 1981 (Wednesday)

7.30— 8.30 a.m.	Lecture Room, Adan Hospital
	Discussion
8.30—10.30 a.m.	Adan Hospital
	Visit
10.30—11.00 a.m.	Break
11.00—12.30 p.m.	Lecture Room
	Seminar
12.30— 1.30 p.m.	Adan Hospital
	Visit

February 19, 1981 (Thursday)

7.30— 8.30 a.m.	Lecture Room, Infectious Diseases Hospital
	Discussion
8.30—10.30 a.m.	Wards, Lab. etc.
	Visit
10.30—11.00 a.m.	Break

11.00—12.30 p.m.	Infectious Diseases Hospital Visit
12.30— 1.30 p.m.	Lecture Room Seminar

February 21, 1981 (Saturday)

7.30— 8.30 a.m.	Al-Sabah Hospital Lecture Room Discussion
8.30—10.30 a.m.	Wards, Lab. etc. Visit
10.30—11.00 a.m.	Break
11.00—12.30 p.m.	Laundry Department Visit
12.30— 1.30 p.m.	Lecture Room Seminar

February 22, 1981 (Sunday)

7.30— 8.30 a.m.	Sabah Hospital, Lecture Room Discussion
8.30—10.30 a.m.	Al-Sabah Hospital Visit
10.30—11.00 a.m.	Break
11.00—12.30 a.m.	Kitchens, Incinerator etc. Visit
12.30— 1.30 p.m.	Lecture Room Seminar

February 23, 1981 (Monday)

7.30— 8.30 a.m.	Orthopaedic Hospital Lecture Room Discussion
8.30—10.30 a.m.	Orthopaedic Hospital Visit
10.30—11.00 a.m.	Break
11.00—12.30 p.m.	Orthopaedic Hospital Visit
12.30— 1.30 p.m.	Lecture Room Seminar
6.00 p.m.	Medical Association Principles of Infection Control

February 24, 1981 (Tuesday)

7.30— 8.30 a.m.	Lecture Room, Jahra Hospital Discussion
8.30—10.30 a.m.	Jahra Hospital Visit
10.30—11.00 a.m.	Break

| 11.00—12.30 p.m. | Jahra Hospital
Visit |
| 12.30— 1.30 p.m. | Lecture Room
Seminar |

Subjects for Seminar

Nurses and Infection Control.
Advisory Role of Infection Control, Nurses in teaching how to do it.
Isolation Techniques.
Control of Catheter Associated Infection.
General Concepts of Surveillance.
General Concepts of Control of Infection.

81C—78/1202
Seminar of Infectious Diseases

Objectives:	The visit of Dr. Richard H. Glew, M.D., Chief, Infectious Disease Service, Worcester, Massachusetts, U.S.A. To teach advances in the field of Infectious Disease Control. To give lectures for MRCP Part I Course for MRCP Part II Course.
Place (Venue):	Department of Medicine (Fever Hospital).
Duration:	6 days, from 4th May to 10th May, 1981.
Organiser:	Ministry of Public Health (Discipline Committee for Medicine).
Programme Director:	Prof. F. F. Fenech.
Participants:	The physicians of the above-mentioned hospital, doctors participating in MRCP Part I Course, MRCP Part II Course and undergraduates.
Programme:	

Monday, 4th May, 1981

| 8.30 a.m. | Visit to Fever Hospital
(Dr. I. Abu Sabra) |

Tuesday, 5th May, 1981

| 9.30 a.m. | Rounds in Ward 5, Al Sabah
(Dr. A. Karnik) |
| 12.00 noon | Medical Grand Rounds, Seminar Room, Chabra, Dept. of Medicine, Al Sabah Hospital. Case presentation—Infections in the Immunosuppressed Hosts |

Wednesday, 6th May, 1981

9.30 a.m.   Rounds in Ward 12, Al-Sabah
                             (Dr. Nasser Hayat)
                             Student Presentation—
                             Extrapulmonary T.B.—Anorexia Nervosa

Thursday, 7th May, 1981

9.00 a.m.   Rounds in Ward 1, Al-Sabah
                             (Dr. Taha)
10.30 a.m.   Student Presentation and Discussion—Case of Staph,
                             Pneumonia and/or Staph, Septicemia

Saturday, 9th May, 1981

8.30 a.m.   Round in Ward 4, Al-Sabah
                             (Dr. Farouk)
10.30 a.m.   Round in Ward 6, Al-Sabah
                             (Dr. Nabillah)
12.00 noon   Student Case Presentation—
                             Meningitis and Brain Abscess

81C—8801
Third Epidemiological Seminar

Objectives: To present results of epidemiological studies conducted
                            in Kuwait.
                            To teach the value of epidemiological research for the
                            management of patients.

Place: Al-Sabah Hospital, lecture room in the old Nursing In-
                            stitute.

Duration: 5 days, from January 11th to January 15th, 1981.

Organiser: Ministry of Public Health
                            Department of Public Health and Planning.

Programme Director: Dr. Philip Brachman.

Coordinator: Dr. Jaffar Ezzat.

Participants: About 50 doctors.

Programme:

Sunday, January 11, 1981

8.00   Dr. Brachman
                            Infectious Disease Update
9.30   Break

Moderator: Dr. Rashed A. Al-Owaish

10.00	Dr. Yousef El-Rakhawai A Study of the Change in the Epidemiological Pattern of Shigellosis in Kuwait during 1970—1980
10.30	Dr. Nibal Kaddah Typhoid Fever—A Review of the Current Status in Infectious Diseases Hospital
11.00	Dr. M. Abo Katwa Typhoid Fever in Geleeb El-Shiokh
11.30	Break

Moderator: Dr. Philip Brachman

12.00 noon	Mrs. Nawal Al-Gassan Investigation of Nosocomial Infections at a Pediatric Surgical Ward
12.30 p.m.	Dr. Nasreen Rafik Ali Nosocomial Infection at the Maternity Hospital Feb.—Aug. 1980
1.00	Dr. Morsi Abo-Chazala, Mrs. Saramma Abraham Nosocomial Infections at the Amiri Hospital, Surgical Ward
1.30	Dr. Abdul Razak Hussein Gastroenteritis in Adan Hospital
2.00	Adjournment

Monday, January 12, 1981

Islamic Conference at Hilton Hotel

Tuesday, January 13, 1981

8.00	Dr. Mustafa Khogali Epidemiology of Heat Stroke during Mecca Pilgrimage 1978—1980
9.30	Break

Moderator: Mr. Virgil Peavy

10.00	Dr. Kamal Al-Zanati Heat Illness Managed by Kuwait Medical Mission during Mecca Pilgrimage 1980
10.30	Dr. Rashid Al-Owaish, Dr. Matthew Zack Risk Factors Associated with the Incidence of Acute Myocardial Infarction in Kuwait, 1978
11.00	Dr. Mostafa K. Mansour Health Problems of International Travellers Arriving Kuwait 1980
11.30	Break

Moderator: Dr. Saleh Al-Kandari

12.00	Dr. Fayek Abdel Hay El-Husseini
	Occupational Accidents among Workers at the Seaport
	of Shuwaikh during June—31 July, 1980
12.30	Dr. Mustafa Fouad
	Epidemiology of Accidents in the Shuwaikh Industrial
	Area
1.00	Dr. Milad Gabriel
	T.B. Drug Resistance—Change in Patterns
1.30	Open
2.00	Adjourn

Wednesday, January 14, 1981

8.00	Dr. James Maynard
	Hepatitis Update
9.30	Break

Moderator: Dr. James Maynard

10.00	Dr. Saleh Al-Kandari
	Hepatitis B Infection among Dentists in Kuwait
10.30	Dr. B. Gheridian, Dr. Hussain Al-Momen, etc.
	Hepatitis in Healthy Girls in Kuwait
11.00	Dr. Ali El-Baz Ibrahim
	Investigation of Hepatitis A among Hawalli Residents
	Returning from Holidays
11.30	Break

Moderator: Dr. Philip Brachman

12.00	Dr. Mohamed Saleh Al-Sai'eed
	Poliomyelitis in Kuwait 1980
12.30	Dr. Safwat Mansi
	Poliomyelitis in Jahra 1980
1.00	Dr. M. A. Dabsha
	A Case Report of Rabies Exposure
1.30	Open
2.00	Adjourn

Thursday, January 15, 1981

Moderator: Dr. Rashed Al-Owaish

8.00	Dr. Abdul Amir Al-Kilidar
	Salmonella in Kuwait, 1979—1980
8.30	Dr. Abdulla Ostaz
	Shigella Carriers and Parasite Data among Food Handlers in Kuwait
9.00	Dr. Helmy Abdul Fatah Mohamed
	Gastroenteritis among Infants below One Year and its
	Relation, the Type of Feeding
9.30	Break

Moderator: Mr. Virgil Peavy

10.00	Dr. Salwa Ahmed Mostafa
	Nutritional Status Assessment of Preschool Children
10.30	Dr. Feryal M. Talat El-Masry
	Eneuresis among School Children in Kuwait
11.00	Closing Comments, Staff
11.30	Presentation of Awards
12.00	Adjourn

81C—8802
Fourth Epidemiological Seminar

Objectives: To present results of epidemiological studies conducted in Kuwait.
To teach the value of epidemiological research for the management of patients.

Place: Conference Room, Ministry of Public Health.

Duration: 5 days, from 17th till 21st January, 1982.

Organiser: Discipline Committee for Public Health.

Programme Director: Dr. Jaffar Ezzat with cooperation of Mr. Virgil Peavy.

Participants: Doctors and other personnel from public health and infectious disease specialities.

Programme:

Sunday, 17th January, 1982

9.00 a.m.	Welcome
	Dr. Na'il A. Al-Naqeeb
9.15 a.m.	Introduction to 1982 Conference
	Mr. Virgil Peavy
10.00 a.m.	New Approach in Measles Control
	Dr. Mounir Guirgis
10.30 a.m.	Assessment of Vaccination Coverage—Hawalli 1981
	Dr. Ali El-Baz
11.00 a.m.	Hepatitis B Antigenaemia and Antibody Prevalence among Kuwaiti Population
	Dr. Saleh Al-Kandari
12.00 noon	An Outbreak of Food Poisoning in Salmiya
	Dr. Ahmed Showki Fangary
12.30 noon	An Outbreak of Gastrointestinal Illness Occurred in a Site of School Construction in Wafra
	Dr. Jalal M. Saad
1.00 p.m.	Clinico Epidemiological Study on a Milkborn Gastrointestinal Outbreak in Quaseem Region, Saudi Arabia, May-June 1978
	Dr. Housein Sabry Nofal
1.30 p.m.	An Outbreak of Typhoid Fever in a Family at Solibia District
	Dr. Abdul Aziz Abdul Hamid

Monday, 18th January, 1982

9.30 a.m.	Incidence and Survival Functions of Lung Cancer Dr. Abdul Aziz Ismail, Dr. Ramzi I. M. Ismail
10.00 a.m.	Epidemiological Approach to Cancer in Kuwait Dr. Safwat Mansi
10.30 a.m.	Trends and Differentials in Congenital Anomalies, Death Rates in Kuwait (1974—1978) Dr. B. R. Kohli
11.00 a.m.	Risk Factors in Diabetes Mellitus Dr. Abdirizack S. Hussein
12.00 noon	An Outbreak of Salmonella Typhimurium in Neonatal Nursery at Farwania Hospital July 1981 Dr. Mohammed Abu Katwa
12.30 noon	Salmonella Outbreak in Bustan Al-Naaem Dr. Zafer Dajani
1.00 p.m.	Salmonella Incidence at Omm-El-Niman District (1977—1981) Dr. Mohammed A. Dabsheh
1.30 p.m.	Salmonella Enteritis in Kuwait (1968—1980) Dr. Fawzi M. Abu El Zein

Tuesday, 19th January, 1982

8.00 a.m.	Update on Statistical Tests for Significance Mr. Virgil Peavy
9.30 a.m.	Typhoid Outbreak in Bahrain Dr. E. L. Ferandes
10.00 a.m.	Contagious Pustular Dermatitis Ecthyma Contagious Dr. Khairy N. Megalla
10.30 a.m.	Haemorrhagic Meningoencephalitis (Anthrax) Dr. Mohammed Abu Katwa
11.00 a.m.	An Outbreak of Enteritis at the Policemen School Kuwait, 1981 Dr. Yousef M. El-Rakhawi
12.00 noon	Heart Diseases Among Students in Hawalli and Jabria Schools Dr. Awatif Harouin, Dr. Farouk El-Saeed
12.30 noon	Defective Vision among Kuwaiti Students Dr. Hegab Samiha M.
1.00 p.m.	Upper Central Incisior Teeth among School Children Dr. Sonia El-Mankabadi
1.30 p.m.	Prevalence of Chronic Diseases with Disability among School Children of Ahmadi District Dr. Fawzi K. Murad

Wednesday, 20th January, 1982

8.00 a.m.	Methodology of Community Survey for Chronic Diseases Dr. Stefan Straka
9.00 a.m.	Epidemiology of Motor Vehicle Accidents in Kuwait Dr. Ahmed Bayoumi

10.00 a.m.	Congenital Lead Encephalopathy Dr. Mohammed Abu Katwa
10.30 a.m.	Obesity Hypertension among Diabetics Mrs. Prasanna Prakash
11.00 a.m.	The Relationship between Fetal Birth Weight and Maternal Glucose Dr. Samir M. Kamel, Dr. Fawzi M. Abu-El-Zein
12.00 noon	Malaria in North Iraq Dr. Saad Nahady
12.20 noon	Wound Infections at Outpatient District Clinics. Mrs. Therese S. Salman
12.40 p.m.	Descriptive Study for the Causes of Death among Foreigners in Kuwait who were Transported Abroad for Burial, 1st Nov.—31st Oct., 1982 Dr. Ezzat Kamel Azab
1.00 p.m.	Health and Medical Services Evaluation at Pilgrim's Rest in Kuwait, 8th Sept.—31st Oct., 1981 Dr. Jamal El-Badawy
1.20 p.m.	Follow up of 10 Cases of Salmonella Typhi and Paratyphi Carriers Dr. Abdulla M. Ostaz

Thursday, 21st January, 1982

8.00 a.m.	Assessment of Immunization Levels in Kuwait Dr. Mounir M. Guirgis
9.00 a.m.	Current Status of Vaccine, Preventable Diseases Dr. Michael Gregg
10.30 a.m.	Solibikhat Nursery Dr. Mohammed S. Azab
10.50 a.m.	An Investigation of Respiratory Illness among Pilgrims to Mecca 1401 A.H. Dr. Saeed Al-Helees
11.10 a.m.	Descriptive Study of Sick Seamen in 1980—1981 Dr. Abdul Aziz Fahmy Hashad
11.30 a.m.	Closing Comments and Presentation of Awards, Staff
12.00 noon	Adjourn

81E—9901
Course for Potential Head Nurses

Objectives:	1. To develop the potential leadership qualities of a staff nurse to a head nurse position.
	2. To teach them the principles of administration in general and of a unit in particular.
	3. To stimulate and sustain interest in professional needs.
Place:	Lecture Room, Nurse Training Unit, Sharq.
Duration:	18 days (31. 1. 81—19. 2. 81).

Organiser:	Nurse Training and Planning Unit, Training Division, Dept. of Public Health and Planning.
Programme Director:	Miss Awatef Quttan, Head of Nurse Training and Planning Unit.
Participation:	25 nurses from different health facilities (names not available).
Course Programme:	The course programme shall include the development of modern administration (scientific management), administrative functions like management, planning, delegation, organisation, decision making and evaluation. General topics on ward policies, ward teaching and general discipline. Field experience in selected hospitals for the particular post (head nurse) and the field visits to various hospitals to get acquainted with modern equipment, personnel and their working system. To evaluate their performance during and at the end of the course, through a system of observation records and examination. A detailed programme will be formed before course begins.

81E—9902
Course for Potential Head Nurses

Objectives:	1. To develop the potential leadership qualities of a staff nurse to a head nurse position. 2. To teach them the principles of administration in general and of a unit in particular. 3. To stimulate and sustain interest in professional needs.
Place:	Lecture Room, Nurse Training Unit, Sharq.
Duration:	18 days (5. 9. 81—24. 9. 81).
Organiser:	Nurse Training and Planning Unit, Training Division, Dept. of Public Health and Planning.
Programme Director:	Miss Awatef Quttan, Head of Nurse Training and Planning Unit.
Participation:	25 nurses from different health facilities (names not available).
Course Programme:	The course programme shall include the development of modern administration (scientific management), administrative functions like management, planning, delegation, organisation, decision making and evaluation. General topics on ward policies, ward teaching and general discipline.

Field experience in selected hospitals for the particular post (head nurse) and the field visits to various hospitals to get acquainted with modern equipment, personnel and their working system.

To evaluate their performance during and at the end of the course, through a system of observation records and examination.

A detailed programme will be formed before the course begins.

81E—9904
Course for Head Nurses

Objectives:
1. To strengthen knowledge on principles of management.
2. To make them aware of the importance of ongoing education.
3. To help them to develop a planned supervisory programme to help the nursing personnel.

Place: Nurse training and planning unit.

Duration: One week from 23. 5. 81 to 28. 5. 81.

Organiser: Nurse training and planning unit.

Participants: 16 head nurses from different health facilities.

Course Programme: A one week course was planned with some management topics to enrich the head nurses knowledge in managing the unit. Topics included head nurses role in health services, leadership qualities, supervision, problem solving, delegation, control of infection and staff appraisal. A workshop was held on the functions of management in which the head nurses took interest in preparing, planning, organising, motivating and controlling.

Course Evaluation: The members expressed that the course was excellent though short. It gave them information and renewed their knowledge in administration and kept them up-to-date. They suggested having a well equiped class room and offering refreshments at 10 a.m.

Conclusion: The course went on smoothly. The members were very cooperative and interested.

81E—9905
Refresher Course for Head Nurses

Objectives:
1. To strengthen knowledge on principles of management.
2. To make them aware of the importance of on-going education.
3. To help them to develop a planned supervisory programme to help the nursing personnel.

Place:	Lecture Room, Nurse Training Unit, Sharq.
Duration:	6 days. From 23. 5. 81 to 28. 5. 81.
Organiser:	Nurse Training and Planning Unit Training Division, Dept. of Public Health and Planning.
Programme Director:	Miss Awatef Quttan, Head of Nurse Training and Planning Unit.
Participation:	26 head nurses from various health facilities (names not available).
Course Programme:	The course programme will include principles of administration, delegation, supervision, leadership, decision making, ward teaching, nursing rounds, assignment and evaluation. Workshops, film shows and visits will also be included.
	A detailed programme will be formed before the course begins.

81E—9906
Course for School Health Nurses

Objectives:	1. To refresh knowledge in general.
	2. To strengthen knowledge on common diseases among school children.
	3. To develop the power of observation and reporting.
	4. To teach them the modern trends and facilities available for an emergency.
Place:	Lecture Room, Nurse Training Unit, Sharq.
Duration:	12 days (28. 2. 81—12. 3. 81).
Organiser:	Nurse Training and Planning Unit, Training Division, Dept. of Public Health and Planning.
Programme Director:	Miss Awatef Quttan, Head of Nurse Training and Planning Unit.
Participation:	50 nurses from school health (names not available).
Course Programme:	The course shall include the growth and development of the school age group, personal and environmental hygiene, common diseases among school children, demonstration on handling emergencies among children and present problems of school age group.
	A detailed programme will be formed before the course begins.

81E—9907
Course for School Health Supervisors

Objectives:	1. To help them to understand the modern trend in school health care.

2. To review the knowledge of common diseases among children, and their management.
3. To acquaint the course members with the present day problems of school children.

Place: Nurse Training and Planning Unit.

Duration: 6 days (16. 5. 81—21. 5. 81).

Organiser: Nurse Training and Planning Unit.

Programme Director: Head of Nurse Training and Planning Unit.

Participation: 27 health supervisors from school health.

Course Programme: The course programme was planned to meet the professional needs of school health supervisors, so that they will be able to manage any problems arising in the care of school children. It included growth and development of school children, hygiene, common diseases in children, psycho-social problems, general observation and annual screening, management of handicapped children, skin handling emergencies and evaluation. Programme included workshop on: Habits of School Children of Different Ages and in Different Areas of Kuwait.
According to their observation the undesirable habits found in Kuwait's school children were lack of personal hygiene and psychosocial problems.

Course Evaluation: Three questions were given to the group:
1. Was the course up to your expectation?
2. Did the course achieve its objectives and if so, how?
3. Give your suggestions to improve future courses.
The following comments were given by them.
1. The course was well planned and organised.
2. The topics were all relevant to their work.
3. They gained knowledge about diseases and psychological problems of students.
4. Timing of lectures was a kind of motivation for them and it helped to keep them interested.

Evaluation: The course was a success. It included most of the needed topics. The group was interested. It was also requested by them that they would like to have such courses in future so as to keep up-to-date with current knowledge and to improve their skills.

81E—9908
Potential Assistant Directors of the Nursing Course

Objectives: 1. To recognise the need for good nursing services within the hospital and other health facilities.
2. To learn the principles of management and to implement them with her own responsibilities in mind.

3. To understand the organisational structure of the Ministry of Public Health and make use of the facilities available for the betterment of nursing services.
4. To learn her job description.

Place: Lecture Room, Nurse Training Unit, Sharq.

Duration: 53 days. From 1. 3. 81 to 30. 4. 81.

Organiser: Nurse Training and Planning Unit, Training Division, Dept. of Public Health and Planning.

Programme Director: Miss Awatef Quttan, Head of Nurse Training and Planning Unit.

Participation: 15 head nurses from different health facilities (names not available).

Course Programme: The course shall include the organisational structure of the Ministry of Public Health and Nursing Division, development of scientific management, the principles of management and the related experience in specific fields, job description, job analysis and the evaluation process for achievement of different functions.
Planning and budgeting in relation to equipment and supplies for short and long terms.
Common problems occurring in the Nursing Division and the management of solving the problem, understanding supervision of the personnel and development of a plan for its implementation.
Evaluation of the different forms and processes in practice in the Ministry.
A detailed programme will be formed before the course begins.

81E—9909
Course for Clinical Instructors

Objectives: 1. To prepare the selected staff nurses to be clinical instructors.
2. To teach them the principles of teaching.
3. To help them to plan, prepare and deliver teaching sessions.
4. To teach in the clinical situation with the interest of the patient and the nurse in mind.

Place: Lecture Room, Nurse Training Unit, Sharq.

Duration: 12 days. From 2. 5. 81 to 14. 5. 81.

Organiser: Nurse Training and Planning Unit, Training Division, Dept. of Public Health and Planning.

Programme Director: Miss Awatef Quttan, Head of Nurse Training and Planning Unit.

Participation: 20 nurses from different health facilities.

Programme:	To meet the requirements of various hospitals. For the post of clinical instructors the course was specially designed to suit their work as instructors. The programme mainly concentrated on teaching aspects. The topics included were:

1. Job description of a clinical instructor.
2. Principles of teaching.
3. Methods of teaching.
4. Learning process.
5. Development of instructional objectives.
6. Audio-visual aids.

There was a visit to Sabah Hospital to see the staff development department. They had to prepare lesson plans and practice teaching during the course. Each one had to take two classes; one theory and the other practical, each lasting for 15 minutes.

Evaluation: There was an interview at the end of the course, during which their lesson plan and practical teaching were discussed with them individually. During the interview all the members expressed satisfaction about the course and its related activities. They all said that the duration of the course was short and there should have been more time for hospital visits to see the staff development department in detail.

81E—9910
Course for Clinical Instructors

Objectives: At the end of the course the members will be able to:
1. Develop instructional objectives for formal teaching in the working area.
2. Create interest in the members to keep current with modern trends in teaching.
3. Recognise the importance of developing bedside teaching.

Place: Post Graduate Medical Centre, Al Adan Hospital.

Duration: 17. 10. 81 — 28. 10. 81.

Organiser: Nurse Training and Planning Unit.

Programme Director: Miss Awatef Quttan.

Course Tutor: Mr. S. Baskaran.

Guest Speaker: Mrs. Evelyn R. Barritt.

Participants: 19 clinical instructors from various hospitals who had undergone a course on clinical instruction and had from two to four years experience.
Educational Background of the Candidate: All the course members are qualified nurses having worked in the nursing field for five to ten years. Most of them are Bachelors in Nursing and some of them are postgraduate in teaching. Though all of them did not have aca-

demic teaching experience, they have attended a clinical instructors' course conducted by this department,
and have had from one to four years experience at present. All of them speak the English language very well.

Course Programme: In order to develop the clinical instructors' talents and
to use them effectively for the improvement of patient
care at their respective working areas, the programme
was developed keeping in mind the objectives set forth.
The programme was centered on preparation of instructional objectives, instructional plan, modern trends in
teaching, use of audio-visual aids and methods of assessment. Professor Evelyn R. Barritt, Dean of School
of Nursing, Miami University, was invited as the main
speaker.

Saturday, 17th October, 1981

8.30—10.30 a.m.	Introduction and Briefing
10.30—11.00 a.m.	Break
11.00— 1.00 p.m.	Learners and Learning

Sunday, 18th October, 1981

8.30—10.30 a.m.	Introduction to Course Members and Free Discussion for the Assessment of Their Needs.
10.30—11.00 a.m.	Break
11.00— 1.00 p.m.	Clinical Teaching as it is Understood by the Members.

Monday, 19th October, 1981

8.30—10.30 a.m.	Library Resources
10.30—11.00 a.m.	Break
11.00— 1.00 p.m.	Who is a Good Teacher?

Tuesday, 20th October, 1981

8.30— 1.00 p.m.	Workshop: How to Improve Clinical Teaching Motivation of the Learners Improving the Clinical Situation Evaluation of Teaching

Wednesday, 21st October, 1981

8.30—10.30 a.m.	How to Develop Instructional Objectives
10.30—11.00 a.m.	Break
11.00— 1.00 p.m.	Exercise: Preparation of Instructional Objectives

Thursday, 22nd October, 1981

8.30—10.30 a.m.	Preparation of Instruction Plan
10.30—11.00 a.m.	Break
11.00— 1.00 p.m.	Film

Saturday, 24th October, 1981

8.30—10.30 a.m.	Concept of Bedside Teaching
10.30—11.00 a.m.	Break
11.00— 1.00 p.m.	Importance of Orienting New Nursing Personnel to the Working Area

Sunday, 25th October, 1981

8.30—10.30 a.m.	Audio-Visual Aids.
10.30—11.00 a.m.	Break
11.00— 1.00 p.m.	Demonstration: Audio-Visual Aids

Monday, 26th October, 1981

8.30—10.30 a.m.	Modern Trends in Teaching
10.30—11.00 a.m.	Break
11.00— 1.00 p.m.	Methods of Assessment

Tuesday, 27th October, 1981

8.30—10.30 a.m.	Measurement of Educational Objectives
10.30—11.00 a.m.	Break
11.00— 1.00 p.m.	Closing Session

Wednesday, 28th October, 1981

8.30—10.30 a.m.	Exercise: Preparation of Instruction Plan Intramuscular Injection Taking Blood Pressure Hand Hygiene
10.30—11.00 a.m.	Break
11.00— 1.00 p.m.	Tour to Adan Hospital (Teaching Area) Discussion on Instruction Plan

81E—9911
Course for Assistant Nurses

Objectives:	1. To understand the patient and his individual needs. 2. To recognise their role in team nursing and to contribute effectively towards patient care. 3. To appreciate the importance of ongoing education.
Place:	Lecture Room, Nurse Training Unit, Sharq.
Duration:	6 days from 16. 5. 81 to 21. 5. 81.
Organiser:	Nurse Training and Planning Unit Training Division, Dept. of Public Health and Planning.
Programme Director:	Miss Awatef Quttan, Head of Nurse Training and Planning Unit.
Participation:	26 assistant nurses from different health facilities (names not available).
Course Programme:	Course programme includes the role of an Assistant Nurse in team nursing, importance of communication,

handling emergencies, nutrition and feeding, aseptic technique, vital signs, observation and recording, hygiene of the patient and control of infection.
A detailed programme will be formed before the course begins.

81E—9912
Course for Assistant Nurses

Objectives:
1. To understand the patient and his individual needs.
2. To recognise their role in team nursing and contribute effectively towards patient care.
3. To appreciate the importance of ongoing education.

Place: Nurse Training and Planning Unit.

Duration: 6 days, from 16. 5. 81 to 21. 5. 81.

Organiser: Nurse Training and Planning Unit.

Participants: 16 assistant nurses from various hospitals and clinics.

Course Programme: This course aimed to meet the learning needs of assistant nurses, to help them contribute effectively to patient care. The programme enlightened their knowledge in aseptic technique, care of seriously ill patients, how to act in emergency, role of the social worker in health care and the psychological needs of patients. Topics also included fire hazards and prevention, job description and evaluation. One day was set apart for a workshop on observation of vital signs, which motivated them to look into the details of vital signs.

Course Evaluation: All the course members expressed satisfaction in the course programme. They gained knowledge in better patient care. The course was short and there were no visits to other hospitals.

Conclusion: The course went on smoothly and it was well appreciated by all the members.

81E—9913
Course for Assistant Nurses

Objectives:
1. To understand the patient and his individual needs.
2. To recognise their role in team nursing and contribute effectively towards patient care.
3. To appreciate the importance of ongoing education.

Place: Lecture Room, Nurse Training Unit, Sharq.

Duration: 6 days from 26. 9. 81 to 1. 10. 81.

Organiser: Nurse Training and Planning Unit, Training Division, Dept. of Public Health and Planning.

Programme Director:	Miss Awatef Quttan, Head of Nurse Training and Planning Unit.
Participation:	26 assistant nurses from different health facilities (names not available).
Course Programme:	Course programme includes the role of an Assistant Nurse in team nursing, importance of communication, handling emergencies, nutrition and feeding, aseptic technique, vital signs, observation and recording, hygiene of the patient and control of infection. A detailed programme will be formed before the course begins.

81E—99/3714
Course for Midwives

Objectives:	1. To implement the modern concept in the care of the mother during antenatal, labour and postnatal periods. 2. To demonstrate scientifically the care of the newborn. 3. To exhibit skill in managing the mother on various obstetrical disorders and the baby with neonatal problems.
Place:	Lecture Room, Nurse Training Unit, Sharq.
Duration:	10 days. From 1. 6. 81 to 11. 6. 81.
Organiser:	Nurse Training and Planning Unit, Training Division, Dept. of Public Health and Planning.
Programme Director:	Head of Nurse Training and Planning Unit.
Participation:	17 nurses from various M.C.H. clinics and from Maternity Hospital (names not available).
Course Programme:	The course programme includes antenatal and postnatal care, normal and abnormal labours, psychological aspects in pregnancy, use of contraceptives, diseases complicating pregnancy, complications of pregnancy, care of newborn baby, premature baby and jaundice in newborn. Film shows, workshops, assignment and visits will be supplemented in the programme. A detailed programme will be formed before the course begins.

81E—99/3715
Course for Midwives

Objectives:	1. To implement the modern concept in the care of mother during antenatal, labour and postnatal periods.

2. To demonstrate scientifically the care of the newborn.
3. To exhibit skill in managing the mother on various obstetrical disorders and the baby with neonatal problems.

Place: Lecture Room, Nurse Training Unit, Sharq.

Duration: 10 days from 31. 10. 81 to 10. 11. 81.

Organiser: Nurse Training and Planning Unit, Training Division, Dept. of Public Health and Planning.

Programme Director: Head of Nurse Training and Planning Unit.

Participation: 17 nurses from various M.C.H. clinics and from Maternity Hospital (names not available).

Course Programme: The course programme includes antenatal and postnatal care, normal and abnormal labours, psychological aspects in pregnancy, use of contraceptives, diseases complicating pregnancy, complications of pregnancy, care of newborn baby, premature baby and jaundice in newborn.
Film shows, workshops, assignment and visits will be supplemented in the programme.
A detailed programme will be formed before the course begins.

81E—99/1216
Refresher Course for Medical Nurses

Objectives: 1. To strengthen knowledge on various medical conditions common in Kuwait.
2. To provide additional information in medical nursing.
3. To develop skill in understanding the patient and to meet individual needs.

Place: Lecture Room, Nurse Training Unit, Sharq.

Duration: 12 days. From 13. 6. 81 to 25. 6. 81.

Organiser: Nurse Training and Planning Unit, Training Division, Dept. of Public Health and Planning.

Programme Director: Head of Nurse Training and Planning Unit.

Participation: 24 nurses from different medical units (names not available).

Course Programme: This course consists of medical topics like common allergic conditions, diabetes mellitus, modern trends in tuberculosis treatment, bronchitis, respiratory failure, C.C.F., anaemia and renal failure, nursing management in admission, E.C.G. reading and interpretation, control of infection, control of communicable diseases, nursing care plan and nurses' notes, and the nurse's role in I.V. fluid administration.

The course shall also include general subjects like employment policy, role of social worker and pharmacology.

A detailed programme will be formed before the course begins.

81E—99/1217
Refresher Course for Medical Nurses

Objectives:

1. To strengthen knowledge on various medical conditions common in Kuwait.
2. To provide additional information in medical nursing.
3. To develop skill in understanding the patient and to meet individual needs.

Place: Lecture Room, Nurse Training Unit, Sharq.

Duration: 12 days. From 14. 11. 81 to 26. 11. 81.

Organiser: Nurse Training and Planning Unit, Training Division, Dept. of Public Health and Planning.

Programme Director: Head of Nurse Training and Planning Unit.

Participation: 24 nurses from different medical units (names not available).

Course Programme: This course consists of medical topics like common allergic conditions, diabetes mellitus, modern trends in tuberculosis treatment, bronchitis, respiratory failure, C.C.F., anaemia and renal failure, nursing management in admission, E.C.G. reading and interpretation, control of infection, control of communicable diseases, nursing care plan and nurses' notes, and the nurse's role in I.V. fluid administration.

The course shall also include general subjects like employment policy, role of social worker and pharmacology.

A detailed programme will be formed before the course begins.

81E—99/3318
Refresher Course for Paediatric Nurses

Objectives:

1. To develop skill and power of observation for better nursing care planning for children.
2. To keep in touch with modern developments through studies and discussions.
3. To revise their knowledge in:
   a) Growth and development of children.
   b) The effectiveness of immunisation.

4. To review and expand knowledge in basic nursing and advanced trends in paediatric nursing.

Place: Lecture Room, Nurse Training Unit, Sharq.

Duration: 8 days. From 1. 7. 81 to 9. 7. 81.

Organiser: Nurse Training and Planning Unit, Training Division, Dept. of Public Health and Planning.

Programme Organiser: Head of Nurse Training and Planning Unit.

Participation: 25 nurses from paediatric units (names not available).

Course Programme: The course programme shall contain embryo development, common communicable diseases in children, immunisation, blood diseases, growth and development, gastro-intestinal disorders, electrolyte balance and I.V. infusion, nursing process care plan, control of infection, acute glomerulonephritis, and bronchopneumonia.
A detailed programme will be formed before the course begins.

81E—99/3319
Refresher Course for Paediatric Nurses

Objectives: 1. To develop skill and power in observation for better nursing care planning for children.
2. To keep in touch with modern developments through studies and discussions.
3. To revise their knowledge in:
   a) Growth and development of children.
   b) The effectiveness of immunisation.
4. To review and expand knowledge in basic nursing and advanced trends in paediatric nursing.

Place: Lecture Room, Nursing Training Unit, Sharq.

Duration: 8 days. From 28. 11. 81 to 6. 12. 81.

Organiser: Nurse Training and Planning Unit, Training Division, Dept. of Public Health and Planning.

Programme Organiser: Head of Nurse Training and Planning Unit.

Participation: 25 nurses from paediatric units (names not available).

Course Programme: The course programme shall contain embryo development, common communicable diseases in children, immunisation, blood diseases, growth and development, gastro-intestinal disorders, electrolyte balance and I.V. infusion, nursing process care plan, control of infection, acute glomerulonephritis, and bronchopneumonia.
A detailed programme will be formed before the course begins.

81E—99/2320
Refresher Course for Surgical Nurses

Objectives:
1. To appreciate the need for specialisation in surgical nursing to meet the changing techniques and increasing demands.
2. To add information to the modern development in surgery and care of the patient.
3. To exhibit skill in giving surgical nursing care.

Place: Lecture Room, Nurse Training Unit, Sharq.

Duration: 12 days. From 8. 8. 81 to 20. 8. 81.

Organiser: Nurse Training and Planning Unit, Training Division, Dept. of Public Health and Planning.

Programme Director: Miss Awatef Quttan, Head of Nurse Training and Planning Unit.

Participation: 26 nurses from different surgical units (names not available).

Course Programme: The course programme will include management of pre- and post-anaesthesia, pre- and post-operative care, emergency surgical admission control of infection, neonatal surgical conditions, osteomyelitis, goitres, tracheotomy, chest and heart surgery, head injury and intestinal obstruction.
A detailed programme will be formed before the course begins.

81E—99/2321
Refresher Course for Surgical Nurses

Objectives:
1. To appreciate the need for specialisation in surgical nursing to meet the changing techniques and increasing demands.
2. To add information to the modern development in surgery and care of the patient.
3. To exhibit skill in giving surgical nursing care.

Place: Lecture Room, Nurse Training Unit, Sharq.

Duration: 12 days. From 12. 12. 81 to 24. 12. 81.

Organiser: Nurse Training and Planning Unit, Training Division, Dept. of Public Health and Planning.

Programme Director: Miss Awatef Quttan, Head of Nurse Training and Planning Unit.

Participation: 26 nurses from different surgical units (names not available).

Course Programme: The course programme will include management of pre- and post-anaesthesia, pre- and post-operative care, emergency surgical admission, control of infection, neonatal surgical conditions, osteomyelites, goitres, tracheotomy, chest and heart surgery, head injury and intestinal obstruction.

A detailed programme will be formed before the course begins.

81E—99/6122
Refresher Course for Psychiatric Nurses

Objectives:
1. For the candidates to understand their role in the psychiatric ward.
2. To stimulate them to be aware of modern trends in psychiatry.
3. To develop their knowledge in human psychology for better nursing care.

Place: Lecture Room, Nurse Training Unit, Sharq.

Duration: 6 days. From 22. 8. 81 to 27. 8. 81.

Organiser: Nurse Training and Planning Unit, Training Division, Dept. of Public Health and Planning.

Programme Director: Miss Awatef Quttan, Head of Nurse Training and Planning Unit.

Participation: 23 psychiatric nurses (names not available).

Course Programme: This course shall include human psychology, classification of mental illnesses, drug dependence, alcoholism, modern trends in psychiatric treatment, causes of insomnia, nursing care of violent patients, addict patients, patients with suicidal tendencies and depressed patients.

A detailed programme will be formed before the course begins.

81E—99/9823
Course for School Health Nurses

Objectives:
1. To help them to understand modern trends in school health care.
2. To review the knowledge of common childhood diseases and their management.
3. To acquaint the course members with the present day problems of school children.

Place: Nurse Training and Planning Unit.

Duration: 12 days (28. 2. 81—12. 3. 81).

Organiser: Nurse Training and Planning Unit.

Programme Director: Head of Nurse Training and Planning Unit.

Participants: 46 nurses from school health.

Course Programme: The course programme was planned to meet the professional needs of school health nurses, so that they will be able to manage any problems arising in the care of school children. It included growth and development of school children, hygiene, common diseases in children, psychosocial problems, general observation and annual screening, management of handicapped children, addiction and habits of school children, skin and dental care, handling emergencies and evaluation.

The programme included a workshop on: Habits of School Children of Different Ages and in Different Areas of Kuwait.

According to their observation the undesirable habits found in Kuwait's school children were smoking, addiction to petrol and drugs, lack of personal hygiene and psychosocial problems.

Course Evaluation: Three questions were given to the group:
1. Was the course up to your expectation?
2. Did the course achieve its objectives and if so, how?
3. Give your suggestions to improve future courses.

The following comments were given by them.
1. The course was well planned and organised.
2. The topics were all relevant to their work.
3. They gained knowledge about diseases and psychological problems of students.
4. Timing of lectures was a kind of motivation for them and it kept them interested.
5. Asked to prolong the course, also requested to plan another course in the summertime so that all the nurses get a chance to attend.

c) International Meetings

81C—13/07/65/15/73/1401
1st Kuwait International Medical Sciences Conference

Objectives: To teach advances in clinical medicine.

Place: Sheraton Hotel.

Duration: 19—21 January, 1982.

Organiser: Honorary Advisory Committee
S. S. Al-Bader
K. A. Gumaa
N. Al-Naqeeb
A. A. Al-Rasheed
A. M. Yousof
National Organising Committee
K. A. Gumaa—Chairman
A. El-Khawad
H. Al-Mahmood

C. Pilcher
N. Al-Zaid

Programme Director: Prof. A. M. Yousof, Dean, Faculty of Medicine.

Participants: All doctors interested in the subjects of the conference.

Programme:

19th January, 1981 (Monday)

Cancer and Immunology

Session I:

Chairman: Y. Omar, Co-Chairman: A. G. White

8.00— 8.35 a.m.	A. M. Jelliffe (Invited Speaker) Approaches to Clinical Immunotherapy
8.35— 8.45 a.m.	Discussion
8.45— 9.00 a.m.	A. S. Ismail and Y. Omar A Clinico-Epidemiological Study of Breast Cancer in Kuwait
9.00— 9.15 a.m.	A. Albader, A. G. H. Al Zuhair, A. A. Ramadan and M. E. Mohammed The Effect of the Anti-Cancer Drug Cis-Acid on the Ultrastructure of Hela Cells
9.15— 9.30 a.m.	G. M. Abouna, A. M. S. Kumar, S. Daddah, E. Lashen, A. G. White and M. Ashkar Acute Renal Allograft Rejection Successfully Treated with Intravenous Antilymphocyte Globulin
9.30— 9.45 a.m.	M. J. Ahmed and M. S. Motawy Multiple Myeloma in Kuwait. Clinical Features as Prognostic Index
9.45—10.00 a.m.	Discussion
10.00—10.15 a.m.	Intermission

Session II:

Chairman: M. Y. Ali, Co-Chairman: Na'il Al Naqeeb

10.15—10.30 a.m.	M. A. J. Al-Mousawi, M. Kadri, M. Salama and A. Salem Screening of Chemical Mutagens in the Marine Environment of Kuwait
10.30—10.45 a.m.	K. Fahmy Colposcopy in Diagnosis of Cervical Dysplasia and Cancer
10.45—11.00 a. m.	A. H. Awaad, M. Y. Yozgi, Y. Omar, M. Barakat and G. M. Abouna Cancer of the Pancreas and Periampullary Region
11.00—11.15 a. m.	G. Abouna, A. G. White, H. A. Youssef, A. Kumar, K. Lubaadah and S. Daddah Kidney Transplantation in Kuwait
11.15—11.30 a. m.	A. M. Karnik, A. Al-Khattrash, M. Barakat and Y. Omar Primary Hepatocellular Carcinoma in Kuwait

11.30—11.45 a.m.

L. G. Lindberg
New Concept of Malignant Non-Hodgkin Lymphoma, More Accurate Prognosis and Treatment Using the Lennert Classification System

Poster Session

12.00—12.45 p.m.

R. Morrison
Recent Advances in Radiotherapy and the Use of Drugs as Radiosensitisers
A. White
A New Assay for Measuring the Bactericidal Capacity of Human Phagocytic Cells
P. S. Sahni, A. M. Abulmajd, F. Bottazzo and T. D. R. Hockadaylslet
Cell Antibodies and C. Peptide Concentrations in Insulin Treated Diabetics in Kuwait
A. A. H. Al-Khars
Bioavailability of Acetylsalicylic Acid Preparations Registered in Kuwait
H. Angelo
The Metabolism of Debrisoquine, a Rare Example in Pharmacogenetics
K. Menon, S. Shuwaikh, M. Barakat, A. Badawi, K. Guman and M. A. A. Moussa
Jaundice in Children, Kuwait Experience
K. Saleh
Injury of the Diaphragm and Associated Involvement of the Liver
M. M. Shaaban, N. M. L. Sharkawy, S. A. Ghaneemah, S. I. Alwan, A. B. Kholeif and Y. H. Ahmed Atef
Urinary Excretion of Oestrogens
17—Oxysteroids and 17—Oxogenic Steroids in Women with Liver Cirrhosis.
W. Al-Nakib, I. L. Chrystie and J. E. Banatvala
Role of Rotavirus in Non-Bacterial Gastroenteritis in Kuwait
V. Bezjak and H. Thorburn
Survey of Kuwait Rat (Rattus norvegicus) Population for Some Human Pathogens
E. E. Al-Sawi, M. Nasser and A. M. Yousof
Sector-Scanning Demonstration
A. G. H. Al-Zuhair, H. Hathout, M. E. A. Ibrahim and M. E. Mohammed
Scanning Electron Microscopic Study of the Human Placenta
M. Abu Hamdiyyah
Molecular Mechanism of Anaesthesia
C. W. T. Pilcher and Sarah M. Jones
Evidence for Some Chemical Substances Role in Nociception and Aversive States

Respiratory Diseases

Session I:

Chairman: F. F. Fenech, Co-Chairman: M. A. Shaaban

14.00—14.35 p.m.	T. J. H. Clark (Invited Speaker) Corticosteroid Treatment of Bronchial Asthma
14.35—14.45 p.m.	Discussion
14.45—15.00 p.m.	P. V. Agius Childhood Asthma
15.00—15.15 p.m.	R. Ellul Mecallef and F. F. Fenech Simultaneous Occurrence of Bronchial Asthma and Diabetes Mellitus
15.15—15.30 p.m.	K. Y. Mustafa, A. El-Khawad, V. Bicik and I. A. Mardini Sympathetic Stimulation Produced Contraction of Tracheal Smooth Muscles in the Rabbit as Demonstrated by a New In Vivo Method
15.30—15.45 p.m.	O. Abdulmajid Pulmonary Hydatid Disease
15.45—16.00 p.m.	Discussion and Concluding Remarks
16.00—16.15 p.m.	Intermission

Session II:

Chairman: T. J. H. Clark, Co-Chairman: P. V. Agius

16.15—16.30 p.m.	M. A. Shaaban Patterns and Trends of Tuberculosis in Kuwait
16.30—16.45 p.m.	F. F. Fenech Endocrine Dysfunction in Bronchogenic Carcinoma
16.45—17.00 p.m.	H. Abdulmajid, H. Bassioum, M. Kalaawi and S. Farwana Pulmonary Complications of Kerosene Poisoning
17.00—17.15 p.m.	K. Y. Mustafa, M. A. Shaaban, C. Ghalayeeni, Nadia M. Noufel Diffuse Pulmonary Fibrosis in Kuwait, Clinicophysiological Study
17.15—17.30 p.m.	Discussion and Concluding Remarks

20th January, 1981 (Tuesday)

Neurotransmitters

Chairman: C. W. T. Pilcher, Co-Chairman: A. O. Elkhawad

8.00— 8.35 a.m.	D. G. Grahame Smith (Invited Speaker) Neurotransmitters. Psychotropic Drugs and Mental Illness
8.35— 8.45 a.m.	Discussion
8.45— 9.20 a.m.	C. W. T. Pilcher—Endorphins in Affective States and Nociception
9.20— 9.30 a.m.	Discussion

9.30— 9.45 a.m.	D. V. Naik
	A New Concept of Neuroendocrine Control of ACTH
	Secretion in Pars Intermedia Transplant in
	Hypophysectomized Rats
9.45—10.00 a.m.	R. Shakir, R. Johnson and D. Lambie
	Treatment of Folate Deficient Epileptics with Folic Acid
	and 5 Formyl Tetrahydrofolate (Folinic Acid)
10.00—10.15 a.m.	Intermission
10.15—10.30 a.m.	O. Thulesius
	Alpha and Beta-Adrenergic Receptors in Human Veins
10.30—10.45 a.m.	A. O. Elkhawad—A Comparative Study of a New
	Dopamine Agonist SK and F 38393
10.45—11.00 a.m.	M. Z. M. Ibrahim
	On the Origin of the Neurolipomastocytoid Cells of the
	Mammalian Central Nervous System
11.00—11.15 a.m.	Discussion and Concluding Remarks
11.15—11.30 a.m.	Intermission
11.30—12.30 p.m.	Poster Session Discussion, Coordinators N. A.
	Mahmoud, M. Y. Ali and H. Hathout

Liver Diseases

Session I:

Chairman: G. M. Abouna, Co-Chairman: B. Al-Nakib

14.00—14.35 p.m.	D. B. McGill (Invited Speaker)
	Progress and Challenges in Liver Disease
14.35—14.45 p.m.	Discussion
14.45—15.00 p.m.	B. Al-Nakib, W. Al-Nakib and A. Bayoumi
	Hepatitis B Virus Indices in Chronic Liver Disease
15.00—15.15 p.m.	M. Barakat, K. Menon, A. Badawi and A. Karnik
	Obstructive Jaundice in Kuwait
15.15—15.30 p.m.	M. H. Alwan, A. T. Menkarios, R. J. Mallick, M.
	Barakat, K. Menon and G. M. Abouna
	Hydatid Disease of the Liver in Kuwait
15.30—15.45 p.m.	J. S. Juggi—Reye's Syndrome
15.45—16.00 p.m.	Discussion and Concluding Remarks
16.00—16.15 p.m.	Intermission

Session II:

Chairman: D. B. McGill, Co-Chairman: M. Barakat

16.15—16.30 p.m.	A. Badawi, M. Shabrawi, K. Menon, M. Barakat, K.
	Gumaa and M. A. A. Moussa
	Jaundice Survey in Adults. The Kuwait Experience
16.30—16.45 p.m.	A. T. Menkarios, H. A. Youssef, A. Awaad, M. H.
	Alwan, M. A. Bassiouni, M. Barakat, A. Badawi, F.
	Al-Addawui and G. M. Abouna
	Distal Spleno-Renal Shunt for Portal Hypertension

16.45—17.00 p.m.	G. M. Abouna, B. A. Z. Barabas, F. Alexander and D. W. Kinninburg—Experimental Models of Fulminant Hepatic Failure
17.00—17.15 p.m.	G. M. Abouna, B. A. Z. Barabas, F. Alexander and D. W. Kinninburg Resin and Charcoal Haemoperfusion in Treatment of Hepatic Coma
17.15—17.30 p.m.	Malak I. Shoukry Extraction of Lipid from Mammalian Liver Using Non-Toxic Solvents
17.30—17.45 p.m.	Discussion and Concluding Remarks

21st January, 1981 (Wednesday)

Epidemiology

Session I:

Chairman: M. Khogali, Co-Chairman: G. Ezzat

8.00—8.35 a.m.	J. A. Dudgeon (Invited Speaker) The Control of Communicable Diseases by Immunization—Present Status and Prospects of the Future
8.35— 8.45 a.m.	Discussion
8.45— 9.00 a.m.	M. Khogali Environmental Heat Illnesses
9.00— 9.15 a.m.	L. S. Deep, G. M. Ezzat, R. I. M. Ismail A Description of Diabetes Mellitus in Kuwait
9.15— 9.30 a.m.	R. Al-Owaish Epidemiological Patterns of Myocardial Infractions in Kuwait (1978)
9.30— 9.45 a.m.	R. Labib, M. Aboutabik, A. S. Ismail and Y. T. Omar Experience with Kuwait Population Based Registry
9.45—10.00 a.m.	Discussion
10.00—10.15 a.m.	Intermission

Session II:

Chairman: J. A. Dudgeon, Co-Chairman: V. Bezjak

10.15—10.30 a.m.	R. I. M. Ismail An Epidemiological Study of Breast Cancer Incidence in Kuwait (1976)
10.30—10.45 a.m.	A. Bayoumi Epidemiology of Motor Vehicle Accidents in Kuwait
10.45—11.00 a.m.	Salwa A. Mustafa Nutrition Status Assessment of Pre-School Children
11.00—11.15 a.m.	K. Elhag Bacteraemia in the United Arab Emirates
11.15—11.30 a.m.	T. D. Chug Drug Resistance of Salmonellae in Kuwait

Cardiology

Session I:

Chairman: A. M. Yousof, Co-Chairman: H. Shuhaiber

14.00—14.30 p.m.	F. Bashour (Invited Speaker) A Decade of Coronary Artery Surgery
14.30—14.35 p.m.	Discussion
14.35—14.55 p.m.	A. M. Yousof Kuwait Contribution to Dye Dilution Research
14.55—15.00 p.m.	Discussion
15.00—15.15 p.m.	M. Nasser Early Experience with Coronary Angiography in Kuwait
15.15—15.30 p.m.	H. Shuhaiber Open Heart Surgery in Kuwait
15.30—15.45 p.m.	Percutaneous Raskind Septostomy
15.45—16.00 p.m.	Intermission

Session II:

Chairman: F. Bashour, Co-Chairman: M. M. Gomaa

16.00—16.10 p.m.	E. E. Al-Sawi, M. Nasser, A. M. Yousof, N. Khan 18 Months Experience in Sector Scanning
16.10—16.20 p.m.	P. Stransky, J. Kvasnicka, A. M. Yousof, J. Endrys and I. Zyka Quantitative Evaluation of the Left Ventricle Motility in Coronary Heart Disease
16.20—16.30 p.m.	N. Khan, P. Stransky, A. M. Yousof and M. Nasser Computer Assisted Processing of Left Ventricular Echocardiogram
16.30—16.40 p.m.	Discussion
16.40—16.50 p.m.	M. M. Gomaa and S. W. Taylor New Technique for the Mapping of the RS-T Segments
16.50—17.00 p.m.	H. A. Majeed, N. Khan, M. Dabbagh, K. Najdi and N. Kaateeb Acute Rheumatic Fever during Childhood in Kuwait
17.00—17.10 p.m.	J. S. Juggi Myocardial Preservation Methods and Functional Assessments
17.10—17.20 p.m.	Discussion
17.20—17.30 p.m.	K. Y. Mustafa, H. Shuhaiber, M. Mustafa Nour, M. A. Shabaan and A. M. Yousof Respiratory Function Status of Patients with Severe Valvular Heart Disease Pre- Post-Operative Evaluation
17.30—17.40 p.m.	O. Thulesius Non-Invasive Evaluation of Arterial Disease

81C—73/01/1302
2nd Kuwait International Medical Conference

Objectives:	To teach advances in clinical medicine.
Place:	Kuwait Hilton Hotel.
Duration:	January 16th to 18th, 1982.
Organiser:	Advisory Committee

President: Prof. A. M. Yousof
Dean, Faculty of Medicine

Dr. A. M. Al-Rifai
Secretary General
Kuwait University

Dr. N. A. Al-Naqeeb
Undersecretary
Ministry of Public Health

Dr. E. Ruzyllo
Prof. A. R. Yousof
Prof. N. A. Mahmoud
Prof. K. A. Gumaa
Dr. M. J. McBroom

Organising Committee
Chairman: Prof. O. Thulesius
Dr. A. O. Elkhawad
Secretary and Programme Chairman

Dr. F. M. Al-Awadi
Social Chairman

Dr. A. A. Al-Bader
Financial Chairman

Programme Director:	Prof. O. Thulesius, Department of Pharmacology, Faculty of Medicine.
Participants:	Doctors interested in subjects.
Programme:	

16th January, 1982 (Saturday)

Section I

Testing Procedures, Physical Factors, Electrolytes
Chairmen: J. Shepherd, U.S.A., and B. Altura, U.S.A.
Secretary: C. Pilcher, Kuwait

9.25— 9.45 a.m.	Testing Procedure for Isolated Blood Vessels R. F. W. Moulds, Australia
9.45—10.05 a.m.	Effect of Cold on the Blood Vessel Wall J. T. Shepherd, N. Rusch and P. M. Vanhoutte, U.S.A.
10.05—10.15 a.m.	Vascular Effects of Hyperthermia on Isolated Blood Vessels A. O. Elkhawad, O. Thulesius and M. M. Khogali, Kuwait

10.25—10.35 a.m.	Vascular Effects of Cardioplegic Solutions J. S. Juggi, O. Thulesius, A. O. Elkhawad and A. M. Yousof, Kuwait
10.35—11.00 a.m.	Discussion

Section II	Autonomic Innervation, Adrenergic and Cholinergic Receptors Chairmen: Ch. Owman, Sweden, and P. Vanhoutte, U.S.A. Secretary: A. Elkhawad, Kuwait
11.20—11.40 a.m.	Autonomic Nerves and Corresponding Receptors in Human Brain Vessels—An Overview. Ch. Owman, Sweden
11.40—12.00 noon	Prejunctional Modulation of Norepinephrine Release P. M. Vanhoutte and J. T. Shepherd, U.S.A.
12.00—12.10 p.m.	Neuronal and Extraneuronal Uptake and Metabolism of Catecholamines K. H. Graefe, Federal Republic of Germany
12.10—12.20 p.m.	The Role of Facilitatory Presynaptic Receptors in Human Digital Arteries R. F. W. Moulds and M. J. Stevens, Australia
12.20—12.30 p.m.	Characterization of Adrenergic Receptors in Hand Arteries and Veins by In Vitro Analysis and Hand Angiography B. Arneklo-Nobin, L. Edvinsson, B. Eklof, D. Haffajee, Ch. Owman and Y. Tylen, Sweden
12.30—12.40 p.m.	Vessel Cholinergic Agonists versus Receptors Groupings C. Concettoni, A. Diotallevi and L. Rossini, Italy
12.40—12.50 p.m.	Sympatho-Adrenal Regulation of Blood Flow in Adipose Tissue in Dog and Man P. Hjemdahl, B. Linde, M. Daleskog and E. Belfrage, Sweden
12.50—13.15 p.m.	Discussion

Section III	Species Differences, Regional Differences and Endothelium Chairmen: J. Bevan, U.S.A., and B. F. Robinson, England Secretary: M. M. Angelo-Khattar, Kuwait
14.30—14.50 p.m.	Differences in Blood Vessels between Species; Relation to Differences in Blood Vessels of Varying Types within the Same Species B. F. Robinson, England
14.50—15.00 p.m.	Species Variations in the Cerebrovascular Response to Neurotransmitters and Related Vasoactive Agents J. E. Hardebo and J. Hanko, Sweden
15.00—15.20 p.m.	Characteristics of Human Blood Vessels Studied In Vitro with Particular Emphasis on their Adrenergic Control J. A. Bevan and R. D. Bevan, U.S.A.

15.20—15.30 p.m.	Human and Rat Resistance Vessels: a Comparison of their Morphological and Pharmacological Characteristics C. Aalkjaer and M. J. Mulvany, Denmark
15.30—15.40 p.m.	Regional Differences in the Response of Isolated Human Vessels to Vasoactive Substances E. Mikkelsen and P. O. Lederballe, Denmark
15.40—15.50 p.m.	Heterogeneity of Post-Junctional a-Adrenoreceptors in Cerebral and Peripheral Arteries from Cat and Man T. Skarby, K. E. Andersson and L. Edvinsson, Sweden
15.50—16.00 p.m.	Control of Vascular Smooth Muscle Function by the Endothelial Cells P. M. Vanhoutte and J. D. Mey, U.S.A.
16.00—16.10 p.m.	Endothelial Cell Dependent Relaxation of Pulmonary and Renal Arteries B. Altura and N. Chand, U.S.A.

Section IV   Posters

Chairmen: O. Thulesius and J. Juggi
Secretary: M. Khogali

16.40—17.15 p.m.   Computer Programme for Dose-Response Curves, Testing Vasoconstrictor and Vasodilator Agents
O. Thulesius and F. X. Stephen, Kuwait
Contractile Response of Different Isolated Human Vessels, with Special Regard to Spontaneous and Pharmacologically Induced Rhythmicity
J. T. Holmberg, O. Thulesius and J. E. Gjores, Sweden
Responses of the Pulmonary Artery to Asthma Drugs
J. Boe, Sweden
Interactions Between Formed Elements and the Pulmonary Endothelium
A. B. Malik, F. L. Minnear and A. Johnson, U.S.A.
Modulation of Sympathetic Activity and Vascular Tone by Peripheral Alpha-2 Adrenoceptors in Man
W. Kiowski, L. Hulthen, P. Bolli, R. Ritz and F. R. Buhler, Switzerland
A Functional Abnormality of the Forearm Resistance Vessels in Men with Primary Hypertension
B. F. Robinson, R. J. Dobbs, S. Bayley and P. Chiodini, England
Pharmacological and Haemodynamic Studies on Flunarizine
N. Gulati, H. Huggel and O. P. Gulati
Effect of Prostaglandin Synthesis Inhibitors on Basal and CO_2-Stimulated Cerebral Blood Flow in Man
A. Wennmalm, L. S. Eriksson, D. Law and J. Wahren, Sweden
Vascular Responses Elicited by Venom of Arabian Gulf Catfish (Arius Thallasinus)
O. Thulesius, J. M. Al-Hassan, R. S. Criddle and Martha Thomson, Kuwait

17th January, 1982 (Sunday)

Section V	Prostaglandins, Substance P

Chairmen: S. Moncada, England, and B. Pernow, Sweden
Secretary: A. Al-Khars, Kuwait

8.30— 8.50 a.m.   Prostacyclin and Thromboxane A_2
S. Moncada, U.K.

8.50— 9.00 a.m.   Nicotine Inhibits Vascular Prostacyclin but not Platelet Thromboxane Formation
A. Wennmalm and P. Alster, Sweden

9.00— 9.10 p.m.   New Group of Prostaglandin-like Compounds in P. Acnes
L. Helligren and J. Vincent, Norway

9.10— 9.20 a.m.   Reduced Platelet Aggregation by Effects of Pentoxifylline on Vascular Prostacyclin Isomerase and Platelet Camp
K. U. Weithmann, West Germany

9.20— 9.30 a.m.   Prostaglandin Metabolism and Prostacyclin in Cerebral Vasospasm
K. E. Anderson, L. Baandit, B. Hindfelt, B. Ljunggren and T. Uski, Sweden

9.30— 9.50 a.m.   Substance P. — A Putative Mediator of Antidromic Vasodilatation
B. Pernow, Sweden

9.50—10.00 a.m.   Modulatory Effect of Substance P on Norepinephrine Induced Vasoconstrictions in the Rat Mesentery
N. Gulati, H. Huggel and O. P. Gulati, Switzerland

10.00—10.10 a.m.   Renal Vascular Effects of Angiotensin II Arginine-Vasopressin and Bradykinin in Rats: Interactions with Prostaglandins
K. G. Hofbauer, H. Dienemann, P. Forgiarini and J. M. Wood, Switzerland

10.10—10.40 a.m.   Discussion

10.40—11.10 a.m.   Coffee Break

Section VI	Calcium Entry Blockers

Chairmen: K. E. Andersson, Sweden, and K. Nakayama, Japan
Secretary: F. Al-Awadi, Kuwait

11.10—11.30 a.m.   Effect of Ca-Antagonists on the Contraction of Cerebral and Peripheral Arteries Produced by Electrical and Mechanical Stimuli
K. Nakayama, K. Ishii and H. Kato, Japan

11.30—11.40 a.m.   The Role of Extracellular Calcium and Effects of Calcium Antagonists in Isolated Human Pial Arteries
K. E. Andersson, L. Brandt, L. Edvinsson and B. Ljunggren, Sweden

11.40—11.50 a.m.	Effects of Nifedipine on Potassium-Induced Contraction and Noradrenaline Release in Cerebral and Extracranial Arteries from Rabbits E. D. Hogestatt and L. Edvinsson, Sweden
11.50—12.00 noon	Effects of Nifedipine on Isolated Human Pulmonary Vessels AM. Sakr. and E. Mikkelsen, Denmark
12.00—12.10 p.m.	Verapamil-Induced Vasodilator Response is Enhanced in Essential Hypertension P. Bolli, U. L. Hulthen, F. W. Amann, W. Kiowski and F. R. Buhler, Switzerland
12.10—12.20 p.m.	On the Mechanism of the Anti-Hypertensive Effect of Ca^{++}-Blockers E. Marmo, Italy
12.20—12.50 p.m.	Discussion of Section IV and VI

Section VII   Vasoconstrictors, Antihypertensive Drugs

Chairmen: B. Clark, Switzerland, and O. Thulesius, Kuwait
Secretary: A. Al-Bader

14.15—14.35 p.m.	Vascular Effects of Ergot Alkaloids E. Muller-Schweinitzer, Switzerland
14.35—14.45 p.m.	Vasoconstrictor Effects of Midodrine, ST 1059, Noradrenaline, Etilefrine and Norfenefrine on Disolated Dog Femoral Arteries and Veins H. Pittner, Austria
14.45—14.55 p.m.	On the Influence of Amezinium on Various Regions of the Dog R. Kretzschmar, H. D. Lehmann, D. Lenke and M. Raschack, West Germany
14.55—15.05 p.m.	Effect of Ruscus Aculeatus Extract on Isolated Canine Saphenous Veins G. Marcelon, H. Lauressergues and P. M. Vahoutte, U.S.A.
15.05—15.15 p.m.	Vascular Effects of Glucocorticosteroids, with Special Reference to Budesonide M. M. Angelo-Khattar and O. Thulesius, Kuwait
15.15—15.25 p.m.	Differential Effect of Hydralazine on the Arterial Bimodal Contractile Response M. A. Khayyal, Cairo F. Gross and V. Kreye, West Germany
15.25—15.35 p.m.	Effects of Pindolol on Vascular Smooth Muscle B. J. Clark and A. Bertholet, Switzerland
15.35—15.40 p.m.	Effects of Beta-Blockers with Intrinsic Sympathomimetic Activity on Isolated Human Blood Vessels J. E. Gjores, Sweden, O. Thulesius, Kuwait, and E. Berlin, Sweden
15.40—16.10 p.m.	Discussion

Section VIII	Pathological Responses of Blood Vessels
	Chairmen: D. Boullin, England, and R. F. W. Moulds, Australia
	Secretary: R. E. Micallef, Kuwait
16.30—16.50 p.m.	Pharmacological Responses of Human and Animal Cerebral Arteries in Health and Disease D. J. Boullin, P. Tagari, G. H. D. Boulay, V. Aitken and J. Beckett, U.K.
16.50—17.00 p. m.	Differences between Human Intra- and Extracranial Arteries in Reactivity to Vasoactive Agents H. E. Hardebo, J. Hanko and Ch. Owman, Sweden
17.00—17.10 p.m.	Variations between Individuals in Cerebrovascular Responsiveness to Different Vasoactive Substances, Human Plasma, and Cerebrospinal Fluid from Patients with Aneurysmal Subarachnoid Hemorrhage K. E. Andersson, L. Brandit, B. Hindfelt and B. Ljunggren, Sweden
17.10—17.20 p.m.	Late Cerebral Arterial Spasm: The Cerebral Arterial Response to Hypercapnia, Induced Hypertension and the Effect of Nimodipine of CBF Autoregulation in Experimental such in Primates N. Aa. Svendgard, J. Brismar, T. Delgado, Ch. Owman, Ch. Sahlin and L. Salford, Sweden
17.20—17.30 p.m.	Inhibition of the Arteriolar Smooth Muscle Na^+-K^+-Pump Induces an Enhanced Vasoconstriction in Borderline Essential Hypertension U. L. Hulthen, P. Bolli, W. Kiowski and F. R. Buhler, Switzerland
17.30—17.40 p.m.	Aortic Coarctation: The Vitro Response to Noradrenaline, Potassium and Prostaglandin F_2 in the Aorta and Intercostal Arteries J. Sehested and E. Mikkelsen, Denmark
17.40—17.50 p.m.	Contractile Responses of Normotensive and Hypertensive Human Arteries O. Thulesius, J. E. Gjores and E. Berlin, Sweden
17.50—18.00 p.m.	Catecholamine-Induced Lung Vascular Injury A. B. Malik and F. L. Minnear, U.S.A.
18.00—18.10 p.m.	Hypoxic and Embolic Pulmonary Vasoconstriction J. Boe, Sweden
18.10—18.50 p.m.	Relations Between Endothelial Factors, Circulation and Disturbances of Autonomic Nervous Function in Diabetes Mellitus L. O. Almer, B. Lilja and G. Sundkvist, Sweden
18.20—18.50 p.m.	Discussion

81C—17/30/54/6903
Bulgarian-Kuwaiti Medicine Week

Place:	Al-Sabah Hospital, Chest Hospital.
Duration:	February 27—March 3, 1982.

Organiser:

Chairman:	Dr. Talib Astarabadi, Training Division, Ministry of Public Health
Secretary:	Dr. Jetchka Vassileva, Dept. of Gastro-enterology, Al-Sabah Hospital.
Members:	Mr. Grozdan Grozdanov, Representative, Bulgarian Embassy.
	Mr. Ali Khuraibat, Chief, Public Relations Dept., Ministry of Health.
	Mr. Saad Al-Nabhan, Vice-Chairman, Training Division, Administration Affairs.
	Mr. Aljosha Todorov, Ministry of Public Health, Bulgaria.
	Dr. Abbas Ramadan, Ibn Sina Hospital.
	Dr. Fahed Al-Mai, Al-Sabah Hospital.
	Mrs. Amal Harb, Secretary, Under-Secretary's Office.

Participants: Doctors interested in topics.

Programme:

27th February, 1982

5.00 p.m.	Opening Ceremony Minister of Public Health Opening Address Bulgarian's Embassy World
5.30 p.m.	Health Care System and Health Services in Bulgaria Prof. Iordanov
6.15 p.m.	Bulgarian Mineral Water and Spa. Resorts Prof. Kostadinov
6.45 p.m.	Slides and Films about Bulgaria Prof. Kostadinov

28th February, 1982

4.30 p.m.	Recent Development in Health and Manpower Prof. Iordanov
5.00 p.m.	Criteria for Determining Insulin Resistency in Patient with Obesity Prof. Izanev
5.30 p.m.	Extracranial Surgical Approach to Hypophysical Adenoma Prof. Karajesov and Dr. Abbas Ramadan
6.30 p.m.	Immunological Problems with Corneal Graft Prof. Konstantinov
7.00 p.m.	Sources of Health—Film Prof. Kostadinov

1st March, 1982

4.30 p.m.	Bulgarian Mineral Water and Balneotherapy Prof. Kostadinov

5.00 p.m.	Surgery of Brain Vessels—Recent Problems and Trends of Development Prof. Karajosov
5.30 p.m.	Treatment of Uveitis Prof. Konstantinov
6.30 p.m.	Recent Advances in Intensive Care—Achievement, Problems, New Perspective Prof. Jordanov

2nd March, 1982

4.30 p.m.	Surgery of Iris and Ciliary Body Tumor Prof. Konstantinov
5.00 p.m.	Surgery of Glaucoma with Film Prof. Konstantinov
5.30 p.m.	Anterior Surgical Approach in Cervical Spondilotic Myelophthisis Prof. Karajosov
6.30 p.m.	Low-Back Pain—Causes and Rehabilitation Prof. Kostadinov
7.00 p.m.	Myocardial Infarction and What Then? Film Prof. Kostadinov

3rd March, 1982

4.30 p.m.	Risk Factors in Patients with Metabolic Disease Prof. Tzanev
5.00 p.m.	Round Table Discussion—Acute Respiratory Failure Moderators—Prof. Iordanov and Dr. Yacob
6.15 p.m.	Treatment of Diabetic Retinopathy Prof. Konstantinov and Dr. Sharif

II. List of Medical Sciences (in Alphabetic Order) Subjects for Postgraduate Studies, Presented by Course Identifying Numbers (see pages 28—33)

Allergology

81C—*07*01	184
81C—*07*02	185
81C—13/*07*/65/15/73/1401	325

Anaesthesiology and Analgesia

81A—23/45/47/51/*69*04	71
81A—*69*/45/2307	77
81A—12/23/33/37/82/*69*/7113	67
81B—*69*/0101	132
81C—*69*10	176
81C—*69*11	178
81C—*69*12	179
81C—*69*13	180
81C—*69*14	181
81C—*69*01	275
81C—*69*/24/4502	278
81C—*69*03	280
81C—*69*/30/4504	282
81C—*69*/3705	284
81C—*69*/4506	286
81C—*69*07	289
81C—17/30/54/*69*03	337

Bacteriology and Virusology

81C—71/08/7903	294

Basic Medical Sciences

81A—*01*/12/23/33/3701	51
81A—*01*/12/23/33/3703	54
81A—*01*04	56
81A—*01*/12/23/33/3706	59
81B—23/*01*01	109
81B—37/*01*01	124
81C—71/*01*02	292
81C—71/*01*04	296
81C—73/*01*/1302	332

Behavioural Sciences
    81A—*6111* 88
    81C—*6101* 264
    81E—99/*6122* 324

Biostatistics
    81A—89/44/*02*/88/78/95/90/8610 85
    81C—*02* 01 183

Cardiac Surgery
    81C—*24* 01 219
    81C—*24* 02 220
    81C—*24* 03 221
    81C—*24* 04 222
    81C—69/*24*/4502 278

Cardiology
    81C—*13* 01 197
    81C—*13* 02 198
    81C—*13* 03 198
    81C—*13* 04 200
    81C—*13*/07/65/15/73/1401 325
    81C—73/01/*13* 02 332

Clinical Laboratory Medicine
    81A—12/56/61/66/*7101* 67
    81A—*71*/1203 70
    81A—*7112* 88
    81A—12/23/33/37/82/69/*7113* 88
    81C—*71*/1801 206
    81C—*71*/0102 292
    81C—*71*/08/7903 294
    81C—*71*/0104 296
    81C—*7105* 298

Community Medicine
    81A—*89*/44/02/88/78/95/90/8610 85

Dentistry
    81B—*76* 01 138

Dermatology
    81C—*56* 01 258
    81C—*56*/7902 258
    81C—*56* 03 259

Dietetics

Education and Teaching Facilities
    81A—*09* 02 53
    81A—*09* 05 58
    81C—*09* 01 187
    81C—*09* 02 188
    81C—*09* 03 189
    81C—*09* 04 189
    81C—65/*09* 03 271

Endocrinology
    81C—*17*01 205
    81C—23/*17*04 217
    81C—*17*/30/54/6903 337

Environmental Health
    81A—89/44/02/88/78/95/90/*86*10 85

E.N.T.
    81A—23/45/47/51/6904 71
    81A—47/2306 76

Epidemiology
    81A—89/44/02/*88*/78/95/90/8610 85
    81C—*88*01 304
    81C—*88*02 307

Family Medicine
    81C—*43*01 247

Gastroenterology
    81C—*14*20 202
    81C—23/*14*01 223
    81C—33/*14*02 241
    81C—33/*14*03 239
    81C—13/07/65/15/73/*14*01 325

Gynaecology and Obstetrics
    81A—01/12/23/33/*37*01 51
    81A—01/12/23/33/*37*03 54
    81A—01/12/23/33/*37*06 59
    81A—*37*09 82
    81A—12/23/33/*37*/82/69/7113 88
    81B—*37*/0101 124
    81C—*37*01 244
    81C—*37*02 246
    81C—69/*37*05 284
    81E—99/*37*14 319
    81E—99/*37*15 315

Health Education
    81E—99/*98*23 324

Haematology
    81C—*18*01 206
    81C—*18*02 208
    81C—*18*03 209
    81C—71/*18*01 290

Hygiene

Industrial Medicine
    81A—89/44/02/88/78/95/*90*/8610 85

Immunobiology
    81C—*07*01 184
    81C—*07*02 185
    81C—13/07/65/15/73/1401 325

Infectious Diseases
    81A—89/44/02/88/78/95/90/8610 85
    81C—*78*01 300
    81C—*78*/1202 303

Intensive Care
    81A—23/*45*/47/51/6904 71
    81A—69/*45*/2307 77
    81C—69/24/*45*02 278
    81C—69/30/*45*04 282
    81C—69/*45*06 286

Internal Medicine
    81A—01/*12*/23/33/3701 51
    81A—01/*12*/23/33/3703 54
    81A—*01*/12/23/33/3706 59
    81A—12/56/61/66/7101 67
    81A—56/*12*02 98
    81A—71/*12*03 104
    81A—*12*/23/33/37/82/69/7113 88
    81B—*12*01 91
    81B—*12*02 98
    81C—*12*01 168
    81C—*12*02 168
    81C—*12*03 170
    81C—*12*/0101 201
    81C—67/*12*01 268
    81C—78/*12*02 303
    81C—99/*12*16 320
    81E—99/*12*17 321

Metabolic Diseases Including Diabetology
    81C—*19*01 211

Nephrology
    81C—*16*01 203

Neurology
    81C—*59*01 261
    81C—*59*02 262
    81C—*59*03 263

Neurosurgery
    81C—69/*30*/4504 282
    81C—17/*30*/54/6903 337

Nuclear Medicine
    81C—*67*/1201 268
    81C—*67*/6502 270

Nursing
    81E—*99*01 309
    81E—*99*02 310
    81E—*99*04 311
    81E—*99*05 311

81E— *99* 06   312
81E— *99* 07   312
81E— *99* 08   313
81E— *99* 09   314
81E— *99* 10   315
81E— *99* 11   317
81E— *99* 12   318
81E— *99* 13   318
81E— *99*/3714   319
81E— *99*/3715   319
81E— *99*/1216   320
81E— *99*/1217   321
81E— *99*/3318   321
81E— *99*/3319   322
81E— *99*/2320   323
81E— *99*/2321   323
81E— *99*/6122   324
81E— *99*/9823   324

Nutrition

Occupational Therapy
81A—89/44/02/88/78/*95*/90/8610   85

Oncology
81C—67/*65*02   270
81C— *65*/0903   271
81C—13/07/*65*/15/73/1401   325

Ophthalmology
81A—54/2305   75
81C— *54*/9601   251
81C— *54* 02   252
81C— *54* 03   254
81C— *54* 04   254
81C— *54* 05   256
81C—17/30/*54*/6903   337

Orthopaedic Surgery
81C— *27*/2801   232

Paediatrics
81A—01/12/23/*33*/3701   51
81A—01/12/23/*33*/3703   54
81A—01/12/23/*33*/3706   59
81A— *33* 08   80
81A—12/23/*33*/37/82/69/7113   88
81C— *33* 04   172
81C— *33* 01   238
81C— *33*/1402   241
81C— *33*/1403   239
81C—63/*33*02   266
81E—99/*33* 18   321
81E—99/*33* 19   322

Paediatric Surgery
    81C—*29* 01 234
    81C—*29* 02 236

Parasitology
    81C—56/ *79* 02 258
    81C—71/08/ *79* 03 294

Pharmacology
    81C—75/ *73* 01 299
    81C—13/07/65/15/ *73*/1401 325
    81C— *73*/01/1302 332

Pharmacy
    81C— *75*/7301 299

Physical Medicine
    81C—54/ *96* 01 251

Plastic Surgery
    81C—27/ *28* 01 232

Preventive Medicine

Primary Health Care
    81A—89/ *44*/02/88/78/95/90/8610 85
    81C— *44* 01 250

Professional Diseases

Psychiatry
    81A—12/56/ *61*/66/7101 67
    81A— *61* 11 88
    81C— *61* 01 264
    81E—99/ *61*22 324

Public Health
    81A—12/23/33/37/82/69/7113 88

Pulmonology
    81C—13/07/65/ *15*/73/1401 325

Radiology
    81C— *63* 05 174
    81C— *63* 06 174
    81C— *63* 07 175
    81C— *63* 08 175
    81C— *63* 09 176
    81C— *63* 01 265
    81C— *63*/3302 266
    81C— *63* 03 267

Radiotherapy
    81A—12/56/61/66/7101 67

Radiation Protection

Rehabilitation
    81C—54/ *96* 01 251

Rheumatology
       81C—*20*01 212

Surgery
       81A—01/12/*23*/33/3701 51
       81A—01/12/*23*/33/3703 54
       81A—01/12/*23*/33/3706 59
       81A—*23*/45/47/51/6904 71
       81A—54/*23*05 75
       81A—47/*23*06 76
       81A—69/45/*23*07 77
       81A—12/*23*/33/37/82/69/7113 88
       81B—*23*/0101 109
       81B—*23*/0102 117
       81C—*23*01 213
       81C—*23*02 216
       81C—*23*03 217
       81C—*23*/1704 217
       81C—*23*/1401 223
       81E—99/*23*20 323
       81E—99/*23*21 323

Thoracic Surgery

Toxicology

Tropical Medicine

Urology
       81C—2601 230
       81C—2602 231

Venerology

Virusology
       81C—71/*08*/7903 294

III. Invited (Foreign) Lecturers

Name	Place of work	Course	Page
1. C. Aalkjaer	Denmark	81C—73/01/1302	332
2. B. Altura	U.S.A.	81C—73/01/1302	332
3. K. E. Anderson	Sweden	81C—73/01/1302	332
4. Dr. J. P. Ballantyne	Consultant Neurologist, Southern General Hospital, Glasgowm U.K.	81B—1202 81C—5902	98 262
5. Prof. Evelyn R. Barrit	Dean of the School of Nursing, University of Miami, Miami, FL 33101, U.S.A.	81E—9910	315
6. M. N. Barton, FRCS	Orthopaedic Surgeon, Nottingham	81C—27/2801	232
7. F. Bashour	England	81C—13/07/65/73/1401	325
8. E. Belfroge	Sweden	81C—73/01/1302	332
9. Dr. H. Berry, MA, DM, MRCP	Consultant Physician, Dept. of Rheumatology, King's College Hospital, Denmark Hill, London, U.K.	81B—1202 81C—2001	98 212
10. J. Bevan	U.S.A.	81C—73/01/1302	332
11. Dr. G. W. Black	England	81B—69/0101	132
12. J. Boe	Sweden	81C—73/01/1302	332
13. P. Bolli	Switzerland	81C—73/01/1302	332
14. D. Boullin	England	81C—73/01/1302	332
15. Dr. Phylip Brachman	—	81C—8801	304
16. Dr. T. B. Brewin	Deputy Director, Institute of Radiotherapy and Oncology, Western Hospital, Glasgow, U.K.	81C—65/0903	271
17. Prof. Phylip R. Bromage	—	81C—69/3705	284

Name	Place of work	Course	Page
18. Mr. Hugh Brown, TD, OHS, FRCS	Plastic Surgeon, Newcastle	81C—27/2801	232
19. Mr. Hy Browne	—	81B—23/0101	109
20. John Bullock, Ph.D.	Associate Professor of Physiology, College of Medicine and Dentistry of New Jersey, New York, U.S.A.	81A—01/12/23/ 33/3706	59
21. Mrs. Julie Carner	Infectious Control Nurse, Centre for Disease Control, Atlanta, Ga., U.S.A.	81C—7801	300
22. Pamela Champe, Ph.D.	Assistant Professor of Biochemistry, Dept. of Biochemistry, Rutgers Medical School, University Heights, Piscataway, NJ 08854, U.S.A.	81A—01/12/23/ 33/3706	59
23. B. Clark	Switzerland	81C— 73/01/1302	332
24. T. J. H. Clark	—	81C—13/07/65/ 15/73/1401	325
25. C. Concettoni	Italy	81C— 73/01/1302	332
26. Dr. Max Cooper, MD	Prof. of Paediatrics and Microbiology, University of Alabama, School of Medicine, Birmingham, Alabama, U.S.A.	81C—0702	185
27. Dr. L. T. Cotton, MCh, FRCS	Dean, King's College Hospital, Medical School, University of London	81C—12/0101	168
28. M. Daleskog	Sweden	81C— 73/01/1302	332
29. Prof. Gordon K. Danielson, MD	Prof. of Surgery, Mayo Clinic, 200 First St Street South West, Rochester, Minnesota, U.S.A.	81C—2401	219
30. Noble J. David, MD	Prof. of Neurology, Dept. of Neurology, University of Miami, School of Medicine, Miami, FL 33101, U.S.A.	81A—01/12/23/ 33/3706 81C—4301 81C—5903	59 247 263
31. Dr. J. T. Davie	—	81B—69/0101	132
32. Dr. Jeff Davies	Consultant Ophthalmic Surgeon, Eye Dept., King's College Hospital, London, U.K.	81C—5405	256
33. Dr. I. Pryse Davies	—	81B—37/0101	124
34. Dr. A. M. Dawson	—	81B—1201	91

Name	Place of work	Course	Page
35. Dr. Thomas Demeester	Professor of Surgery, University of Chicago Medical School, Chicago, Ill., U.S.A.	81C—23/1401	223
36. Sir J. Dewhurst	England	81B—37/0101	124
37. Dr. Z. Dienstbier	Director, Institute of Biophysics and Nuclear Medicine, Charles University, Prague, Czechoslovakia	81C—65/0903	271
38. Dr. R. Dinwiddie	—	81B—37/0101	124
39. Dr. Adrian C. Douwes	Paediatrics Gastroenterologist, Children's Department, Free University Hospital, Amsterdam, Netherland	81C—33/1402	241
40. Prof. G. Doyle	—	81B—23/0101	109
41. Dr. I. T. Draper, MD, FRCP	Consultant Neurologist, Southern General Hospital, Glasgow	81B—1201 81C—5901	91 261
42. J. A. Dudgeon	—	81C—13/07/65/ 15/73/1401	325
43. Dr. Terence A. H. English, FRCS	Consultant Cardio Thoracic Surgeon, Pappworth (near Cambridge), England	81C—2402	220
44. L. Edvinsson	Sweden	81C— 73/01/1302	332
45. Prof. Uno Erickson	Head of Dept. of Diagnostic Radiology, Uppsala University, Sweden	81C—6301	265
46. Dr. Jim Finucane	— — —	81B—23/0101 81B—23/0102 81B—7601	109 292 138
47. Dr. William Fitch	Senior Lecturer, Royal Infirmary, University of Glasgow, Scotland	81C— 69/30/4504	282
48. Prof. P. Fitzpatrick	—	81B—23/0101	109
49. Prof. T. Foster	University of Kentucky Medical Center, Lexington, Kentucky, U.S.A.	81C—75/7301	299
50. Latifa Ghandur Mnaymneh	Associate Professor of Pathology, University of Miami, School of Medicine, Miami, FL 33101, U.S.A.	81A—01/12/23/ 33/3706	59
51. Dr. Richard H. Glew, MD	Chief, Infectious Disease Service, Worcester, Massachusetts, U.S.A.	81C—78/1202	303

Name	Place of work	Course	Page
52. Burton J. Goldstein, MD	Vice-Chairman, Dept. of Psychiatry, University of Miami, School of Medicine, Miami, FL 33101, U.S.A.	81A—01/12/23/33/3706 81C—4301 81C—6101	59 247 264
53. K. H. Graefe	Germany	81C—73/01/1302	332
54. Prof. Malcolm Greaves	Prof. of Dermatology, The Institute of Dermatology, St. John's Hospital for Disease of the Skin, London, England	81C—5603	259
55. Prof. J. M. Greep	Prof. of Surgery, Dean, Faculty of Medicine, Rijksuniversiteit, Limburg, Netherlands	81C—23/1401	223
56. N. Gulati	Switzerland	81C—73/01/1302	332
57. M. Hamer	—	81B—69/0101	132
58. Dr. A. Hayward	—	81B—7601	138
59. Prof. P. D. J. Holland	—	81B—7601	138
60. INH J. N. Horton	—	81B—69/0101	132
61. Dr. Robert Hume, MD, FRCP, FRCPG	Consultant Physician, Southern General Hospital, Glasgow	81C—1802	208
62. Dr. Timothy S. Harrison	Prof. of Surgery and Physiology, The Milton S. Hershey Medical Center, Pennsylvania State University, U.S.A.	81C—23/1401	223
63. Dr. J. T. Harries	Reader in Paediatrics, Hon. Consultant Physician, Institute of Child Health, Hospital for Sick Children, Great Ormond Street, London	81C—33/1403	239
64. Dr. Henry	—	81C—3701	244
65. W. M. Haining	—	81C—5403	254
66. Dr. Richard Heller	Prof. of Paediatric Radiology, Director of Paediatric Radiology, Vanderbilt University, Nashville, Tennessee, U.S.A.	81C—63/3302	266
67. Dr. M. G. Hanna	Director, Frederick Cancer Research Centre, Frederick, Md., U.S.A.	81C—65/0903	271
68. P. Hjemdahl	Sweden	81C—73/01/1302	332
69. K. G. Hofbauer	Switzerland	81C—73/01/1302	332

Name	Place of work	Course	Page
70. J. E. Hardebo	Sweden	81C—73/01/1302	332
71. J. T. Holmberg	Sweden	81C—73/01/1302	332
72. Dr. B. Hoffbrand MD, FRCP, FRCPG	Consultant Physician, Whittington Hospital, London, U.K.	81B—1202	98
73. Prof. P. D. F. Holland	—	81B—23/0101	109
74. L. Helligren	Norway	81C—73/01/1302	332
75. Prof. J. Howell, B. Sc., MB, Ph.D., FRCP	Dean, Southampton University Medical School, Southampton	81B—1202	98
76. Dr. R. Hume, MD, FRCP, FRCPG	Consultant Physician Haematologist, Southern General Hospital, Glasgow, U.K.	81B—1202	98
77. Dr. W. J. Irvine, B. Sc., MD, CHB, D. Sc.	Consultant Physician Endocrine Unit, Immunology Laboratory, Royal Infirmary, Edinburgh, U.K.	81C—0702	185
78. Dr. Abdul H. Islami, MD	Director, Dept. of Graduate Medical Education and President of Medical Staff at St. Barnabas Medical Centre, U.S.A.	81A—01/12/23/33/3706 81C—2303	59 217
79. Prof. Paul H. Jacobs, MD	Professor of Clinical Dermatology, Stanford University, School of Medicine, Stanford, California, U.S.A.	81C—56/7902	258
80. Dr. Keith James, Ph.D., MRCPath., FRS (E)	Reader, Dept. of Surgery, University of Edinburgh, Teviot Place, Edinburgh, Scotland, U.K.	81C—0702	185
81. Prof. S. Jeffcoate	—	81B—37/0101	124
82. A. M. Jelliffe	—	81C—13/07/65/15/73/1401	325
83. Mr. Wibfried de Jong	—	81C—0702	185
84. Dr. David Johnston	Professor of Surgery, University Dept. of Surgery, The General Infirmary, Leeds, U.K.	81C—23/1401	223
85. Mr. George W. Johnston	Consultant Surgeon Royal Victoria Hospital, Grosvenor Road, Belfast, U.K.	81C—23/1401	223

Name	Place of work	Course	Page
86. Prof. Jordan Jordanov	Professor of Anaesthesia and I.C.U. and Vice President of the Bulgarian Medical Academy, Sofia, Bulgaria	81C—6901 81C—69/4506 81C—17/30/54/ 6903	275 286 337
87. Prof. Martin H. Kalser, MD	Chief, Division of Gastroenterology, Dept. of Gastroenterology, University of Miami, School of Medicine, Miami, FL 33101, U.S.A.	81A—01/12/23/ 33/3706 81C—1420	59 202
88. Dr. Zigmund C.Kaminski	Associate Prof., Depts. of Microbiology and Pathology, New Jersey Medical School, College Hospital, Newark, NJ 07103, U.S.A.	81A—01/12/23/ 33/3706	59
89. Prof. Karajasow	Bulgaria	81C—17/30/54/ 6903	337
90. Prof. Robert Kistner	University of Hawaii, Honolulu, Hawaii, U.S.A.	81C—2404	222
91. Prof. G. Kock, MD, Hon. FRCS (Engl.)	Professor of Surgery, University of Göteborg, Dept. of Surgery, Sahlgrenska Sjukhuset, S-413 45 Göteborg, Sweden	81C—23/1401	223
92. Prof. Nobuhiko Komi, MD	Prof. of Surgery, School of Medicine, University of Tokushima, Japan	81C—2901	234
93. Prof. Kostadinow	Bulgaria	81C—17/30/54/ 6903	337
94. Mr. D. W. Lamb, FRCS (E)	Orthopaedic Surgeon, Edinburgh	81C—27/2801	232
95. Kenneth F. Lampe, Ph.D.	Senior Scientist: Division of Drugs, American Medical Association, 535 N. Dearborn, Chicago, Illinois, U.S.A.	81A—01/12/23/ 33/3706	59
96. Mr. B. Lane	—	81B—23/0102	117
97. Miss Antonia Lant	Royal Postgraduate Medical School, Various Ancillary Staff, London	81C—0901 81C—0902 81C—0903 81C—0904	187 189 189 189
98. Prof. M. H. Lessof, MD, FRCP	Dept. of Medicine, Guy's Hospital Medical School, London	81B—1201 81C—0701	91 205

Name	Place of work	Course	Page
99. Dr. Harvey Lincoff, MD	Ophthalmic Surgeon, Retina Service, New York Hospital, Cornell School of Medicine	81C—5404	254
100. B. Linde	Sweden	81C—73/01/1302	332
101. Doris B. Linder, MD	Associate in the Practice of Internal Medicine, 85 Woodland Road, Short Hills, NJ 07077, U.S.A.	81A—01/12/23/33/3706	59
		81C—1304	200
		81C—4301	247
102. Dr. J. G. Lloyd, MBBS, MRCP (U.K.)	Senior Medical Specialist, Ahmadi Hospital, Kuwait	81B—1201	91
		81B—1202	98
103. Dr. F. Loeffler	—	81C—3701	124
104. J. N. Lunn	—	81B—69/0101	132
105. Prof. Lynch	—	81B—23/0101	109
		81B—23/0102	117
		81B—7601	138
106. Prof. M. C. McCnaughton	Prof. of Obstetrics and Gynaecology, University of Glasgow, U.K.	81C—3701	244
107. Dr. M. N. Maisey, MD, FRCP	Director, Dept. of Nuclear Medicine, Guy's Hospital, London	81B—1201	91
		81C—67/1201	268
108. A. B. Malik	U.S.A.	81C—73/01/1302	332
109. W. W. Mapleson	—	81B—69/0101	132
110. E. Marmo	Italy	81C—73/01/1302	332
111. Dr. James Maynard	—	81C—8801	304
112. Mr. R. J. McCormack	—	81B—7601	138
113. D. B. McGill	—	81C—13/07/65/15/73/1401	325
114. Dr. John Maxwell McKenzie, MD	Prof. and Chairman, Dept. of Medicine, University of Miami, School of Medicine, Miami, FL 33101, U.S.A.	81A—01/12/23/33/3706	59
		81C—1701	205
		81C—4301	247
115. Dr. Allen McLeod, MD	Professor and Vice Chairman, Dept. of Obstetrics and Gynaecology, University of Miami, School of Medicine, Miami, FL 33101, U.S.A.	81A—01/12/23/33/3706	59
		81C—3702	246
		81C—4301	247
116. Prof. Henry Menn	—	81C—5601	258
117. E. Mikkelsen	Denmark	81C—73/01/1302	332
118. S. Moncada	England	81C—73/01/1302	332
119. Prof. E. Moorehause	—	81B—23/0102	117
		81B—7601	138

Name	Place of work	Course	Page
120. Dr. A. R. Moosa, B. Sc., MD, FRCS (Eng. and Edin.) FACS	Prof. of Surgery, Dept. of Surgery, 950 East Fifty-Ninth Street, University of Chicago, Chicago, IL 60637, U.S.A.	81C—23/1401	223
121. R. F. W. Moulds	Australia	81C—73/01/1302	332
122. Prof. Phylip Myerscough	—	81C—3701 n	244
123. K. Nakayama	Japan	81C—73/01/1302	332
124. Dr. F. Nally	—	81B—7601	138
125. Dr. Haruo Nakamura	Aoto Hospital, Tokyo, Japan	81C—1901	211
126. Prof. H. M. Newsome	Prof. and Vice Chairman, Dept. of Surgery, Virginia Commonwealth University, Richmond, Va., U.S.A.	81C—2301	213
127. B. Arneklo-Nobin	Sweden	81C—73/01/1302	332
128. Dr. G. O'Conor	Director, International Affairs, National Cancer Institute, Bethesda, Maryland, U.S.A.	81C—65/0903	271
129. Dr. Chisholm S. Ogg, B. Sc., MB, ChB, MRCS	Renal Physician, and Director of Dialysis and Transplant Unit, Guy's Hospital, London	81B—1201 81C—1601	91 268
130. Dr. Marshal Orloff	Professor and Chairman, Dept. of Surgery, University of California, U.S.A.	81C—23/1401	223
131. Ch. Owman	Sweden	81C—73/01/1302	332
132. Mr. Virgil Peavy	U.S.A.	81C—8801 81C—8802	304 307
133. Rafael A. Penalver, MD	Director, Office of International Medical Education, University of Miami, School of Medicine, Miami, FL 33101, U.S.A.	81A—01/12/23/33/3701 81A—01/12/23/33/3706	51 59
134. Dr. M. Webb Peplee	—	81B—1201	91
135. B. Pernow	Sweden	81C—73/01/1302	332
136. Prof. J. Pinkerton	U.K.	81C—3701	244
137. Dr. L. Price	Consultant Medical Oncologist, Institute of Cancer Research, London, U.K.	81C—65/0903	21
138. H. Pittner	Austria	81C—73/01/1302	332

Name	Place of work	Course	Page
139. Mr. Guy Pulvertaft, FRCS	Emeritus Consultant Hand Surgeon, Derby, U.K.	81C—27/2801	232
140. Dr. Eric Reiss	University of Miami, Miami, FL 33101, U.S.A.	81A—01/12/23/ 33/3706	59
141. Prof. John Richmond, MD, FRCP	Prof. of Medicine, University of Sheffield, U.K.	81B—1201 81C—1801	91 206
142. B. F. Robinson	England	81C— 73/02/1302	332
143. Dr. Donald Ross	National Heart Hospital, U.K.	81C—2403	221
144. Edward Russell, MD	Professor and Director, Diagnostic Radiology, University of Miami, School of Medicine, Miami, FL 33101, U.S.A.	81A—01/12/23/ 33/3706 81C—4301 81C—6303	59 247 267
145. Dr. Witold Ruzyllo, MD	Head, Dept. of General Cardiology, State Institute of Cardiology, Alpejska 42, 04-628 Warsaw, Poland	81C—1302	198
146. Sami I. Said, MD	Chief, Pulmonary Disease and Critical Care Section, Prof. of Medicine, University of Oklahoma, U.S.A.	81A—01/12/23/ 33/3706 81C—4301	59 247
147. Prof. Atef Sallam	Prof. of Surgery, Emory University, Atlanta, Georgia, U.S.A.	81C—23/1401	223
148. Dr. Scholtz	University of Miami, Miami, FL 33101, U.S.A.	8A— 01/12/23/33/ 3706	59
149. Dr. John Scott, FRCS	Consultant Paediatric Surgeon, Newcastle Upon Tyne, England	81C—2902	236
150. Mr. J. D. Scott, FRCS	Director of Retina Service, Adenbrooks Hospital, Cambridge, U.K.	81C—5402	252
151. J. Shepherd	U.S.A.	81C— 73/01/1302	332
152. Dr. John Simpson, FFARCS	Senior Consultant Anaesthetist, National Heart Hospital, London, U.K.	81C— 69/24/4502	278
153. Mr. Doig Simmonds	Chief Medical Artist at the Royal Post-Graduate Medical School, Hammersmith Hospital, London	81C—0901 81C—0902 81C—0903 81C—0904	187 188 189 189

Name	Place of work	Course	Page
154. T. Skarby	Sweden	81C—73/01/1302	332
155. D. G. Graham Smith	—	81C—13/07/65/15/73/1401	325
156. Dr. Vernon Smith FRCS	Consultant Ophthalmic Surgeon, Birmingham Eye Hospital, U.K.	81C—54/9601	251
157. Dr. John Soothill	—	81C—0702	185
158. Mr. S. J. Steele	—	81B—37/0101	124
159. J. D. Stephens, MD, MRCP	Consultant Cardiologist, The London Hospital (Whitechapel), Whitechapel, London, U.K.	81B—1202 81C—1303	168 198
160. Dr. M. Le Swiet	—	81B—37/0101	124
161. Prof. Akram Tamer, MD	Associate Professor of Paediatrics, University of Miami, School of Medicine, Miami, FL 33101, U.S.A.	81A—01/12/23/33/3706 81C—3301 81C—4301	59 238 247
162. James C. Thompson, MD	Professor and Chairman, Dept. of Surgery, University of Texas Medical Branch, Galveston, TX 77550, U.S.A.	81C—23/1401	223
163. Dr. Ron Thompson, B. Sc., MBBS, MRCPath., FRCP	Consultant Immunologist, Regional Immunology Lab., East Birmingham Hospital, Bordesley Green East, Birmingham, B9 5ST, U.K.	81C—0702	185
164. Dr. J. Thompson, FRCP (Glas), FRCP (Ldn)	Consultant Physician, University Medical Unit, Glasgow, U.K.	81B—1202	168
165. Prof. J. A. Thornton	—	81B—69/0101	132
166. Prof. Sten Tiblin	Dept. of Surgery, Malmö, University of Lund, Sweden	81C—23/1704	217
167. Joseph H. J. Timmes, MD	Professor of Surgery, Director of Surgery, Jersey City Medical Center, U.S.A.	81A—01/12/23/33/3706 81C—2302	59 216
168. Dr. J. G. Turcotte	Prof. and Chairman, Dept. of Surgery, University of Texas Medical Branch, Galveston, TX 77550, U.S.A.	81C—23/1401	223
169. Y. Tulen	Sweden	81C—73/01/1302	332
170. Prof. Tzanew	Bulgaria	81C—17/30/54/6903	337

Name	Place of work	Course	Page
171. Dr. Humberto B. Valdes	Adjunct Asst. Prof. of Anatomy, University of Miami, School of Medicine, Miami, FL 33101, U.S.A.	81A—01/12/23/ 33/3706	59
172. Dr. Vang	Chairman, Dept. of Surgery, Central Hospital, Eskjo, Sweden	81C—65/0903	271
173. P. Vanhoutte	U.S.A.	81C— 73/01/1302	332
174. Dr. U. Veronesi	President, U.I.C.C., Director, Istituto Nazionale per lo Studio e la Cura dei Tumori, Milan, Italy	81C—65/0903	271
175. Prof. M. D. Vickers	Prof. of Anaesthetics, Welsh National School of Medicine, Cardiff	81B—69/0101 81C—6903 81C—6907	132 280 289
176. Dr. P. Watkins, MD, FRCP	Consultant Physician Diabetologist, King's College Hospital, London, U.K.	81B—1202	98
177. Dr. M. M. Webb Peplee, FRCP, MD	Consultant Cardiologist, St. Thomas Hospital, London	81C—1301	197
178. A. Wennmalm	Sweden	81C— 73/01/1302	332
179. Dr. A. White, B. Sc., Ph.D.	Associate Prof., Dept. of Surgery, University of Kuwait	81B—1202	98
180. Mr. Arthur Williams	—	81C—3701	244
181. Prof. Wilkinson	University of Connecticut, Storrs, Conn., U.S.A.	81C—75/7301	299
182. Dr. Abel A. Yunis, MD	Prof. of Medicine and Biochemistry, Director, Divn. of Haematology, University of Miami, School of Medicine, Miami, FL 33101, U.S.A.	81A—01/12/23/ 33/3706 81C—1803 81C—4301	59 209 247

IV. Annual Reports of Committees

1. Area Executive Committee for Professional Medical Training

The committee has nominated coordinators for the various disciplines in all the hospitals. A special meeting was arranged with all the nominated coordinators, and in this meeting the functions and responsibilities of the coordinators were explained. Then a discussion of the problems and ways of improving the implementation of the programmes in the various hospitals was carried out.

It is hoped that after meeting with the coordinators, enthusiasm with regard to the professional training programme will be fostered, and implementation of the programmes of training will be more successful in future.

However, there are certain problems which need urgent solutions.

Generally it has been found that trainees are usually allocated to the Sabah and Mubarak Hospitals leaving other hospitals with very few trainees attached to them. The Area Executive Committee for professional training recommends that the number of trainees in each discipline should not be less than six, otherwise trainers will lose interest and will find it difficult and irritating to give lectures to two or three trainees. The Jahra Hospital cannot take trainees because there are no residential rooms for trainees to stay in when they are on duty. We think this should be rectified immediately.

The professional training programme is aimed at doctors who have recently qualified for it. However, a lot of hospitals receive doctors who are appointed to the clinics and are sent to various departments through the Director of Hospital Administration. At the present time these doctors usually join the professional training programmes, and on the whole this leads to a crowding of the departments with junior doctors which, at the same time, interferes with the professional training programme. We feel that since these doctors are appointed to the clinics, a special training programme should be made for them which should be different from the professional training programmes in general.

Finally, it is felt that the implementation and success of the professional training programme will depend on two factors. Firstly, the accreditation of units for participating in this programme. Secondly, the enthusiasm and successful relationship of the coordinators with the chairmen of various departments.

2. The Area Executive Committee for Medical Speciality Training

Structure and Organisation

The Area Executive Committee on Medical Speciality Training was made up of the following members:

Professor F. F. Fenech   Chairman
Dr. Abdulla Rashid
Professor G. N. Abouna
Professor H. Hathout
Professor S. Roy Choudhury
Dr. M. Khogali
Dr. A. M. Abdul Malek   Secretary

Activities of the Committee

The committee held its first meeting on the 28th November, 1981 and has met three times since. It is next due to meet on Sunday, 25th April when the proposals for the Medical Postgraduate Training Programme submitted by the Discipline Committee of Medicine will be discussed.

The V.Q.E. Course was discussed and a fruitful meeting took place with Dr. Martin Kalser, Chairman, Curriculum Committee of the V.Q.E. Course, Miami University. It was felt that the course should be made more relevant to the V.Q.E. Examination, and there was a very frank discussion of the difficulties experienced during the first course. Local coordinators had been nominated by the various disciplines in all subjects. The role of local faculty in subsequent courses remained, however, unclear.

The special postgraduate courses e.g. FRCS, MRCOG, FDS and MRCP 1 and 2 run by the Faculty jointly with the Ministry of Health were discussed and evaluated. It was felt that these courses should be continued and further evaluation carried out at the end of the year.

The letter from Professor McGowan about Part 2 FRCS (I) was discussed and it was decided to refer it to the Discipline Committee for Surgery for their consideration and recommendations. A reply from the Discipline Committee for Surgery is awaited.

The committee also reviewed and approved the criteria for recognition of Hospitals and Clinical Staff. As a result a special Accreditation Committee has been set up by the Joint Board.

The committee discussed the Surgical Postgraduate Training Programme submitted by the Discipline Committee of Surgery. After a thorough discussion this was approved, however, there are still a few minor issues to be decided which will be discussed at the next meeting due to be held on 25th April. The recommendation of the Discipline Committee for Anaesthesiology and Intensive Care that the course and examination of the Primary FFARCS be repeated in the year 1982—1983 was approved.

3. Area Executive Committee for Continuing Medical Education

The activities of Continuing Medical Education can be seen, though indirectly, through the accomplishments and organisations of the varied medical education programmes, symposia, and seminars which have taken place in the field of surgery, medicine, gynaecology, etc.

Meetings at the rate of one a month have been going on. Of particular importance was the meeting held with the chairmen of the Discipline Committees dated
8th March 1982. At this meeting the chairman of Continuing Medical Education
repeated and emphasized two points: one concerning the submission of bi-annual
reports to the Continuing Medical Education Committee by the Chairmen of Discipline Committees, which to our regret and disappointment were not done (with the
exception of a report from the chairman of Medicine Discipline), despite the fact
that several reminders have been sent by the secretariat of Continuing Medical Education. It would be an underestimation to consider such reports of secondary or
minor importance because they are the only channels through which Continuing
Medical Education can supervise, monitor and finally evaluate the implementation
of the policies laid down by the Joint Board for Postgraduate Medical Education.
Moreover, they would help in the formation of the conceptual rearrangement for
prospective planning, if necessary.

The other point dealt with the procedure to be observed by committees requiring visitor participants for the educational programme. The Continuing Medical
Education Committee was always presented with a request for inviting a visitor participant without and almost before the necessary submission of a relevant programme for the committee's consideration. Such practice was considered inconsist-
ent with the stipulation laid down by the Joint Board, and lead to turbulence and
many times caused difficulties in running the desired activity.

The Medical Discipline Committee reviewed and assessed the activities of the
Pan Arab Board Committee Examination. Our Area Executive Committee is in receipt of a Postgraduate Training Programme in general surgery prepared by the
Discipline Committee for Surgery and unanimously approved by the Area Executive for Speciality Training. It is interesting that the prepared programme was iden-
tical to the one prepared by the Pan Arab Board for Surgical Specialities.

The Committee for Continuing Medical Education was given the charge to arrange for the Bulgarian-Kuwait Medical Project by the Ministry of Public Health.
The endeavour was considered successful and it was conducted without a hitch.

4. Accreditation Committee

During the last academic year the committee have had eight meetings. The
committee decided to accredit first the hospitals and later on the clinical staff in
those hospitals. The Accreditation Committee decided to fully examine and study
the situation in one hospital at a time and Farwania Hospital was chosen for this
purpose.

The committee in full visited the hospital and had a meeting with the director
and other administrative staff of the hospital. Based on learned experiences the
committee formed sub-committees to inspect the departments in all hospitals beginning again with Farwania Hospital.

A sub-committee for each of the major disciplines, namely Medicine, Surgery,
Paediatrics, Gynaecology and Obstetrics and also for Medical Records was established to inspect and accredit corresponding departments/units in all hospitals.

The following sub-committees were chosen:

i) Medical Records

Professor Edward Ruzyllo	Convenor
Dr. Youssof T. Omar	Member
Mr. John Davies	Member

ii) Medicine

Dr. Basil Al Naqeeb	Convenor
Professor F. Fenech	Member
Dr. Abdul Razzak Al Yousof	Member

iii) Surgery

Professor G. M. Abouna	Convenor
Dr. Mehmoud Al Bader	Member
Professor Bo Eklof	Member
Dr. Ahmed Abu Gabal	Member

iv) Paediatrics

Dr. Mehmoud Al Bader	Convenor
Dr. Abdulla Rashied	Member
Dr. Hassan Abdul Majed	Member
Dr. L. Devarajan	Member

v) Gynaecology and Obstetrics

Dr. Samir Mustafa Kamel	Convenor
Professor Hassan Hathout	Member
Dr. Nelly Fernando	Member

Reports of the subcommittees were discussed at the meeting of the Accreditation Committee and accreditation of the Farwania Hospital was finally completed. It was conditionally accredited as a teaching hospital for postgraduate medical education. The following report has been accepted:

The Accreditation Committee examined the Report of the Director of the Hospital and took into consideration the findings of the Committee which carried out the site visit and made the following decision:

That the hospital as an institution be approved for postgraduate training purposes in the following areas:

> Surgery
> Medicine
> Paediatrics
> Gynaecology and Obstetrics

However, full accreditation of each of the above departments is subject to the recommendations received from the appropriate subcommittees of the Accreditation Committee as below:

Surgery

The Accreditation Committee on the advice of the Surgical Subcommittee recommends that:

a) the Surgical Department of Farwania Hospital be fully approved for professional training in surgery;

b) the department also be approved for "postgraduate speciality training in general surgery" subject to the following conditions:

    i) better and easier access to the departmental library be made;

    ii) a senior casualty officer (Sr. Registrar or Consultant level) be appointed to the accident and emergency department;

    iii) clinical meetings and teaching be more structured and better organised.

The number of accredited training posts for each of the postgraduate "professional training" and "speciality training" unit should be 2 candidates per each surgical unit.

A structured programme for "professional training in surgery" as well as a programme of "postgraduate speciality training in general surgery" will be in accordance with those laid down by the Discipline Committee for Surgery as approved by the Joint Board.

The Surgical Subcommittee will review the Department of Surgery at Farwania Hospital in September 1982, to ensure fulfilment of the above requirements.

Medicine

The Accreditation Committee on the advice of the Medical Subcommittee recommends that:

a) The Medical Department of Farwania Hospital be fully approved for professional training in internal medicine.

b) Accreditation for Speciality Training in Medicine has been deferred until another site visit is carried out by the appropriate sub-committee.

The number of accredited training posts for each of the postgraduate "professional training" and "speciality training" units should be 2 candidates per each medical unit.

A structured programme for "professional training in medicine" as well as a programme of "postgraduate speciality training in general medicine" will be in accordance with those laid down by the Discipline Committee for Medicine as approved by the Joint Board.

Paediatrics

The Accreditation Committee on the advice of the Paediatrics Sub-Committee recommends that:

a) The Paediatrics Department of Farwania Hospital be fully approved for professional training in Paediatrics.

b) Accreditation for Speciality Training in Paediatrics has been deferred until another site visit is carried out by the appropriate sub-committee.

The number of accredited training posts for each of the postgraduate "professional training" and "speciality training" units should be 2 candidates per each paediatric unit.

A structured programme for "professional training in paediatrics" as well as a programme of "postgraduate speciality training in paediatrics" will be in accordance with those laid down by the Discipline Committee for Paediatrics as approved by the Joint Board.

Gynaecology and Obstetrics

The Accreditation Committee on the advice of the Gynaecology and Obstetrics Subcommittee recommends that:
a) The Gynaecology and Obstetrics Department of Farwania Hospital be fully approved for professional training in Gynaecology and Obstetrics.
b) Accreditation for Speciality Training in Gynaecology and Obstetrics has been deferred until another site visit is carried out by the appropriate subcommittee.

The number of accredited training posts for each of the postgraduate "professional training" and "speciality training" units should be 2 candidates (at most 4) per each gynaecology and obstetrics unit.

A structured programme for "professional training in gynaecology and obstetrics" as well as a programme of "postgraduate speciality training in gynaecology and obstetrics" will be in accordance with those laid down by the Discipline Committee for Gynaecology and Obstetrics as approved by the Joint Board.

Medical Records

The Farwania Hospital is expected to make appropriate improvement in the records system as recommended by the Sub-Committee for Medical Records.

5. Discipline Committee for Medicine

The Discipline Committee met six times since October 1981 and as in the previous years its activities were related to matters affecting General Professional Training as well as Continuing Medical Education. Moreover, the Committee was also involved in preparation of a programme for Speciality Training. The General Professional Training was brought up to date. The Committee approved the amended programme of General Professional Training which was submitted to the Area Executive Committee for General Professional Training and subsequently approved by them. It also recommended to this Area Executive Committee some changes in the second year of this Professional Training Programme in Psychiatry and Dermatology for those doctors intending to specialise in Internal Medicine. The Committee appointed coordinators for the Professional Training Programme in the various hospitals in Kuwait.

The various postgraduate courses were evaluated as in previous years. The MRCP Part I course lasted four months and there were two weekly sessions of two hours each. A Mock examination will be held on May 13th to choose the 25 Kuwaiti candidates. In October 1981 the MRCP Part I examination was held in Kuwait and out of the 25 Kuwaiti candidates, 8 passed, giving a pass rate of 32%. The MRCP Part II course was again organised. As in the previous years, local faculty members and visitors to the Ministry of Health participated in both programmes, with local staff being involved in at least two-thirds of the activities for these courses. Symposia on Immunology, Chest Pain, Mycology and Oncology were held throughout the year.

The Discipline Committee also approved a programme of postgraduate training in Medicine whose objectives are to provide a broad based structured training programme in Internal Medicine spread over a period of four years. The training will take place in units accredited for this purpose by the Accreditation Committee. Activities of the Pan Arab Board Speciality Committee Examination in Internal Medicine were reviewed and progress in this field was assessed by the committee throughout its year of activities.

The Discipline Committee again made up a list of visitors to be invited by the Ministry of Health in conformity with the objectives laid down by the Joint Board. The committee also reviewed a number of applications for the consultant post and gave appropriate advice to the Ministry of Public Health.

6. Discipline Committee for Surgery

Introduction

The Committee for the Discipline of Surgery is a subcommittee of the Joint Board for Postgraduate Medical Education and is delegated to organise and supervise the Postgraduate Professional and Speciality Training in the various subspecialities of Surgery as directed by the Board. The committee also recommends the number and type of symposia and postgraduate courses to be held in Kuwait in the field of Surgery and nominates suitable candidates for scholarships and study periods abroad. This committee has been functioning for the past three years during which many important developments have taken place in the area of postgraduate and professional surgical training in Kuwait, in which the Discipline Committee for Surgery has played a very important role. The membership of the committee which is determined by the Joint Board was initially for the term of two years and this term was renewed for another two years in May 1981. Recently, additional members were added to the committee in order to make its function more comprehensive and the membership representative of most of the surgical subspecialities.

Organisation and Meetings

At the first meeting of the committee which was held in October 1982, Dr. John McCallum was elected as Vice-Chairman and Dr. Abdulla Behbehani as Secretary. The committee has since held monthly meetings; the 8th and last was held on May 18th, 1982.

Activities

1. The committee recommended, at the request of the Joint Board, that the primary F.R.C.S. Course which has been held in Kuwait by the Royal College of Surgeons of Ireland for the past five years should be continued since this course has served a very useful purpose as a method of speciality training as well as continuing medical education for young surgeons in training.
2. The committee recommended, also at the request of the Joint Board, that the final examination for the fellowship should be held in Kuwait since the Registrar of the Royal College of Surgeons of Ireland and the past President of the College had expressed their interest in holding the examination locally. The membership of the Discipline Committee for Surgery is of the opinion that this would be advantageous to Kuwait from scientific, financial and personnel availability points of view.

3. The committee recommended the following surgeons as coordinators for the Professional Training Programme in general surgery for the various hospitals for the year 1981—1982.

Dr. Majeed Alwan for Sabah Hospital
Dr. Joseph Cherian for Adan Hospital
Dr. Ghazali for Farwania Hospital
Dr. Abu Nema for Mubarak Hospital
Dr. Hemayun for Jahra Hospital.

4. A suggested evaluation sheet for the trainees in their rotation to general surgery was worked out by Dr. Abdel Malek at one of the meetings of the subcommittee.

5. An agreed protocol was worked out for the invitation of visitors and information about Postgraduate Programmes by all the Chiefs of Services that all such information be directed to the Chairman and the Secretary of the Discipline Committee from whose offices the information will be transmitted to the Joint Board and disseminated to other hospital departments of surgery.

6. Recommendation of visitors for the various subspecialities in Kuwait for the year 1981—82.

7. At the request of the Joint Board the Committee considered the proposal by Mr. Abdel Reda Abbas, Head of Emergency Medical Services in Kuwait to hold a training course for the management of trauma for a selected number of Kuwait doctors sponsored by the American College of Surgeons, Section of Trauma. The committee recommended to the board that this training course would be of great advantage to the country in view of the volume of trauma and the lack of training in its management. It recommended that this course should be held in collaboration with other ministry departments and representatives of the American College of Surgeons.

Postgraduate Programme in Surgery

1. The committee reviewed the previously approved programme for professional training in general surgery in the various hospitals and after some amendments it was approved. This was distributed to all the departments of surgery in the various hospitals for implementation in the training of residents during their six months of rotation to surgery.

2. Postgraduate Speciality Training Programme in general surgery. At the request of the Joint Board and the Ministry of Health, the Discipline Committee formulated the Working Party in November 1981 to work out a comprehensive Postgraduate Training Programme in General Surgery for Kuwait. After several weeks of discussion and consultation, a four year speciality training programme was prepared with specific objectives, proposals for the methods of application and selection of candidates, precise periods of rotation through the different surgical subspecialities, a proposed syllabus for training both in the basic sciences and in clinical surgery, definitive procedures for acquisition of operative skills and for evaluation. The programme was designed in such a way as to be applicable to all the hospitals in Kuwait, to be acceptable as a requirement for training by the Royal Colleges of Surgeons of Great Britain, by the Arab Board for Surgery or by any local examining body that may be established in Kuwait. This programme was subsequently discussed at various meetings and also with representatives of the Royal Colleges of Surgeons before it was put in the final form. After further discussion and approval by the Area Executive Committee for speciality training the programme was put to the Joint Board at its Sixth

Meeting on April 20th, 1982. The board approved the programme as the formal training programme in general surgery for Kuwait. At the direction of the Joint Board the programme was recently distributed to all the departments, heads of units and coordinators in the various hospitals. The implementation of this programme is being worked out and applications will be considered from eligible candidates who, after appropriate interview by the subcommittee of the Discipline Committee for Surgery, will be taken on the programme. The number of candidates will depend on the available facilities in the approved departments and units of Kuwait hospitals, and also on the needs of the country for specialists in general surgery. It is proposed that at the next meeting of the Discipline Committee for Surgery precise details of the procedure of implementation will be finalised and the information disseminated to the various hospitals so that the programme can be put into effect in September—October 1982.

3. Two members of the committee, Prof. George M. Abouna and Dr. Sudad Sabri, who are members of the Arab Board for Surgical Specialities have been actively involved in the development of the surgical clinic programme for the Arab Surgical Board which is very much on the same lines as those worked out by the Discipline Committee for Surgery in Kuwait. The programme for the Arab Board for Surgery is also due to start in October 1982.

Postgraduate Courses and Symposia Held in 1981—82

1. Instructional course in Hand Surgery:
   This course was organised by Prof. J. P. James in collaboration with five invited participants from outside Kuwait and several others from within Kuwait and was held at Sulaibhikat Orthopaedic Hospital during November 1981. About 50 participants attended the course but only about 10 could be accommodated for the full instructional part of the course. The course dealt with most of the common conditions of the hand, both emergency and elective, and it proved very useful for those concerned with the treatment of hand injuries and hand abnormalities in Kuwait.

2. The first postgraduate symposium on the Surgery of the Alimentary System was held in Kuwait on February 1—5, 1982. This symposium, with international representation, was organised by the Discipline Committee for Surgery and the following were members of the Organising Committee:

   Dr. G. M. Abouna   Chairman
   Dr. Nael Al-Naqeeb
   Dr. Youssef Oomer
   Dr. Basil Naqeeb
   Dr. Abdulla Al-Behbehani
   Dr. Edward Ruzyllo

   The following international faculty participated in this symposium:
   Dr. Thomas Demeester, University of Chicago; Prof. J. M. Greep, Professor of Surgery and Dean, University of Limberg, Maastricht, Holland; Prof. David Johnston, Professor of Surgery, Leeds; Dr. George Johnston, Surgeon, Royal Victoria Hospital, Belfast; Prof. Nils Kock, University of Göteborg, Sweden; Prof. A. R. Moussa, University of Chicago; Prof. Marshall Orlaff, University of California, San Diego; Prof. Atef Salam, Amory University, Atlanta; Prof. James Thompson, University of Texas, Galveston; Prof. J. V. Turcotte, University of Michigan; Prof. Timothy Harrison, Pennsylvania State University.

In addition to the invited faculty there were 19 local faculties contributing to the symposium. There were 43 major papers delivered at the symposium which covered the entire gastrointestinal system together with liver, pancreas and the biliary duct.

The symposium was attended by more than 140 doctors and surgeons from Kuwait and from other parts of the Middle East. The general evaluation of the symposium was rated by most as excellent, and requests were made by many of the participants for more symposia to be held in Kuwait in the future.

Visitors

The following visitors were invited at the recommendation of the Discipline Committee for Surgery for 1981—82:

1. *E.N.T.:*   Dr. R. Percy, London; Dr. W. M. S. Ironside, Herdress-field, U.K., and Dr. A. G. M. Maran, Edinburgh.
2. *Ophthalmology:*   Dr. Hall, Birmingham, Dr. J. Davies, London, Dr. H. Lincoff.
3. *Cardiac Surgery:*   Dr. Donald Ross, London; Dr. Terrence English, Cambridge, England, and Dr. Dr. Gordan Danielson, Mayo Clinic, U.S.A.
4. *Orthopaedic Surgery:* Dr. J. A. Chalmers, Edinburgh; Dr. Han Blen, Glasgow. Dr. H. Brattstrom, Lund, Sweden.
5. *Plastic Surgery:*   Dr. Dale Birdsel, Calgary University, Canada.
6. *Surgical Oncology:*   Dr. Elias George Elias, University of Maryland, U.S.A.
7. *Paediatric Surgery:* Dr. J. E. Scott, University of Newcastle, England; Dr. Nobuhiko Komi, Tokushima University, Japan.

General Visitors

The following representatives of the Royal Colleges of Surgeons visited Kuwait and met with the Discipline Committee for Surgery to discuss Postgraduate Training in Kuwait and its support by the Royal Colleges in Britain:

Prof. Gillingham, President, Royal College of Surgeons of Edinburgh; Dr. Allan, Dean, Secretary of Royal College of Surgeons of Edinburgh; Prof. W. A. L. MacGowan, Registrar, Royal College of Surgeons of Ireland; Dr. Harry O'Flanigan, Former Dean, Royal Colleges of Surgeons of Ireland.

Future Plans and Goals

In addition to the above two symposia the Discipline Committee for Surgery hopes that the Postgraduate Training Programme in General Surgery which has been approved by the Joint Board will start next October and will be supported by the Ministry of Health and the Faculty of Medicine. They hope that it will meet a very urgent and important need in postgraduate training in surgery in this country. The Discipline Committee for Surgery is hopeful that the initiation and the maintenance of such a programme will help to raise the standards both of the surgical services and of surgical education in Kuwait.

If the recommendations of the Discipline Committee for Surgery that the final examination of the surgical fellowship be held in Kuwait are accepted, this too will go a long way towards raising the standard, improving the quality and generating enthusiasm and interest in surgical training in this country.

The Discipline Committee for Surgery plans to work with the department of Anatomy and other basis science departments of the Faculty of Medicine towards implementing the part of the training programme relating to the basic sciences, so that the primary fellowship course is held not in one "lump sum" of a period of 8 weeks, which disrupts hospital services, but over a more protracted period which will allow more time for the trainees to assimilate the basic sciences and without them having to leave the hospital services.

The Discipline Committee for Surgery plans to improve the organisation of postgraduate lectures, courses and many symposia that are so often held in Kuwait but poorly attended because of a lack of information and because they are poorly organised. At its last meeting the committee decided that all programmes in postgraduate medical education in surgery should be channeled through the office of the Discipline Committee for Surgery where proper documentation, announcement and dissemination of information will take place.

The Discipline Committee for Surgery is also concerned about the training of Senior Registrars and it intends at its subsequent meetings to work out a programme where present fellows of the Royal College holding Senior Registrar status will go through a form of higher surgical training to enable them to assume ultimate responsibilities as consultants in the future.

The Discipline Committee for Surgery intends to work in closer collaboration with the Executive Committee for Continuing Medical Education and with the training division of the Joint Board to improve the organisation and the selection of all its postgraduate symposia, lectures and postgraduate courses.

The Discipline Committee hopes to assist the departments of surgery of the hospitals in Kuwait to obtain recognition of their training facilities both by the local accreditation committee and by other international accreditation committees. This will enable the trainees, in those departments qualified for the certifying examinations that they will be taking at the completion of the training programme, to be able to compete.

Recommendations

From the experience of the past 3 years of developing surgical training programmes and surgical continuing education in Kuwait the following recommendations are worthy of consideration:

1. There is a great need for maintaining continuity. The Discipline Committee for Surgery has embarked on a very important project: the initiation of the Postgraduate Training Programme in Surgery. In order that this be successful and become the nucleus for other training programmes to be developed in the other subspecialities, continuity of the momentum now generated within the Discipline Committee is essential.

2. There is still great difficulty in the communication between one department of surgery and another and between these departments and the training division of the Ministry of Health. Notices of meeting, not infrequently, arrive after the meeting has taken place. It is recommended that the Discipline Committee for Surgery should have assigned to it a mailman (Murasil) with adequate means of

transportation whose function will be to see that correspondence, announce-
ments, information and programmes are distributed to the various departments
and hospitals within 24 hours.
3. A part of the training and education of a surgeon, trainer and trainee, is the opportunity to meet colleagues and peers, at the international level to discuss problems and to see how others manage to solve them. This requires that surgeons in
this country are given the opportunity to attend one symposium or international
meeting a year, and it is recommended that every consultant and senior registrar
be given this privilege by the Ministry of Health through the training division
and the Joint Board regardless of whether or not an individual has a scientific
paper to deliver.
4. In the training of senior registrars and subspecialists it is also necessary that a
period of study leave be given to promising and outstanding surgeons at the consultant and senior registrar level to go abroad for periods of 3—6 months in order to develop expertise in one of the rapidly developing areas of surgery. It is
recommended that this principle be accepted and that a limited number of
candidates should be selected at the recommendation of the discipline committee for surgery to go for a study leave with a full salary for a limited period.

Summary

In summary, the Discipline Committee for Surgery has made in its third year
some important progress in the development and implementation of postgraduate
training in surgery in this country. The structure of the committee at the present is
diverse, the enthusiasm among its members is increasing, and the general atmosphere of work for the objectives of postgraduate surgical education and training in
surgery is positive and friendly. There is every reason to believe that this encourag-
ing trend will continue. The Discipline Committee managed to achieve a number of
important projects in the development of good postgraduate surgical training and
education in this country such as the development of the postgraduate training programme in general surgery, the organisation of postgraduate symposia and its improved procedures and programmes for the many visitors that come to Kuwait
from abroad. The role of the Discipline Committee in postgraduate training in surgery will undoubtedly increase and become more detailed and diverse with the
implementation of a postgraduate training programme and with better streamlining
and organisation of more postgraduate symposia in the various developing or con-
troversial areas in surgical practice. There are however a number of problems and
obstacles which stand in the way of establishing effective and stable postgraduate
training programmes and continuing surgical education. Some of these have already been alluded to while others are beyond the control of the Discipline Committee and even the Joint Postgraduate Board. The Discipline Committee for Surgery is appreciative of the increasing support which is given to it for the implementation of its programme by the Chairman and Secretary of the Joint Board, by the
Undersecretary of the Ministry of Health, by the Medical and Secretarial staff of
the Training Division, by the Chairman of the Area Executive Committee for Continuing Medical Education, and by the Public Relations Department of the Ministry of Health. The future plans and goals of the Discipline Committee for Surgery
in the future are positive and ambitious but are quite realistic and with the kind of
support it has hitherto received, its future programmes can be brought to fruition.

7. Discipline Committee for Obstetrics and Gynaecology

A Summary of the Main Happenings:

1. General Professional Training proceeds normally and it seems to have attained reasonable stability. However, I would like to issue the reminder about the allowances due to the organisers. In a recent meeting of the Gynaecology Council, it was thought optimal to send one trainee per unit. The maximum should not exceed two, if proper exposure and training are to be ensured.

2. The C.I.N. for visitors to the department during 1982/83 in various hospitals has been prepared and I trust your office has by now received it.

3. The process of accreditation of various departments has started but is not over yet. You will be receiving relevant reports from Dr. Samir Kamel, convener for our visiting team.

4. The intensive course oriented to the Part 2 MRCOG examination has been a success. Clinical rounds started in the late morning after the doctor candidates had carried out their essential daily work. Lectures were given in the afternoon and were open to general attendants. In this way the course members did not have to lose their summer vacation, and all doctors could avail themselves of the benefit of the afternoon lectures. We strongly recommend this course format.
Unfortunately, some misunderstandings blemished the preparatory phase of the course. In view of the short notice we urged the training division to give us a green light and proceed to make the necessary contacts and arrangements in Britain. We got the green light in a written message from your department. It was therefore to our great horror and dismay that a short while before the course was due, we simultaneously received word that the British team were anxiously awaiting visas and tickets, and word from your department that there were local obstacles in Kuwait, and a hint that the matter was not finally settled. Fortunately the confusion was successfully sorted out in due time. I was much hurt, however, when the matter was pictured as if the fault was ours, claiming that we had bypassed the training division straight to the ministry. The experience is forgiveable but not forgettable.
We are proposing to repeat the same course with some alterations in personnel next year, if we have your solid approval.

5. The part I MRCOG examination results showed that seven candidates from the Kuwait centre have passed. All are from Kuwait. One candidate attended the course given this year and one attended last year's course (and failed last year). Five candidates never attended the course.

6. The part I Arab Fellowship examination was given in Kuwait this year. Four candidates from Kuwait passed the examination. The overall result of the examination was a passed rate of 20%.

8. Discipline Committee for Paediatrics

For the continuing medical education (CME) of the doctors in service, including those doing their professional training programme in Adan Hospital, a variety of clinical paediatric and neonatal problems, procedures, and the basic science needed to understand these were provided. Different members of the staff did this by means of case presentation and discussion, analysis of a collection of cases, formal dissertation including recent knowledge, or journal clubs.

Paediatricians in the area were also invited to attend these sessions. However, since it was difficult to arrange a time that would ensure adequate attendance by hospital and clinic staff, it was decided to schedule the meetings to suit the hospital staff and to provide CME of the Area Paediatricians by other means.

For this purpose an exchange programme has been arranged whereby 2 paediatricians from the MCH clinics of the area transfer to the Hospital for 2 months and are replaced by 2 paediatricians from the hospital staff for this period. This provides the 2 incoming doctors with full exposure to acute problems at the inpatient level, and gives them the opportunity to refresh and expand their knowledge.

An extension of this step, which not only provides CME but also contributes towards the goal of Integration of Hospital and Regional Services, was the introduction of a specialist clinic once per week at Fahaheel Polyclinic. A few MCH doctors who were free to attend these sessions did so on a few occasions. For the next year it is planned to arrange compulsory attendance at these sessions in such a way that each MCH Paediatrician will have 1 attendance per 4 to 5 weeks.

Unfortunately, due to the late receipt of notices of the CME programmes organised by different Discipline Committees, it was not possible for our staff to participate in as many of the programmes as was desired.

Attached is a list of Subject Titles with names of doctors responsible for the presentations.

General Paediatric Subjects

1. Chronic diarrhoea in infancy — Dr. Asad Abd Bari
2. Gastrointestinal allergy — Dr. N. Fernando
3. Case of myositis ossificans progressive — Dr. Ghazi Kandil
4. Mechanisms of host defense — Dr. Mohsen Abd Salam
5. Urinary tract infections (MCH service) — Dr. Jinan Towfiq
6. Salmonellosis — Dr. Ipe John
7. Tuberculosis in childhood 1 — Dr. Galal Mirghani
   2
   3 — (Slides / lecture)
8. Case of lymphoedema — Dr. Suhad Yaish
9. Failure to thrive—Marfan's syndrome managed by hyperalimentation — Dr. Osama Al-Agamawi
10. Complement system — Dr. Mohsen Abd Salam
11. Rickets — Dr. Abd Hameed Al-Sayed
12. Case of metabolic acidosis due to inherited abnormality — Dr. N. Fernando
13. Adreno genital syndrome — Dr. Nagla Falaki
14. Hypernatremia—management — Dr. Danuta Fedechko
15. Vitamin responsive disorder presenting as metabolic acidosis — Dr. N. Fernando
16. Diagnostic approach to patient with metabolic acidosis — Dr. N. Fernando
17. Acute asthma in childhood (journal club) — Dr. Nagla Falaki
18. Case with multiple nutritional deficiency metals— essential and toxic — Dr. N. Fernando

19. Anaemia—diagnosis   Dr. Kamel Dudin
20. Clinical approach to child with vomiting   Dr. Intissar Salah (MCH)
21. Immunity in protein energy malnutrition   Dr. Mohsen Abd Salem
22. WBC function in protein energy malnutrition   Dr. Mohsen Abd Salem
23. Iron metabolism   Dr. Nagla Falaki
24. Pyrexia of unknown origin   Dr. Abd Hameed Al Syed
25. Cardiac arrhythmias   Dr. Nagla Falaki
26. Serum electrolytes in diabetic   Dr. Suhad Yaish
    hyperlipidemia—case and discussion
27. Pyrexia (journal club)   Dr. Sayid Wajid
28. Analysis of 14 cases of hypernatremic   Dr. Ipe John
    dehydration—discussion of management
29. A case of marasmus, responding well to lead   Dr. N. Fernando
    chelation
30. Water and electrolyte balance   Dr. Danuta Fedechko
31. Case of short stature changes—   Dr. Ghazi Kandil and
    Morquio's disease   Dr. Saeed Al Mohtaseb
32. Acute iron poisoning (journal club)   Dr. Ipe John
33. Congenital chloride losing in diarrhoea   Dr. Hassan Daban
                                                         (MCH)
                                                         Dr. Danuta Fedechko
34. Protracted diarrhoea (journal club)   Dr. N. Fernando
35. Journal club, role of zinc in newborn   Dr. Sayid Wajid
    oral rehydration
36. Abdominal tumour   Dr. Sayid Wajid

Lectures by Visiting Experts

1. Intestinal obstruction in the newborn   Dr. John Scott
                                                         Paediatric surgeon, U.K.
2. Congenital bilary malformation   Prof. Nobuhiko Komi,
                                                         Japan

Neonatal Problems and Procedures

1. Exchange transfusion in neonatal period   Dr. Ahmed Fouda
2. Neonatal statistics—meaning and value   Dr. Abraham Kurilla
3. Neonatal infection   Dr. Kawser El Hamy
4. Neonatal jaundice   Dr. Adnan Khayyat
5. Meconium staining   Dr. Omer Hassan Ibrahim
6. Birth injuries   Dr. Adnan Khayyat
7. Umbilical vessel catheterisation   Dr. Mansoor
8. Oxygen therapy of newborn   Dr. O. N. Bhakoo
9. Neonatal hypoglycemia—prevention and   Dr. Viswanathan
   management
10. Hypocalcemia and hypomagnesemia in   Dr. Ahmed Fouda
    neonatal period
11. Neonatal resuscitation (specially for   Dr. O. N. Bhakoo
    MCH doctors)
12. Prolonged hyperbilirubinaemia in newborn   Dr. M. N. Mansoor

13. Temperature control in newborn   Dr. O. N. Bhakoo
14. Thyroid status in perinatal period, 3 sessions   Dr. Kawser El Hamy
15. A case of neonatal hyperammonemia discussion   Dr. Galal Mirghani
    of urea cycle disorders
16. Intracranial haemorrhage in newborn   Dr. Omar Hassan Ibrahim
17. Perinatal hypoxia—ischemic injury of CNS   Dr. Omar Hassan Ibrahim
18. Pathophysiology of perinatal asphyxia   Dr. M. N. Mansoor
19. Neonatal jaundice—case and discussion   Dr. Kawser El Hamy
20. Neonatal septicaemia—case and discussion   Dr. Omar Hassan Ibrahim
21. Hypernatremia in septicaemic newborn—   Dr. N. Fernando
    case and discussion
22. Plasma aminoacid levels in newborns   Dr. Ipe John
    admitted to ICU (journal club)

9. Discipline Committee for Public Health

No Report

10. Discipline Committee for Family Medicine

No Report

11. Discipline Committee for Radiology

The Activities of the Medical Discipline Committee covered the following:
1. Regular meetings.
2. Establishment of the policy for different aspects of medical training such as professional training, specialisation and the Continuing Medical Education Programme.
3. Lectures delivered on different topics.
4. Suggestions regarding Diploma Degree Course or fellowship Part I Course in Radio-Diagnosis in Kuwait.
5. Invitation to foreign visitors.

1. Regular meetings almost monthly have been held in Mubarak-Al-Kabeer Hospital, during which the different functions of the Committee have been discussed. Opinions and different proposals were also presented by each member concerning the fulfilment of the different aims.
2. Establishment of programmes regarding participation and responsibility of different members in the general professional training and continuing medical education programmes have been approved by all members, and the curriculum has been sent to the secretary of the Joint Board of Postgraduate Medical Education. It was the goal of the Discipline Committee to cover all fields of radiology and medical imaging which they feel is suitable for the candidates to whom the syllabus will be delivered.
3. The following lectures have been delivered:
   A. Medical Ultrasound   — Dr. H. Bassiony
   B. Radio-Isotopic Bone   Prof. Abdel-Dayam
      Scanning
   C. Intervention Radiology   — Prof. Steinhart

4. A suggestion regarding having a Diploma-Degree in Radio-Diagnosis or Fellow-ship Part I in Kuwait has been discussed, and effective steps will soon be taken to fulfill this goal.
5. The following professors visited Kuwait, delivered lectures and shared in final discussions concerning their opinions and suggestions for achieving a higher standard of radiological services, especially in the field of Postgraduate Medical Education.

1. Prof. Uno Erikson, Uppsala University, Sweden
2. Prof. Edward Russel, Miami University, U.S.A.
3. Prof. R. Hellar, U.S.A.

12. Discipline Committee for Anaesthesiology and Intensive Care

According to the bylaws of the Joint Board for postgraduate training and teaching, biannual reports should be submitted to the head of the Training Division in the first week of November and of May every year to be distributed to the Area Executive Committees.

As a matter of fact, the Discipline Committee of Anaesthesiology and Intensive Care was formed recently in September, 1981 and we did not have the chance to send a report in November, 1981 simply because there was nothing to report except two meetings of the committee.

Referring to the last meeting with the Chairman of the Area Executive Commit-tee for Continuing Medical Education, the head and the two assistant heads of the Training Division, which was held in the Training Division on the 8th of March, 1982, it was decided that for this year one report should be submitted to the Head of the Training Division to be distributed to all area executive committees during the second half of April, 1982.

The Discipline Committee for Anaesthesiology and Intensive Care have already held six meetings, in which the following decisions were taken.

1. Postgraduate Training in Anaesthesiology and Intensive Care

Programmes were established for the three divisions of postgraduate training including Professional Training, Postgraduate Speciality Training and Continuing Medical Education. These programmes were distributed to the head of the Training Division and all members of the Discipline Committee. A programme is enclosed.

2. Activities Accomplished During the Last Year

a) As regards the field of Professional Training, I am submitting a list (enclosed with this report) with the numbers and names of trainees who came to the Depart-ment of Anaesthesiology and Intensive Care covering Sabah, Chest and Infectious Diseases Hospitals. Professional Training as well is taking place in Adan and Mu-barak Hospitals. Unfortunately, no reports were received from the heads of the de-partments regarding the numbers and names of the trainees.

b) No single Kuwaiti trainee has joined any anaesthesia department for post-graduate speciality training despite the encouragements and efforts to attract doc-tors to the speciality.

Primary FFARCS, Course and Examination

A course for the Primary FFARCS Examination has been established in Kuwait for the Gulf area through the Ministry of Public Health, Kuwait University, Faculty of Medicine, and in agreement with the Welsh National School of Medicine. Dr. Mohamed M. Motaweh was appointed as the Coordinator of the course and Dr. H. A. El-Fattah Yousef as Assistant Coordinator. This FFARCS Course was approved by the Postgraduate Committee in the Kuwait Faculty of Medicine, the Joint Board and the Royal College of Surgeons of England. This course started on the 14th of April and will continue for six weeks. It is an afternoon day release course from 4—7.30 p.m. every day of the week except Thursday when a tutorial for one hour is held. 29 candidates applied for this course and 20 candidates were selected by a selection committee formed of:

Prof. A. M. Yousof	Dean of the Faculty of Medicine, Kuwait University.
Prof. Olav Thulesius	Professor and Chairman Pharmacology Department, Kuwait University.
Prof. Roy Choudhury	Professor and Chairman, Anatomy Department, Kuwait University.
Dr. Mohamed M. Motaweh	Chairman of the Discipline Committee of Anaesthesiology and Coordinator of the Primary FFARCS Course and Examination.
Dr. Hussein A. Youssef	Assistant Prof. of Anaesthesia, Faculty of Medicine, Kuwait University and Assistant Coordinator of the Primary FFARCS, Course and Examination.

Letters were sent from the Chairman of the Joint Board to all Gulf States to nominate one of their candidates to attend the course for the examination. Only Iraq responded and their candidate had already joined the course. After an agreement with the Royal College of Surgeons of England, it has been decided that a board of three examiners and one administrator will come to Kuwait to start the examination on the 19th of June, 1982. Nasr El-Din Mahmoud, Prof. of Physiology in Kuwait, Faculty of Medicine, will participate as external examiner.

Three observer examiners will share in conducting the examination, namely:

1. Prof. Olav Thulesius
2. Dr. Mohamed M. Motaweh
3. Dr. Hussein A. Fatah

The syllabus and timetable of the course is attached.

Continuing Medical Education

1. *Scientific Activities:*
All of the anaesthesia departments in different hospitals are holding their scientific meetings on Thursday of each week. Usually it is a discussion of some scientific topic concerning the speciality, followed by group discussion. Some departments are holding journals club meetings and clinical morbidity and mortality meetings. The objectives of those meetings is to improve the working conditions in the departments and the efficiency of the working staff members and to keep them up to date in their work. Discussion rounds are held every day in the theatres and departments having an I.C.U. to discuss the management and progress of the critically ill patients. Orientation classes for staff nurses are held weekly in some departments to improve their efficiency and to refresh their knowledge. The scientific programmes

for the Anaesthesia Departments of Sabah, Maternity, Farwania, Orthopedic and Mubarak Hospitals are enclosed with this report.

Some departments have got their libraries which have a regular supply of recent books, journals and periodicals from the Training Division. Measures have already been taken to supply the hospitals lacking libraries with books and periodicals.

2. *Visitors:*

During the last year, 1981, visitors in Anaesthesiology and Intensive Care have visited Kuwait. Their programme included lectures and tutorials and visits to different anaesthesia departments in different hospitals.

The Discipline Committee of Surgery made up a list of visitors invited last year by the Ministry of Health with the objectives laid down by the standing committee of anaesthesia at that time before the formation of the Discipline Committee for Anaesthesiology.

Visitors who came for other objectives were invited to deliver lectures for continuing medical education in Anaesthesia, namely:

1. Prof. Hassan Aly, Professor of Anaesthesia, Harvard University, U.S.A.
2. Prof. W. W. Mapelson, Professor of Physics Applied to Anaesthesia, Welsh National School of Medicine.
3. Prof. M. D. Vickers, Professor of Anaesthetics, Welsh National School of Medicine.
4. Prof. Kenneth Messeler, Professor of Anaesthesiology, Lund University, Sweden.
5. Dr. J. N. Horton, Tutor, F.F.A.R.C.S., England.

13. Discipline Committee for Clinical Medical Laboratory

No Report

14. Training Committee for Dentistry

This is an overview report on the training programmes performed during the year 1981—82.

I. A training programme run by the Eastman Dental Hospital for 24 dentists that entailed
  1. clinical
  2. theoretical
  components.
  1. 4 overseas lecturers were invited during the period 30th January—11th February, 1982.
     Subjects discussed were Prosthodontics, Conservative Dentistry, oral and maxillo-facial surgery and Pedodontics.
     Working hours were from 7.00 a.m.— 1.00 p.m. for two successive weeks.
     The morning sessions were mainly clinical and each 6 candidates affiliated to the lecturer for 1¼ hours and the four specialities were covered on a rotation basis during the day.
  2. Afternoon sessions entailed 30 lectures; 12 of them were assigned to all dentists in Kuwait. This activity has been performed in the dental centre.
     The course evaluation was submitted to your office on the 27th of February, 1982.

II. A training programme for dental technicians in the Dental Centre.
Concomitant to the No. I program, 2 senior dental technicians from the East-man Dental Hospital arrived along with the 4 Consultants in Dentistry and they performed on-job training of dental technicians in Kuwait that entailed acrylic work, metal work, gold castings and ceramics. Eight dental technicians were in close association with the overseas technicians, and during the period, both clinical and laboratory procedures were discussed with the dental technicians in full details.

III. A 2-week program for dental nurses started on the 28th February, 1982 and entailed lectures, demonstrations and on-job training of 20 dental nurses working in the dental department.
11 local doctors, 6 local staff nurses and 1 technician participated.

IV. The F.F.D. Course.
The course was conducted from the period of 30th January 1982—25th March 1982, which 12 candidates have attended.
The course has been the total responsibility of the coordinator, Dr. M. R. El-mostehy and it was planned to be dovetailed with the course of the FRCS running yearly for the last 5 years. This is the first time that such a course in the dental speciality has been acknowledged by the R.C.S. Dublin.
The course was intensive and condensed, with tutors both from the local faculty and overseas.
The course entailed basic teaching in Anatomy, Physiology, Pathology, Dental Anatomy and Dental Physiology.
12 candidates finished the examination that started on May 1st, 1982 and only 1 candidate satisfied the examiners in all subjects. By launching this course, one should state that those courses to be repeated yearly will eventually raise the level of excellence among the dental personnel in Kuwait.
A full report on the running of the course and the examinations will be submitted to your office under separate cover.

V. Anatomy; Postgraduate in Head and Neck Anatomy.
This was a course to augment the knowledge of anatomy for the dental profession in Kuwait and it included weekly sessions of 2 hours each beginning 31st December, 1981 to 23rd March, 1982. The course included orientation lectures, anatomy slides, movies in the development of the head, neck and face. It included as well surgical anatomy of various parts of the head and neck. A course evaluation of these orientation lectures was submitted to your office on the 24th of March, 1982.

Recommendations:

1. High standards of excellence of all dental personnel and auxiliaries is anticipated by repeated programs of such a nature.
2. Overseas lecturers should be invited from all disciplines.

V. Preparatory Steps for a New Programme for Postgraduate Medical Education for the Academic Year 1982—1983

26th January, 1982

CIRCULAR NO. 1

Regarding the Programme of Education for 1982—1983

To

Chairmen,
All Discipline Committees,
and
All Training Committees

Dear Doctor:

According to the decision of the Joint Board for Postgraduate Medical Education, Kuwait, the postgraduate medical education programmes should be formed for the fiscal year which begins on the 1st of July and ends on the 30th of June.

Past experience shows that delay in the proper management of the organisational preparations delays a programme of teaching and in many instances forces a change of projected activities.

In some instances we were overloaded by the time pressure and urgent administrative requests.

To escape from that I kindly request you to discuss now the topics and form of postgraduate medical education in 1982/83 in all fields of activities, i.e. professional, speciality and continuing medical education.

All instructions for programming are included in the Organisational Document of the Joint Board for Postgraduate Medical Education. Detailed information about it you may find on pages 6, 7, 8, 9, 10, 37 and 38 of the above-mentioned Organisational Document.

I would especially like to ask you to send us names of the invited lecturers with the provisional programmes included for them, in the form which you are obliged to use by Joint Board decision (see page 38).

Please find enclosed copies of the above-mentioned pages.

Yours sincerely,

Dr. E. Ruzyllo
Secretary of the Joint Board

Encl.: as above.
cc: Chairman, Joint Board.
cc: Ex-Officio Members of Joint Board.
cc: Chairman, Postgraduate Committee of the Faculty of Medicine.
cc: Chairman, 3 Area Executive Committees.

7th February, 1982

CIRCULAR NO. 2

Regarding the Programme for Postgraduate
Medical Education for 1982—1983

To

Chairmen,
All Area Executive Committees.

Dear Professor / Doctor:

According to the decision of the Joint Board for Postgraduate Medical Education, Kuwait, programmes for postgraduate medical studies should be prepared for the fiscal year (academic year). All instructions for programming are included in the Organisational Document of the Joint Board for Postgraduate Medical Education. Relevant pages of this document please find enclosed.

Secretariat of the Joint Board for Postgraduate Medical Education has sent Circular No. 1 dated 26. 1. 1982 to the Chairmen of 10 Discipline Committees requesting them to study the proposals for the new postgraduate academic year 1982—83. A copy of this letter has been sent as information to the Chairmen of the Area Executive Committees.

Having in mind that the Area Executive Committees are in fact executive bodies of the Joint Board in given fields of training and education, it is important that the general policy has to be thought of and discussed by these bodies.

It would be the first year that the Area Executive Committees have the possibility of forming a proper programme in each field of training: professional, speciality and continuing medical education (see pages 4 and 5). The Secretariat of the Joint Board is fully prepared to cooperate in this important task (see page 13).

All Discipline Committees will form an outline of their three programmes: professional, specialisation and continuing medical education, which should be sent to the relevant Area Executive Committee not later than the second half of March. The programmes sent to the relevant Area Executive Committee by the Discipline Committee should be arranged according to principles given by the Joint Board (see pages 7, 8 and 30).

May I call your attention to the fact that foreign lecturers should be invited at a proper time and in a proper form. In the past it gave us a lot of trouble and inconvenience in inviting foreign lecturers. So from the very beginning we request that the Discipline Committees should go along with the principles given on pages 37, 38 of the Organisational Document of the Joint Board for Postgraduate Medical Education.

Just for your information: in 1980/81 we invited 80 foreign lecturers, in 1981/82 we invited 79 foreign lecturers (these numbers are not exact as many of the lecturers were not invited through our Secretariat and those foreign lecturers who did not arrive in Kuwait, the Secretariat was not informed about).

For 1981/82 doctors were invited in the following specialities:

Medicine	12
General Surgery	28
Cardiac Surgery	3
Orthopaedic Surgery	3
Dermatology	2
Radiotherapy	5
Psychiatry	1
Gynaecology and Obstetrics	5
Paediatrics	4
E.N.T.	3
Ophthalmology	3
Anaesthesia	4
Immunology	6
Total	**79**

It is up to each Area Executive Committee to keep a proper balance of the number of invited lecturers.

A number of courses should be carefully thought of, taking into consideration different subspecialities and priorities for national health care system requirements.

The courses should be arranged chronologically in such a way that they should not conflict with each other, allowing doctors to participate in each of them.

The Area Executive Committee for Continuing Medical Education may also like to discuss in detail the Programme of Accreditation of Postgraduate Medical Studies. Having in mind the principles given in the Organisational Document on page 34, the whole problem of credit hours may finally be settled.

All Area Executive Committees may also discuss problems of full utilisation of tutor-coordinators of education so that more detailed programmes or instructions to the tutor-coordinators may come out of the discussions (see page 28). This problem is most important for the Area Executive Committee for Professional Training and Specialisation.

Special attention should be paid to Important Courses (I.C.) (see pages 9—11). Each Area Executive Committee may not have more than 1 or 2 such courses during one academic year. The I.C. should be organised at least 9 months before the scheduled time of performance to allow us to invite international participants from neighbouring countries.

Area Executive Committees having propositions from the Discipline Committees may see to the proper coding (Code Identifying Numbers) of the course, according to instructions from the Organisational Document pages 41—44. Consecutive numbers of the courses could be given in each speciality or could be given to all consecutive courses of each Area Executive Committee.

May I suggest that the following procedure be accepted for your consideration:

1. Each Area Executive Committee may like to invite to the meeting of the Committee all Chairmen of Discipline Committees to discuss its policy and requirements (see pages 4 and 5). The proper time for meeting the Chairmen of Discipline Committees would be at the end of February and the beginning of March.
2. During the discussion a general outline may be formed of the teaching programme for each Area Executive Committee and then discussed as to how it should be implemented (see pages 14 and 15).
3. To discuss a particular subject, Area Executive Committees may form subcommittees giving them concrete task to be fulfilled.

Please find enclosed copies of above-mentioned pages.

Yours sincerely,

Dr. E. Ruzyllo
Secretary, Joint Board

Encl.: as above

cc: Chairman, Joint Board.
cc: Ex-Officio Members of Joint Board.
cc: Chairman, Postgraduate Committee of the
    Faculty of Medicine.
cc: Secretaries of the Area Executive Committees.

5th June, 1982

CIRCULAR NO. 3

Regarding the Programme of
Education for 1982—1983

To

Chairmen,
All Discipline Committees,
and
All Training Committees

Dear Doctor:

With reference to my Circular No. 1 dated 26. 1. 82 and Circular No. 2 dated 7. 2. 82, I would like to inform you that the majority of the Discipline Committees gave their educational programmes for the 1982—83 teaching fiscal year.

Please find attached the Memorandum on these programmes. These programmes have been discussed and accepted by the Area Executive Committees and should be implemented.

I kindly request all Discipline Committees to send to the Joint Board up to the end of June, 1982 detailed programmes for courses, seminars and other forms of teaching activities in the teaching year 1982—83.

All instructions for programming are as detailed on pages 6, 7, 8, 9, 10, 11, 12, 37 and 38 of the Organisational Document of the Joint Board of Postgraduate Medical Education.

Yours sincerely,

Dr. E. Ruzyllo
Secretary of the Joint Board

Encl.: as above.

cc: Chairman, Joint Board.
cc: Ex-Officio Members of the Joint Board.
cc: Chairmen, Area Executive Committees (3).
    Chairman, Postgraduate Committee of the Faculty of Medicine.
cc: Secretaries, Area Executive Committees.

Memorandum

Area Executive Committee for Continuing Medical Education

A.   The following symposia/seminars have been suggested by the various Discipline Committees to take place in the fiscal year 1982—83.

1. *Discipline Committee for Clinical Laboratory:*
   a) Seminar on *Nutritional Support*

Programme Director	:	Dr. P. C. Reavy
Period	:	October—November, 1982
Duration	:	5 days
Guest speakers	:	5 from U.K.

   b) Symposium on *Deep Venous Thrombosis and Pulmonary Embolism*

Programme Director	:	Dr. S. Lopaciuk
Period	:	March—April, 1983
Duration	:	4 days (in the afternoons)
Guest speakers	:	6—7 (2 from USA and the rest from Europe)

2. *Discipline Committee for Surgery:*
   a) Symposium on *Renal Transplant and Renal Surgery*
       (Postponed from Budget for 1981—82)

Programme Director	:	Dr. George M. Abouna
Period	:	Middle of November, 1982
Duration	:	Not specified
Guest speakers	:	8—10

   b) Symposium on *Surgical Metabolism, Endocrinology, and Critical Care as Applied to the Middle East*

Programme Director	:	Dr. George M. Abouna
Period	:	February—March, 1983
Duration	:	Not specified
Guest speakers	:	10—12

   c) International Symposium in *Ophthalmology*
       (i) Management of the Vitreo-Retinal Diseases
       (ii) Photocoagulation

Programme Director	:	Dr. S. M. M. Sheriff
Period	:	Some time in mid part of 1983
Duration	:	3 days
No. of Faculty (suggested)	:	8—10.

3. *Discipline Committee for Medicine:*
   a) Seminar on *Chest Pain*
       (Postponed from Budget for 1981—82)

Programme Director	:	Dr. Abdul Razzak Al Yousof
Period	:	October 1982
Duration	:	Not specified
Guest speakers	:	3

   b) *Radiotherapy*
       Intensive Course on High Energy Photons and Electron Therapy

Programme Director	:	Dr. Y. T. Omar
Period	:	October—November, 1982
Duration	:	5 days
Guest speakers	:	5

4. *Discipline Committee for Anaesthesiology:*
   Only Programme for the Primary Fellowship Examination. (This is a diploma-oriented course. There is no suggestion for a symposium / seminar programme for continuing medical education.)

5. *Discipline Committee for Gynaecology:*
   Part II M.R.C.O.G. Course in 1983. (This is a diploma-oriented course. There is no suggestion for a symposium / seminar programme for continuing medical education.)

There is no response from the following Discipline Committees:
   1. Discipline Committee for Paediatrics.
   2. Discipline Committee for Public Health.
   3. Discipline Committee for Family Medicine.

B. Reports of activities were received from the following Discipline Committees:
   1. Discipline Committee for Surgery.
   2. Discipline Committee for Anaesthesiology.
   3. Discipline Committee for Clinical Laboratory.

Part Three

A Short History of Postgraduate Medical Education in Kuwait

The Constitution of the State of Kuwait contains 4 Articles which relate to the provision of health care and 2 Articles specifically to the provision of education:

Article 9: The family is the corner-stone of society. It is founded on religion, morality and patriotism. The law shall preserve the integrity of the family, strengthen its ties and protect under its auspices, motherhood and childhood.

Article 10: The State cares for the young and protects them from exploitation and from moral, physical and spiritual neglect.

Article 11: The State ensures aid for citizens in old age, sickness or inability to work. It also provides them with the services of social security, social and medical care.

Article 13: Education is a fundamental requisite for the progress of society, assured and promoted by the State.

Article 14: The State shall promote science, letters and the arts to encourage scientific research therein.

Article 15: The State cares for public health and for the means of prevention and treatment of diseases and epidemics.

Since the Fifties, the Government encourages Kuwaitis to make use of the facilities and to support the Government in providing for University study, postgraduate study and training programmes.

Any Kuwaiti completing his secondary education can go to any university in the world at the State's expense.

Any Kuwaiti in the service could have a full-paid leave to complete his Secondary School Education and go to any university immediately after completion of the Secondary School Certificate.

Any Kuwaiti University Graduate should be appointed by the State soon after graduation and he shall be entitled to full-paid leave and a scholarship immediately after appointment (some non-Kuwaitis were included in the postgraduate scholarship programme).

This policy has been amended several times, the last of which was by the Regulations of the 1980 General Services Function Council. Medical Education received particular attention and encouragement.

Postgraduate Medical Education could be considered in two stages:

A) Before 1970, when Kuwaiti doctors were eligible to have scholarships abroad. The outcome was very poor and economically and scientifically not feasible— some activities were done in some hospitals or departments but with no clear objectives or plans, and were dealt with according to individual consultant's ideas.

It was as early as 1965 when a group of Kuwaiti doctors worked on establishing medical education in Kuwait, having in mind that establishing a local Faculty of Medicine would solve the problem of shortages of well trained doctors and medical allied personnel. By these means and by involving the academic staff in the service, we could improve the quality and standard of the health care delivery system. They were successful in 1973 when an Amiri Decree was issued to establish the Faculty of Medicine in the University of Kuwait, and the University appointed a Dean elect in 1973. The Faculty took its first intake of 84 students in September, 1976, and they should be graduated in 1983.

The other marked changes happened in 1970 when a Kuwaiti doctor was appointed to be a Minister of Health and three other doctors were appointed as assistant under-secretaries for Technical Affairs, Curative Health Services and Preventive Health Services. Since then more Kuwaiti technical people have been involved in administration and very rapid development of health services in quantity and quality. By the year 1974, a new Minister who is medically qualified was appointed and all organisations of the Ministry have been changed. Since then the job of Under-Secretary has become a job for technical people.

The need for Postgraduate Medical Education was considered seriously and we always upheld the principle that successful Postgraduate Medical Education in a country is that system developed and organised in the country itself. This is because it should be based on the country's health care delivery system, its health problems, culture and tradition. Several models and attempts were tried until we successfully put the efforts of both the Ministry of Public Health and the Faculty of Medicine in a combined body.

A joint Postgraduate working party from the Ministry of Public Health and the Faculty of Medicine was established in January, 1976 to study Postgraduate training in Kuwait.

The working party determined that, before such graduates could obtain full registration to practice medicine here, they must undertake a postgraduate training programme with approved units in Kuwait. This must ensure some uniformity of coverage of clinical medicine and strengthen ethical principles in relation to patient care. An adequate evaluation of teaching and of learning must be built into this training.

As such, the first Postgraduate Joint Board, established in November, 1976, gives the detailed organisational structure and functions of that Joint Board. Its total membership was eight, four from the Ministry and four from the Faculty of Medicine. (For an original text of the organisational documents of the first postgraduate Joint Board see page 3.)

It comprised one Executive Postgraduate Committee and twelve Curriculum Committees as infrastructure. The Board should communicate its decisions to the Executive body. The Board Secretary should be the Chief Executive Officer of the Postgraduate Training Programme. The Chairman of the Executive Committee should be a member and secretary of the Board. The Head of the Training Division of the Public Health and Planning Department was supposed to be the Chairman of that Executive Committee.

To date, the routine implementation and supervision of the Postgraduate Training Programme has been mainly in the hands of the Department of Public Health and Planning. The nature of the training and the general rules governing the programme have remained the responsibility of the Joint Board which represents Faculty and Ministry equally.

The programme which was formulated by late 1976 demanded that the doctor in training must perform all the duties of a resident doctor for two years, namely during a first year of six months each in medicine and surgery, and during a second year of three months each in Gynaecology and Obstetrics, Paediatrics, Community Medicine / Primary Health Care and with two months in Psychiatry. This two year period is followed by a third year in which he is employed as an Assistant. Registration to practise in Kuwait is accorded after satisfactory completion of the initial three years.

A working paper on Postgraduate Medical Education has served its purpose. During the following 6 years it served as a postgraduate base and as functional principles for further development of the postgraduate medical studies.

Dr. Nouri Al Kazemi

Postgraduate Medical Education Programme in Kuwait "Working Paper" Contents

I. Organisational Structure and Functions

1. The Board
2. The Board Secretary
3. The Executive Postgraduate Committee
4. The Curriculum Committee
5. The Coordinators

II. General Rules

III. Attachments

1. Board Members
2. Executive Postgraduate Committee Members
3. Curriculum Committees
4. Coordinators
5. Postgraduate Professional Training Programme (A, B, C)
6. Curriculum of the First 3 Years.

I Organisational Structure and Functions

1. *The Board: Joint Postgraduate Medical Board.*—Responsible for the postgraduate training programme in Kuwait.

   a) *Membership:*
   The total membership shall be eight, four from the Ministry of Health, and four from the Faculty of Medicine.
   The members shall be nominated by the Dean of the Faculty of Medicine and the Undersecretary of the Ministry of Health from their respective institutions. The members so nominated shall be mutually acceptable to both parties.
   The membership shall be for a period of 2 years, but renewable.
   The Chairman of the Executive Committee shall be chosen from among the members and secretary of the Board.

   b) *Meetings:*
   The meeting of the Board shall be convened at least once a month (on the first Saturday of the month, at 6.30 p.m. in the Ministry of Public Health). Extra meetings may be held at the request of the Chairman.

c) *Voting:*

All decisions of the Board shall be reached by consensus. Where there is no consensus, decisions shall be taken by simple majority vote.

d) *Functions of the Board:*
  (i) Approving the postgraduate training programme.
  (ii) Approving the curriculum of postgraduate training programmes.
  (iii) Approving the procedures and criteria for appointment of tutors.
  (iv) Approving the appointment of tutors.
  (v) Approving the guidelines for accreditation of training posts.
  (vi) Approving the accreditation of training posts.
  (vii) Approving the regulations for admission of candidates.
  (viii) Approving the admission of candidates.
  (ix) Approving the completion of the course of a candidate and his acceptance to the next course.
  (x) Reviewing the regulations for licensing.
  (xi) Reviewing the regulations for postgraduate degrees.
  (xii) Reviewing the yearly progress report.
  (xiii) Approving the yearly budget.
  (xiv) Evaluation of the program and the people responsible for conducting the programme.

e) *Communications:*

The Board shall communicate its decisions to the Executive Body, the Undersecretary of the Ministry of Health, and the Dean of the Faculty of Medicine.

2. *Board Secretary*

He shall be the Chief Executive Officer of the Postgraduate Training Programme.

a) *Functions and responsibilities of the Board Secretary:*
  (i) The Secretary shall chair the Executive Committee, and shall remain an ex-officio member of all Subcommittees.
  (ii) He shall be responsible for keeping the records of regulations related to Postgraduate Training Programmes, i.e. he is the Head of the Training Division of the Planning Department.
  (iii) He shall keep records of all training posts, trainees and tutors involved in the training programme.
  (iv) He shall be responsible for drawing up the agends for Board meetings and for implementing the decisions.
  (v) He shall receive periodical reports from the Course Coordinators, and prepare yearly reports for submission to the Board.
  (vi) He shall prepare the yearly budget for submission to the Executive Postgraduate Committee and for approval by the Board.

3. *The Executive Postgraduate Committee.*

a) *Membership:*
  — The Head of the Training Division in the Public Health and Planning Departments—Chairman.
  — The Director of Postgraduate Training Programme of Faculty of Medicine—Vice Chairman.
  — Coordinators of Courses—Members.

b) *Meetings:*

The Executive Postgraduate Committee will meet twice every month (on the 2nd and 4th Saturdays of the month at 6.30 p.m. in the Ministry of Public Health).

c) *Functions and Responsibilities:*

 (i) Reviewing and recommending the postgraduate training programme to the Board for approval.
 (ii) Reviewing and recommending the curriculum for approval by the Board.
 (iii) Recommending admission policy.
 (iv) Recommending admissions.
 (v) Recommending entrants to a new course on satisfactory completion of the preceding course.
 (vi) Recommending procedure and criteria for appointment of tutors.
 (vii) Recommending the appointment of tutors.
 (viii) Recommending regulations for accreditation of posts.
 (ix) Recommending accreditation of posts.
 (x) Reviewing yearly reports before submission to the Board.
 (xi) Reviewing the yearly budget before submission to the Board.

4. *Curriculum Committee*

 a) *Membership*

No rules regarding membership of curriculum subcommittees have been specified to date.

 b) *Meetings*

The Curriculum Subcommittees shall meet as often as necessary to develop and revise curriculum for their respective training programmes.

 c) *Functions and Responsibilities of the Curriculum Committee*

Developing and revising curriculum for their respective training programmes as requested by the Board.

5. *Coordinators:*

The coordinators supervise the implementation of the training programme approved by the Board and their departments.

 a) *Functions and Responsibilities of Coordinators:*

 (i) Preparing the timetable, allocating teaching responsibilities and making other essential arrangements to effectively implement the programme.
 (ii) Meeting with the tutors on a regular basis to evaluate the progress of the programme.
 (iii) Meeting with the residents to obtain their evaluation of the programme.
 (iv) Conducting an evaluation of the tutors.
 (v) Guiding the Residents in the selection of their courses and career.
 (vi) Preparing and submitting assessment reports at the end of each course.
 (vii) Preparing the budget for his course.
 (viii) Keeping the Hospital Director informed of the training programme and notifying him in advance of any changes which may encroach upon the hospital services.

II. General Rules

(Applicable to doctors working in the Ministry of Public Health in relation to the postgraduate training programme.)

(i) The newly qualified medical graduates who apply to work in the Ministry of Health must undergo three years of compulsory professional training.

(ii) The newly qualified graduates are advised not to do the Imtiaz as this in most circumstances will not be recognised.

(iii) The Kuwaiti Graduates will have first preference for the training posts.

(iv) Non-Kuwaiti doctors will be considered if vacancies are available in the training programme.

(v) The Resident after his appointment in the Ministry of Health should consult the Head of the Training Division, who will allocate to him the training rota.

(vi) New doctors will be given provisional registration. Full registration can be granted after satisfactory completion of three years' training.

(vii) No doctor will be allowed to go abroad for clinical training on scholarship either from the Ministry of Health or from the Faculty of Medicine unless he is fully registered.

(viii) After satisfactory completion of two years of general professional training the candidate is eligible for promotion to Assistant Registrar status.

(ix) On achieving full registration, the candidate is eligible for a junior registrar post.

(x) A candidate who satisfactorily completes the three year professional training programme will be eligible for the Part I Doctor of Medicine (D.M.) examination conducted by the Faculty of Medicine.

(xi) During the first and second year, the trainees will work as Residents. During the third year they will work as Asst. Registrars in the Dept. of the Speciality selected by the candidates and accepted by the Board.

(xii) After the 3rd year, Asst. Registrars can proceed to their speciality and can sit for the Part II examination in the Faculty of Medicine according to the arrangements made by the Faculty of Medicine, who will grant them the Diplomas. Scholarships may be granted to some of the trainees (if arrangements are not made) but all arrangements for sending them abroad should be done by the Board and the Ministry of Public Health.

Note: The Ministry of Public Health should inform the Board of the job description of the Residents and Asst. Registrars according to the system of the Ministry of Public Health.

III. Attachments

1. *Board Members:*
As per the attached Ministerial Order No. 293/76 dated Nov. 3, 1976, the Postgraduate Medical Board consists of:

Dr. Na'il Al Naqeeb	Chairman
Dr. Nouri Al Kazemi	Member
Dr. Abdullah Rasheed	Member
Dr. W. N. Adams Smith	Member
Dr. Hassan Hathout	Member
Dr. Ismail Sallam	Member
Dr. Abdul Razzak Al Yousof	Member
Dr. Tahsin Muallah	Secretary

2. *Executive Postgraduate Committee* (formed by decision of the Joint Postgraduate Medical Board):

Dr. Nouri Al Kazemi	Acting Chairman
Dr. Abdul Razzak Al Yousof	Vice Chairman

Dr. Hassan Al Awady   Member
Dr. Abdullah Rasheed   Member
Dr. Eddie Burke   Member
Dr. Hassan Hathout   Member
Dr. Joseph K. Cherian   Member
Dr. Hussein Darwish   Member

3. *Curriculum Committee* (formed by decision of the Joint Postgraduate Medical Board):

a) Medicine Sub-Committee:
Dr. Eddie Durke (Chairman)
Dr. Abdul Razzak Al Yousof
Dr. Wilson
Dr. Barakat
Dr. Basil Al Naqeeb

b) Surgery Sub-Committee:
Dr. Hassan Al Awady (Chairman)
Dr. Joseph K. Cherian
Dr. Ismail Sallam
Dr. Mahmoud Al Bader
Dr. Jacob Oomen

c) Gynaecology and Obstetrics:
(Subject to change)
Dr. Hassan Hathout (Chairman)
Dr. Ahmed Naim
Dr. A. Abuzekri
Dr. Kamal Fahmi
Dr. Samir Kamel

d) Paediatrics:
Dr. Abdullah Rasheed (Chairman)
Dr. Nilli Fernando
Dr. Hassan Abdul Majid
Dr. Devarajan

e) Psychiatry:
Dr. Hussein Darwish (Chairman)
Dr. Adel Al Damerdash
Dr. Mohamad Arif

f) Community Medicine:
Dr. Richard Kurtz (Chairman)
Dr. Pritam Singh
Prof. Bayoumi
Dr. Jaffer Izzat
Dr. Fahim Nasser

g) Dermatology:
Dr. Mohamed Mohideen Salin (Chairman)
Dr. Alexandre Rehal
Dr. Ahmed Mohamed Moosa
Dr. Ibrahim Abdul Hameed

h) Orthopaedics:
Dr. Mahmoud Kamel Al Bous (Chairman)
Dr. Mohamed Refat Hassanin
Dr. Jamaluddin Hosni
Dr. Pulbert Taft

i) Ophthalmology:
Dr. Mohamed Shareef (Chairman)

j) E.N.T.
Dr. Mohamed Hassan Safuri (Chairman)
Dr. B. C. Patel
Dr. S. D. Parekh

k) Anaesthesia: Dr. Mian Mohamed Yacoob (Chairman)
                                   Dr. Hussein Abdul Fatah Al Sayd
                                   Dr. (Mrs.) Josephine Candy

l) Radiology: Dr. Mohideen Al Tammami (Chairman)
                                   Dr. Mohamed Husammuddin Basyoum
                                   Dr. Mohamed Ahmed Radwan.

4. *Coordinators* (formed by decision of the Joint Postgraduate Medical Board):

Member/Coordinator	Department
1. Dr. Hassan Al-Awady	Surgery/Amiri
2. Dr. Joseph K. Cherian	Surgery/Sabah
3. Dr. Abdul Razzak Al Yousof	Medicine/Sabah
4. Dr. Eddie Bourke	Medicine/Amiri
5. Dr. Hassan Hathout	Gyn. and Obst./Maternity
6. Dr. Abdullah Rasheed	Paediatrics/Sabah
7. Dr. Hussein Darwish	Psychiatry
8. Dr. Richard Kurtz	Community Medicine

5. *Postgraduate Professional Training Programme*

A. General Professional Training
B. Prespeciality Training
C. Speciality Training

A. *General Professional Training:*

   a) First Year   — 6 months medicine and
                      6 months surgery.
   b) Second Year — 3 months Gynaecology and Obstetrics
                      3 months Paediatrics
                      2 months Psychiatry
                      3 months Community Medicine.

B. *Prespeciality Training:*

Third year program (as for each specialisation)

	6 months	6 months
1. Medicine		
a) General	General	General
b) Cardiology	General	General
c) Nephrology	General	General
d) Neurology	General	General
e) Gastroenterology	General	General
f) Chest	General	General
g) Endocrinology	General	General
h) Haematology	General	General
i) Psychiatry	General	Psychiatry
j) Dermatology	General, or Fever or Paediatrics	Psychiatry Dermatology

	6 months	6 months
2. *Surgery*		
a) General	General	General
b) Neurosurgery	General	General
c) Cardiovascular	General	General
d) Plastic	General	General
e) Urology	General	General
f) Orthopaedics	General	Orthopaedics
g) E.N.T.	General	E.N.T.
h) Ophthalmology	General	Ophthalmology
3. *Paediatrics*	Paediatrics	Paediatrics
4. *Gynaecology and Obstetrics*	Gynaecology and Obstetrics	Gynaecology and Obstetrics
5. *Public Health*	(Fever Hospital)	Public Health
6. *Radiology*	Medicine	Radiology
7. *Anaesthesia*	Medicine or Paediatrics	Anaesthesiology
8. *Basic Sciences*	Basic Sciences	Basic Sciences

C. *Speciality Training:*

6. *Curriculum of the First 3 Years:*
   a) First Year   — Medicine and Surgery
                      (Enclosure 1)
   b) Second Year — Gynaecology and Obstetrics
                      Paediatrics
                      Psychiatry and
                      Community Medicine
                      (Enclosure 2)
   c) *Third Year*   — (being compiled)

Teaching and Learning Processes

Teaching is one of the most difficult and most important factors in which mankind is involved. Teaching is a necessity of modern society. A great deal of knowledge is necessary for a contemporary human being to fulfil the requirements of his everyday life, as well as very sophisticated professions which require extensive study.

The teaching of medicine on all levels of education should be considered as a science, because the human body is a biological science machine, and medicine is the biological science.

Learning is the natural obligation of everybody who wants to fulfil his duties as a member of society, or of a specified profession.

In different professions, the process of teaching and of learning is composed of professional training and educational instructions explaining how the professional and social duties should be performed. It is not to be underestimated that this problem plays a special role in the education of doctors, which requires the roots of responsibility to develop flowers of good ability of practicing medicine. It is not proper to give credit to physicians who attend many seminars but in actual professional performance ignore most of what they know. It is to be realised that postgraduate medical education helps the doctor and serves the patients.

Most traditional, almost atavistic, learning is done by imitation. This factor still plays a very important role in the education of doctors. This is one of the reasons why in teaching hospitals all teachers should be very carefully chosen. Their behaviour, their philosophy and their attitudes will subsequently be imitated by doctor-students. But in postgraduate medical education formal teaching is necessary. This teaching requires a proper balance between practical training and formal teaching. It is why the teaching hospital for postgraduate education should be staffed with properly trained educators, who usually are members of the faculty of medicine or postgraduate medical institutes. Too often, teaching hospitals twist the principle that the focus and first priority of medical education is the patient, toward manual execution and the use of technological procedures.

Well-presented and inspiring lectures may stimulate the doctor-students' enthusiasm and thinking. In the Universities of Central Europe the art of teaching (Latin, *"ars legendi"*) was and still is developing and controlling. The right of teaching (Latin, *"venia legendi"*), may be received from the University after a certain period of work and studies and after presenting to the Faculty of Medicine meetings, a lecture on the theme described by the members of the Faculty. After the lecture of the candidate the members of the Faculty discuss the way and the level of the lecture given and its teaching purposes and during secret voting they decide whether the lecture is satisfactory or unsatisfactory. In case of a positive judgement by members of the Faculty, the candidate receives the title of *"docent"* which means that he is legally and academically eligible to be university teacher. In those universities professors could be chosen only from those persons who have this academic title. This old academic tradition has its deep and sound justification.

From my experience, a number of hedonistically acculturated young doctors usually request that the educational process be made easier and less demanding. By approving such requests, the educators take a big responsibility towards the medical profession and patients. We could change the attitude of these doctors if we conduct the training in such a way that they have input into their own education.

Good teaching involves more than just clear exposition of points. The true measure of teaching is the whole effect it has on the learner. Therefore one has to take account of the interest, attitude and motivation aroused by one's teaching. All learning is to some purpose. The teacher's task is to identify the learner's purpose and to harness the interest inherent in that purpose by presenting his teaching appropriately. The question of securing the proper motivation of students is obviously important in postgraduate teaching.

Teaching and learning possess the same purpose, that of acquiring knowledge. A reason for teaching by lecture is given as evidence that owing to their immaturity young students of medicine learn more readily by listening to lectures than by reading. But the real purpose of teaching by lecture is the possibility of presenting immediate explanations if necessary. In postgraduate teaching the traditional lecture is seldom necessary and in clinical subjects it should rather be considered as an initiation of discussion and interpretation. When basic teaching is given by lecture it is to give doctor-students a framework for their reading and guidance on what to read, or to provide them with information or to show them a point of view which for whatever reason is not available in a suitable form in the literature.

The art of teaching requires study and a psychological predisposition. So far as lecturing is concerned some basic principles should be know and applied. The following generally accepted *principles of lecturing* are recommended.

The lecturer has to select a set of aims or objectives towards which his teaching is directed, and has to select a set of methods or techniques which will enable him to achieve these objectives.

Clearly these two aspects of the teacher's function are closely related. The kind of aims selected will determine the methods used and the effectiveness of any method will be determined by the extent to which it achieves the desired aims. In considering postgraduate teaching methods therefore, it is essential to establish in the first place what we are seeking to achieve.

While emphasizing that there is no betrayal of values when institutions of postgraduate education teach what will be of some practical use, we must postulate that what is taught should promote the general powers of the mind. Similarly, it is not the latest developments in a corpus of knowledge that are the most valuable. It is the development of a mind and its training in method and attack that are important.

Teaching requires systematic programming for each branch of science and the use of simplified classifications. To achieve synthesis, which is the highest level of learning, it is necessary first to carry out careful analysis. The ability to analyse facts and synthesise the results is one of the basic objectives of teaching as well as of learning during the period of basic studies. Whereas the student can develop his analytical faculties to a high degree of perfection, he will probably commit many errors in synthesis because of the lack of acquaintance with all the facts, and insufficient experience.

These statements suggest that it is the purpose of a university education to develop certain habits of mind and thought, and that factual information should be taught in such a way that it does not lie inert but is synthesised and made part of a doctor-student's mental attitudes.

The discussion class must be considered in the light of these aims. The distinguishing feature of the discussion class—the term includes the one-to-one tutorial, the group tutorial, the seminar, the practical, the clinic and the "example" class—is that it demands the active participation of the doctor-student. He has to make a response. In doing so he clarifies his own mind and commits himself on the issues presented, thereby reducing the danger that ideas and information learned from books and lectures will lie inert and unrelated in his mind. Through the exchanges of the discussion class doctor-students are stimulated to think, made aware of vagueness and inconsistencies in their own thinking and forced to commit themselves to that particular position on an issue which appraisal of the evidence and logical analysis justify. The chairman's role in such a class is not to announce the truth but to guide the doctor-students so that they reach it by their own efforts. The discussion class is a learning situation.

Discussion will not proceed freely until the various individuals become a group. It is the chairman's responsibility to create an atmosphere in which doctor-students will feel free to discuss. For many the occasion of the discussion class is an uncomfortable one: it thrusts a completely new role onto many of them and they need first of all to be put at ease.

If doctors of the class have been appointed to lead the discussion they should be advised to keep their introductory remarks as brief as possible. Their purpose is to raise a number of questions the answers to which should emerge during the discussion. Care has to be taken that the discussion does not become an extended dialogue between the two introductory speakers. The chairman should direct his questioning towards other members of the group so that everyone contributes. If the problem has been circulated in advance there is no need for any introductory remarks, not even by the chairman. He should direct attention at once to the problem—the case history, the experimental technique, or the passage for translation. It is this type of discussion that needs to be carefully structured. The chairman should have prepared a number of questions designed to lead the class into the problem. A question can be addressed to the class as a whole and if there is no response it can be rephrased and addressed to a specific member of the class. The response given is then made the basis for the next piece of interaction: either another member takes up the running or another is invited to do so by the chairman.

As has been mentioned already the personality of a lecturer and his style of lecturing means very much for the success of teaching. Roughly we may distinguish the formal and informal style of *lecturing*.

Formal: systematic orderly presentation, precise instructions to the class, teacher-controlled instruction. Informal, or "warm climate": use doctor-students' names, invite questions and discussion, extemporise, larger ratio of illustrative material to precise notes.

Formal lecturing satisfies intellectual needs; informal lecturing satisfies emotional needs. The blending of style of approach, size of class and type of doctor-student is needed.

The teacher plays a crucial role in medical education.

Learning is a natural process of knowledge acquisition. There is constant confusion about both the physician-learners and educational principles involved. The overwhelming majority of physicians have continued to learn in many ways—by reading journals, by attending educational meetings, by the collegial and consultative process, and by participating in formal programmes of continuing education. By reading journals and seeking all forms of consultation the physician is more prompt to translate his knowledge into action than by attending passively organised courses.

Learning is more efficient when there is a knowledge of results. That is why during postgraduate medical education different kinds of assessments should be conducted and discussed. The sense of achievement stimulates learning and serves professional well-being. In terms of the physician-learners, or audience, one may be talking about the medical profession at large, the medical profession arranged along disciplinary boundaries or the individual practitioner himself.

Most of a doctor's learning during postgraduate medical education takes place outside the lecture-room or the discussion class. Learning by doing and learning by reading are the most important way of getting professional skill and professional knowledge. This should be done under the general guidance of teachers of postgraduate education.

The doctor-student also learns a lot in the course of informal discussions with his fellow doctor-students. Sometimes this is the most valuable part of his study experience. For the above-mentioned reason organised postgraduate medical education in the form of courses, etc. is useful and proves to be important.

Clinical competence represents a synthesis of the physician's medical knowledge, his ability to collect data, his clinical judgement and his attitudes.

Continuous learning by practising doctors is then the necessity. To fulfil the requirements of modern life this fact has to be observed. For years, many in the profession have questioned the assumption that once qualified the physician will always be qualified. We all agree now that quality control of the physician's competence should be required as long as he practices medicine. It should be recognised that standards set for licensing are only minimal standards and that these are presently based mainly on the physician's factual knowledge. The issue should not be one of pure knowledge but one of performance—the latter may have little relationship to the former.

From the perspective of the competent physician, certification programs are insignificant. From the point of view of public interest in the quality of care or control of the incompetent physician, certification programs are inadequate. It should be demonstrated that the care of patients is as good as possible.

The aim of postgraduate medical education is to ensure that the right number of personnel with the right skills are provided at the right time and place for the delivery of national health care services.

L. W. Edima developed from his experience eight basic principles of medical education (L. W. Edima—Medical School Education, The New England Journal of Medicine, 1980, Vol. 303, No. 13, p. 72):

1. The focus and first priority of medical-school education is the patient.
2. The profession of medicine is a science, humanely conducted.
3. Learning is a thinking, problem-solving process that requires time.
4. Medical education is a continuum, binding college education, medical-school education and postgraduate education into a unifield whole.
5. Learning medicine requires a proper balance between apprenticeship (practical) training and formal teaching in lectures and seminars.
6. Education requires evaluation procedures that correctly assess progress and competence.
7. Medical-School education requires adherence to a standard of excellence.
8. The profession of medicine demands at all levels the highest ethical conduct.

These principles should be generally accepted and implemented.

Dr. Edward Ruzyllo

Methodology of Self-Education of Doctors

It is a truism today to state that medical studies are whole life studies. Constant progress of science, ever increasing requirements on the part of society, intensive development of the problem of prophylaxis and rehabilitation, ever growing necessity of the doctor's committal to resolving environmental and social problems, increase considerably the framework of former conceptions of medicine.

Conditions in which all matters concerning the disease were resolved between two people, doctor and patient, belong to the past. Today the doctor is only an important element in the complex organisational structure of the process of medical care, within which framework he must learn to work. It means that a contemporary doctor must know and understand all scientific, social and organisational elements comprising the system of prophylaxis, treatment and rehabilitation of the patient.

In order to perform these tasks, doctors—according to the honourable tradition of their profession—constantly supplement and enlarge their knowledge. In view, however, of the extent of the problem and today's great involvement of every doctor in his professional work, there must be a system which would ensure the best conditions without so many time-consuming commitments. The character of the work of every doctor, his personal qualities and environmental conditions may essentially influence his method of self-education. In view of this, no one method binding for all doctors can be accepted. It seems, however, that it is advisable to discuss certain basic problems and principles of procedure as regards these conceptions.

I believe there exist three basic conditions necessary for correctly conducted education:

1. understanding the need of education—aim,
2. finding the right way of learning—method,
3. fixing time and place for learning—organisation.

Understanding of these basic conditions and appropriate attitudes to them characterises particular periods of study, through which modern man must pass.

In *primary school* the degree of conscious commitment of the pupil in these problems is minimal. There is no understanding of the need of learning. This takes shape very gradually, mainly as a result of the educational influence of home and school. It may be assumed that in this period enforced learning predominates without an understanding of its necessity.

The method of learning in the primary school is imitation. A child learns this method under the teacher's direction. Having no experiences of his own in this respect, he learns those that are shown to him. The organisation of the process of learning in the primary school is traditionally established and the pupil has no conscious part in it.

In the *secondary school* there is a marked increase of the degree of committal of the pupil both as to understanding of the purpose of learning and his conscious participation in grasping the method and organisation of education. Imagination of his own future professional work is taking shape, and consequently a personal interest in particular subjects he is learning. The understanding of the necessity of learning in this group of children is not general and not equally developed in all of them. As regards the whole group it may be assumed that this understanding is not general and mature and that compulsion of learning still plays a considerable role in this period of education.

As to methods of learning, a pupil of the secondary school is usually more committed. He has already had some experience and consequently either isolates himself for the purpose of learning or learns collectively. He learns, reading aloud or speaking, making notes, statements or imaginary drawings. Dependent on his ability of concentration, and type of visual and auditory memory, each pupil begins to develop his own method of learning.

The organisation of study in a pupil of secondary school is more conscious. The leading role in this respect is, however, played by school and home. An organised system of school occupations, constant instruction as to when and under what conditions he must study, help him in his efforts. There is a small percentage of school children who, in this respect, have their own full insight, who know and are able to organise their own study. This, of course, mainly concerns the youth of the older groups.

In the *higher school* (university, academy) there is an essential change in methods of learning. Mental maturity at the time of leaving secondary school and the necessity of making a decision as to the choice of profession, force the youth to consider all problems connected with the process of learning. Deciding to take up higher studies, the real purpose of learning is to him quite obvious. It is shaped out of the liking of the chosen subject and the will to attain a suitable position—professional and social—and an understanding of the material base of his future life. In this group of learners the purpose of study is on the whole finally understood and generally acknowledged.

The method of study in a higher school is the evolution of methods applied in secondary school. A student develops his memory and visual ability of learning. He independently organises his studies, being committed in varying degrees to the general organisational system of study. On his enterprise and organisational ability depends getting hold, at the right time, of scrips, notes and textbooks, and accurate calculation and correct utilisation of time necessary to studying particular subjects or their sections. A student already begins to have social commitments. Time for this should be so calculated as not to interfere with the process of learning. This equally concerns sports and other forms of pastime, often already professional.

A higher school student must fully understand the purpose of learning and acquire the ability to organise his studies. Full maturity in this respect has a great social importance, as it gives an insight into the manner and level of his future professional work.

These so different three periods of learning have one common trait, namely that each of them is a definite stage of learning. The completing of primary, secondary or higher school learning is terminated with getting a certificate, maturity certificate or diploma. Dependent on further decisions, the formal duty of learning ends at a definite stage.

A doctor (by analogy it concerns all health service workers with higher education) beginning his professional work is to a large extent committed to matters connected with the organisation of the new period of his life. To these belong living conditions, family involvements and problems of adaptation to his new professional environment. This period is often too long and has a negative influence on his further professional development. In the first period of independent professional work he doubtless realises more and more the tasks and difficulties facing him. Confrontation of his own abilities with professional requirements is a strong and constant stimulus to further learning. The purpose of study in this situation is most understandable.

The full recognition of the necessity of further learning is hindered by the above mentioned familiy and other involvements. No less part is also played by mental attitude, strengthened by the tradition that having obtained the diploma, there is no necessity for a doctor to continue his studies. Often a subconscious wish to free himself from the obligation of learning hinders a beginning doctor from systematic activity in this respect.

For every doctor there is a certain period of time from the moment of receiving his diploma to the moment of starting self-education. This period differs very much in time. It is a very important period in professional life, a period which often influences professional position and even the future fate of a doctor. If during studies, he appreciates the weight and importance of sound knowledge, if the degree of his sense of professional responsibility and prestige are considerable, then the period is short. It is, however, often long and even too long.

There are many factors that may shorten this period. Among the basic factors may be counted:

— the necessity of constantly working on the consciousness of the student in a higher school, that receiving a diploma does not mean the end of studies,
— organisation of postgraduate studies,
— characteristic traits of every doctor.

The first two factors are socially regulated, but social influencing of the third factor is only indirect and on the whole very slight.

A doctor's professional work is full of problems carrying responsibility. Medical sciences are so extensive, that every doctor has some gaps in this respect. In view of this there is a constant stimulus resulting from everyday professional work, to supplement his knowledge. Non-professional life problems of a doctor and man's innate indolence are the hindering agents. Only appropriate traits of character may outweigh the decision of a doctor to pursue consistent self-education. Often some professional experience, some failure, or sometimes a success brings about such a decision.

A doctor's self-education often hinders his professional success which results from the right approach to patients and skillful application of diagnostic and therapeutic means. If a doctor's work becomes routine, it is a grave obstacle to his education. He then loses the conviction that there is a need to supplement his knowledge, and develops the ability of finding ways and means of avoiding a possible responsibility. This professional selfconfidence is sometimes broken by a major mishap, which brings to mind the value of medical action on a scientific basis.

In this way, generally speaking, there is developing in doctors the understanding of the purpose of professional self-education. There is not and cannot be a uniform method of doctors' self-education, for it depends on many factors, often individual.

Generally speaking most *methods of doctors' self-education* may be divided into individual and collective. The individual methods include: 1. use of medical books and periodicals and 2. treating each patient as a source for medical considerations and as a stimulus to immediate studies of his pathological problems.

Collective methods of postgraduate education include:

— active participation in the doctor's own professional environment (medical societies, in-service hospital training etc.) and
— participation in organised continuing postgraduate education.

The *medical textbook* is and will probably ever remain the basic method of self-learning. Its role is different in pregraduate and postgraduate studies. In postgraduate studies a book is not a source of new information, but should be treated as a base of acquired information and as a pointer in searching and resolving definite problems. To fulfil these conditions every doctor should have his "own" book constantly at hand. The choice of such a basic book is very important for every doctor. Once the book has been chosen it should serve the doctor a long time not only with its contents, but also with its system. Such a doctor's "own" book should constantly be supplemented with notes, remarks and references to other sources of literature. It is most important for a doctor to search for a problem—freely and widely. For beginning in this way he will always find the required details. It seems also that the doctor's "basic" textbook should above all serve as a direction indicator. A doctor's "basic" book should be supplemented with his remarks and notes. The form of these notes may be varied. The best perhaps will be that which would refer the problem he is studying to some new good literature. A doctor should constantly consult his "basic" book. This habit plays a very important part in the methodology of self-education. The book handled in this way and supplemented with notes becomes, as it were, a map of his "medical territory", helping him to move on it freely. Whereas the book plays the role of an extensive thematic base in which its entire system is most important, the role of medical periodicals is quite different.

Medical journals deal with current scientific and casuistic problems. They constantly supplement and enlarge textbooks and medical monographs. Periodicals are therefore, for a doctor, a new source of information not contained in textbooks and monographs. They constitute together the whole body of accurate and up-to-date scientific information. In view of this, the learning doctor must read medical periodicals. Nobody today is able to read all medical journals. Therefore every doctor should systematically, dependent on his needs and possibilities, read selected periodicals. It is imperative that every *doctor should constantly read at least one medical periodical.*

Reading medical periodicals suggests to the doctor medical problems, correct diagnosis and correct treatment of his own patients; finally they bring confirmation of his diagnostic and therapeutic decisions. In this way they may bring satisfaction and ensure that the medical procedure is correct. Reading descriptions of medical problems in medical periodicals establishes contact with other medical centres or units. It also creates the possibility of a direct contact, if that is necessary, for explanation of a given problem. Finally, reading periodicals gives a sense of belonging to the profession and permits finding out where certain important problems are being dealt with in this country.

In order to benefit freely and accurately from scientific sources every doctor should have his *own medical library*. Books should be bought for this library only after they have been well looked over and found suitable for the individual needs of a doctor.

A doctor should regularly (once a week or once a month) visit the nearest medical library in order to get acquainted with and study books, monographs and periodicals. He should go to the library with his "basic" book and his own notebook. Studies in the library should add to the notes in the "basic" book and should be appropriately registered in the doctor's accepted system of general note-making. This second problem may be the subject of a separate detailed consideration.

Studies in the library give the possibility of a wide orientation in various problems and so bring the doctor up to the right level, enabling him to follow the progress of medicine. They will not, however, create the conditions provided by a doctor's own library at home. Books and periodicals available at home consolidate his required knowledge. Human memory is fallible and requires constant exercise and consequently, constant refreshing of the acquired knowledge. It is necessary to remember or check things out in daily work. The possibility of consulting scientific sources immediately often conditions successful activity.

However, the most important *doctor's own book is every patient*. A patient who is the subject of a doctor's activity is the most natural source of scientific problems. Studying a disease of particular patients means searching in books and periodicals for explanations of its causes and the mechanism of its course. A doctor should find as clearly as possible, the picture of the disease of the studied patient in literature sources. The quicker he finds it and the clearer he sees it, the greater is the certainty of correct diagnosis and treatment. A patient is a much richer source of medical problems than the most exhaustive monograph. Finding the patient's problems in books and locating appropriate chapters of the books are the best methods of self-education. For this purpose only should serve his "own" book, periodicals, house library and public library. Only this system as a whole will shape a method fully adequate to postgraduate education.

The organisation of self-education may also be individual and collective. *The first* depends on the personal qualities of a doctor, conditions of his life, and above all on the satisfactory organisation of his work, rest and non-professional duties. In all circumstances, however, he must find time and place for self-education. Not necessarily much time will be needed for that. Much more important is systematic activity in this respect and the forming of a habit of reading books and medical periodicals. If 15 minutes daily can be found for it, that is the indispensable minimum. This time can be found after a meal, before going to bed etc. Many doctors do it while travelling in a train, bus etc. In addition to this suggestion or parallel to it, a doctor should find for this purpose several hours on any day of the week. This day should be so organised that full benefit from the hours of study can be obtained. It seems that it would be best to so organise professional work as to be able to find a few hours on a fixed day of the week. Generally speaking, the organisation of individual self-education is mainly based on forming a habit of reading professional information.

Organisation of *collective education* depends above all on the activity of the medical environment, but also to a large degree, on the doctor himself. Sessions of specialist medical societies, conferences organised by local hospitals and postgraduate medical collective conferences are the organised forms of this education. However, individual benefit drawn from these forms will only be full when a doctor takes an active part in these meetings. The activity means that he should be prepared to take part in discussions on the one hand, and on the other to study at home, problems discussed at these meetings.

The organisation of collective local and institutional studies may be the subject of a separate paper. Postgraduate studies of doctors and other health service workers with higher education are conducted throughout the world, and this country also has its own achievements in this field. The professional effect, however, of these studies depends on the work of every doctor. Responsibility is too great for the studies to be abandoned, and science is too extensive to devote to its study only a certain period of a doctor's life.

Dr. Edward Ruzyllo

The Importance of Subjective Examinations in the Diagnosis of Disease

We are in a period in which technical advances and achievements are amazing not only to laymen but also to professionals. In medicine, which is a humanistic science, this fact has special importance. From one side some doctors prepare to be narrow specialists, using sophisticated diagnostic methods and instruments; from the other side the patients are amazed by the technical advances and expect more from heavily armed doctors, appreciating less doctors with a humanistic approach.

The medical examination is a very intimate connection between doctor and patients bringing them closer together.

The well-established clinical method of approaching patients is composed of two parts:

— history taking examination—*subjective examination* and
— physical findings—*objective examination* which includes laboratory methods and other tests used in the modern process of diagnostics.

The first part of the clinical examination is very humanistic and brings doctor and patient closer to each other, giving them possibilities of gaining confidence and esteem. This subjective examination is an integral part of a medical examination, its most traditional form and permanent element of our daily professional activity.

It is doubtless quite obvious that the subjective examination, talk with the patient, careful and thoughtful analysis of his complaints constitute a basic and important element of medical procedure.

At the beginning of the development of medicine including the period of the Middle Ages, the subjective examination was the main method of medical investigation, and for many centuries diagnosis was based on this method. The importance of the subjective examination was somewhat devaluated in the period of the Renaissance when the patient was stripped at last and the method of physical examination introduced. Today, in the period of Technical Development, subjective examination has not lost its value and is still an important and basic part of a medical examination. Physical and biochemical examinations are not sufficient if they are not accompanied by medical thought which strives to find the cause of illness and connects into a logical whole the syndrome of pathological symptoms. Subjective symptoms disconnected logically from the thinking process of a doctor will be valueless, and may even be the source of diagnostic errors.

Subjective examination is important mainly because it helps to direct the course of procedure in the diagnostic process, revealing, moreover, early symptoms of the disease and supplying much information concerning pathological states caused by functional disorders. In these two aspects the subjective examination not only has not lost its importance, but continues to gain it. Today when we have very well developed general pathology and clinical physiology, we understand better certain subjective symptoms, and can better and faster draw diagnostic conclusions from the subjective examination. The achievements in the sphere of technical sciences also emphasize the importance of subjective examinations, not confining or narrowing this method. A headache, a typical symptom of a subjective nature may have different interpretations. If we approach this symptom methodically and begin to analyse the causes and circumstances of its incidence, we shall find that a headache may be the symptom of many serious disorders, which in objective examinations are difficult to detect. Therefore a subjective symptom is often a leading symptom in the diagnostic process. The diagnosis of the disease and its treatment is based on the cooperation of doctor and patient; it cannot be realised by the doctor alone or by the patient himself. If there is no such cooperation, there can be no speaking about the effects and results of treatment. On the doctor's part, is needed above all a consistent striving to explain every pathological symptom, the sequence of phenomena, time of their incidence and intensification in relation to time of day, year, rest etc.

Systematic examination is of basic importance. In order to quickly and correctly conduct a subjective examination, a doctor must have the ability to analyse and synthesise the observed phenomena. The ability of analysing phenomena and drawing correct conclusions is one of the basic qualities of a doctor and one of his most important needs. A doctor—in my estimation—learns these things by the craftsman's method of imitating the master. We are not always sufficiently prepared in this respect. A doctor, if he is responsible and ambitious, striving to achieve good results in his work, and therefore prompt and correct diagnosis, systematically supplements his knowledge in this sphere. Doctors mainly develop their abilities of medical thinking, learning on their errors and also observing other doctors whose example in medical procedure they attempt to follow.

Subjective examination is the foundation of the whole construction on which the diagnosis of the disease is based. If subjective examination is superficial and not fully valuable, any further detailed and often time consuming examination will not contribute to the strengthening of the diagnostic construction and will not come up to expectations, with a loss to the patient and to the detriment of the activity of the doctor.

The problem of subjective examinations is particularly important in the work of out-patients clinics. It constitutes 80% of our professional work. We do not always realise its importance. In the social scale it is most important both in its qualitative and quantitative aspect. In his work in out-patient units a doctor has very little time, limited possibilities of objective examination or conducting additional tests; this forces him to rely mainly on the results of subjective examinations. In order to conduct correctly subjective examinations, a doctor must apply a suitable method of examination, think logically, draw correct conclusions, know symptomatology of the observed phenomena, and have a good professional memory. Without these qualities a doctor will not be able to benefit fully from the possibilities provided by subjective examinations. During pregraduate studies much time is devoted to subjective examination in medical diagnostics. Unfortunately, not all colleagues realise then the importance of subjective examination; fascinated by great technical achievements they often think lightly of this part of medical examinations. In the majority of cases, however, they supplement these shortcomings later. A doctor cannot fully benefit from subjective examination if he does not know symptomatology, if the symptoms have no meaning for him, if a given symptom does not bring to mind any physical organ. Its peculiarity and its psychological outline play a direct part, and may be a manifestation on the part of various organs. No possibility can be overlooked in correctly analysing its importance.

Professional memory must be trained. It is important to train such professional memory, which records not only name, appearance, or other purely physical features of man, but also pathological traits observed in him. Without professional memory, without reaching back to his own experiences, to well known cases, which by analogy may facilitate drawing of correct and right conclusions, subjective examination will not be fully utilised.

Subjective examination would not be complete, if we confined ourselves to symptomatology alone and did not think about man as a whole, about his biological outline, his meaning in the environment, the values he represents. The cognisance of biological conditions is essential in the methodology of medical procedure. Man cannot be understood only in his physical aspect; his personality, his psychological outline, plays a very important part not only in purely organic complaints, but also in the occurrence of functional disorders. The patient's manner of representing or way of describing his complaints, may lead the doctor who lacks the ability of psychological evaluation to draw erroneous conclusions, diagnosing pathological conditions non-existent in this patient. The doctor must know how to evaluate the psychological outline of the patient, because only then will he estimate correctly, complaints described by him. Social conditions of the patient, his family environment, his work conditions and his place in society are essential components of the problem.

The treatment of the patient may be another example of subjective doctor-patient relationship.

The treatment is a function which arises between the physician and the patient. The treatment is established by the physician, but is carried out by the patient himself. A proper report by the patient on the courses of his treatment and on its results gives the physician a chance to modify and properly improve the treatment. It is the very character of the diseases met with nowadays, that increases the role of the patient himself in the treatment process.

Such a situation explains why both the physician and the patient must be trained for such an often difficult collaboration. The physician must be very intelligent, perfectly acquainted with various conditions of life and with various types of people. He should be able rightly to evaluate the information given him by the patient, and must find a proper manner of speaking with him, depending on his mental development and the individual features of his character. Finally, the physician must know how to speak logically and convincingly. All this is the reason why a modern physician should develop his knowledge and abilities in philosophy (logic), psychology and sociology.

On the other hand, the patient should be better prepared to understand the problems of health and disease. And just as the notion that everybody should be something of a technician has become generally accepted, so it is also necessary to teach everybody about the notions and principles of physiology, pathology and hygiene. Without improvement of the education of the population in this respect, we shall not be able to overcome the development of degenerative diseases.

The influence of environment on the occurrence of illness and its course plays an ever increasing pathogenetic role. To the foreground come problems of a psychic and a neurotic nature. In each subjective examination the patient should describe what he feels frankly, directly and coherently. In practice it is often otherwise.

The doctor should correctly estimate each patient. The estimation may not be to the detriment of the patient nor to the detriment of the diagnosis. This depends on the doctor, on his experience and training. The nervous endurance of the doctor, his self-control and right attitude in examining the patient, patience in listening to his complaints and gaining his confidence are absolute conditions of the subjective examination. It is a fact that one of the difficulties we are faced with in subjective examinations, is the low intellectual level of the patient and his psychic disposition unfavourable to establishing the right contact.

There are many types of patients. There are those who know everything, are expert in many spheres and speak authoritatively. To get out of them some important details is very difficult, they willingly generalise, they often make their own diagnosis. The attempt of the doctor to correct this diagnosis meets with discontent and results in their refusal to answer questions so that their complaints cannot be accurately assessed. Applying suitable tactics we must bring these people to give a simple description of each symptom. Another type of patients are those intellectually deficient, who cannot describe their complaints. When examining uneducated and unintelligent people we must use very simple questions and try to understand the meaning of words used by them and to find out all we can about their complaints.

It appears therefore that a doctor should have much wisdom, ability and tact in order to make subjective examination effective as a diagnostic help and its results to form a real foundation on which the construction of the final diagnosis can be based. For that it requires not only professional skill. Medicine is a vocational profession and doctors motivated by a proper understanding of their activities have to develop more friendly and more direct approaches to the patient, in this way gaining his confidence, friendliness and esteem. In such an atmosphere the patient talks about himself freely and fully and the doctor may gain all necessary explanations and conditions which may be linked with the symptoms of the disease. Doctors have to see the patient in his environment and his condition of life which will allow him to understand much of the problem which may concern the patient's health complaints. Ambulatory examination, in which 90% of patients complained of functional disorders rather than organic disorders, is of special value.

A patient represents also the small community in which he is brought up and is living in. To understand these conditions gives a doctor better possibilities of getting good diagnostic results. Finally, subjective examination gives a doctor full understanding of the common symptoms and important differences between community medicine and individual medicine and in the case of family medicine gives him possibilities to introduce both approaches to his activities.

Dr. Edward Ruzyllo

Organisational Forms of Postgraduate Medical Studies

Postgraduate medical education must satisfy the requirements of the whole system of health care of the population as well as the needs of particular doctors. In view of this, postgraduate medical education must be multidirectional in substance and diverse in form.

Scientific direction and essential substance of postgraduate medical education are provided by teaching hospitals. Determination of practical aims of this education belongs to the Ministry of Public Health.

In the realisation of this task it is necessary to determine and accept certain conceptions and definitions. These conceptions and definitions should be identically understood by all concerned, and identically defined. In these circumstances all vagueness or even misunderstanding will be avoided.

Generally speaking, a certain study of postgraduate education is usually defined by the name of the course. By this name is understood a definite programme of education conducted at a definite time in a definite place.

We may distinguish the following organisational forms of postgraduate education:

1. Basic Course
2. Perfecting Course
3. Informative Course
4. Unification Course
5. Verification Course
6. Specialisation Course
7. Non-Continuous Course
8. Seminar
9. Conference
10. Correspondence Course
11. Lectures and Clinical Rounds

Please note the following short definitions or descriptions of such forms of Postgraduate Studies.

1. Basic Course

Basic courses may last from 3 months to 1 year and, dealing with certain spheres, even longer.

This is a form of education in which doctors master basic knowledge pertaining to their professional interests. As regards internal medicine one would repeat the whole of it simultaneously with medical practice. As regards surgery, the doctor gets acquainted with all basic methods of surgery preparing himself to take up or improve his professional work not only in the sphere of his narrow specialised ability.

The basic course will therefore be for some doctors as the recollection and ordering of well-know information and for others, supplementation of gaps in possessed theoretical or practical abilities. This is caused either by the character of professional work hitherto performed (lack of contact with large medical centres, limited possibilities of work), or by a doctor's inability to follow the new achievements of medical science.

The Basic Course may be organised in every medical speciality, it may also be a course which will enable doctors to acquire new abilities, for example, training for work in industrial medicine. The programme of the Basic Course should be worked out in such a way as to ensure acquaintance with the entirety of materials in a methodical and exact manner. On conclusion of the basic course a doctor should be evaluated as to his being of service in a further defined professional work.

2. Perfecting Course

This is a course of relatively short duration, for instance, a period of 1 to 6 weeks.

The aim of the course is to teach doctors definite theoretical or practical knowledge. Thus the perfecting course has as its aim the improvement of accomplishments of doctors, of a good general professional level, in chosen lines or spheres. An example of a perfecting course may be a course on: "Functional Tests in the Clinic of Internal Diseases", and in surgery, a course devoted to gastric surgery etc. A perfecting course is therefore intended for consultants of hospital wards and their counterparts in the professional hierarchy, who would like to train in a particular section of medical knowledge. It appears from the estimation of the needs of health services, that certain doctors should be educated in an appropriate section of medical science. This type of education is therefore a course which should be attended by doctors previously selected for this purpose. The programme of the perfecting course should include all the most modern achievements in this sphere.

3. Informative Course

Informative courses usually last only a short time and should not be longer than 1—4 weeks.

The course may be attended by different doctors of different specialities simultaneously, if problems of an organisational or general medical nature are the subject of the course. Informative courses may also be organised for a definite medical speciality and then the subject of the course will concern an appropriate branch of medical science. The programme of the course may be so diverse that it is difficult to put in into a framework; it may, for example, be a course for heads of district outpatient clinics, where organisational and methodological problems will be the subject. Another example may be endocrinologic, bacteriologic etc. courses for doctors with definite medical specialities, or else for doctors with various medical specialities.

4. Unification Courses

Courses of this type have as their aim the improvement of the efficiency standard of professional work of particular sections of social health service. Therefore doctors with definite professional functions are encouraged to attend these courses. Unification courses are intended for doctors of one speciality or those with various specialities. Problems important in every day professional work, with which a doctor did not get acquainted during medical studies, or did so superficially, are the subject of the course. At these courses current organisational matters of health services, principles of the functioning of its sections, technique of professional work etc. will be discussed.

Further topics of these courses are problems such as: sanatorium treatment, development of the pharmaceutical industry, medical diagnostics, a doctor's duties as an expert in court, infections in hospital, complications in treatment with antibiotics etc.

Apart from these problems, at unification courses current scientific progress will also be discussed, in the branch of medicine for representatives of which the course has been organised.

5. Verification Course

Verification courses are intended for foreign doctors, who wish to work as specialists in Kuwait. The programme of these courses ensures supplementation of knowledge and permits an estimate as to whether a doctor participating in the course fulfils the conditions permitting him to be recognised as a specialist in the country concerned.

6. Specialisation Course

Specialisation courses are either the initiation of specialisation, or are foreseen in the specialisation programme.

7. Non-Continuous Course

To enable the training of local doctors in a definite programme, the so-called non-continuous courses are organised. Such a course may be basic, informative or perfecting, with a monthly programme. This programme, however, takes place only once a week on the same day (for example Wednesday).

In this way 26 days of the training programme are realised in the course of 26 weeks. The participants of such a course do not stop their professional work, devoting to training only one day a week. They receive, however, all benefits to which participants of continuous courses are entitled (training certificates), and are equally bound by the discipline of studies, tutorials and final examinations.

8. Seminar

A seminar lasts from 1—7 days. Seminars are attended by doctors of the same or different speciality, dependent on the subject of the seminar, but on the same level of professional background. The aim of the seminar is to discuss an appropriately worked out subject in order to agree and accept common principles in the estimation of pathological phenomena and medical procedure. The seminar requires very careful preparation on the part of its organisers, and active participation on the part of attending doctors. Foreign guests may also participate in the seminar.

9. Conference

A conference is a one day meeting of an appropriate number of doctors, at which will be discussed a certain subject according to the accepted custom. The conference may bear the character of a round table conference, or the so-called panel discussion. It may also assume more traditional forms, namely, several lecturers may present aspects of a definite topic, creating an atmosphere for further discussion of participants. The conference may also be attended by foreign guests.

10. Correspondence Courses

Correspondence training is organised to provide training for doctors who cannot participate in the organised courses and who would like to continue their education in some form.

11. Lectures and Clinical Rounds

The Head of a Hospital Department organises from time to time a lecture on a definite subject. The subject of the lecture considers programmed didactic tasks of the Chair and discusses the achievements of medical science. Information concerning the lecture is inserted in the medical press, and the lecture itself should take place at such time and in such hours, as to permit the greatest number of doctors to participate. The Head of the Department leads the so-called clinical round, whose time and place are previously given in the medical press. To such clinical round come doctors interested in problems discussed on the round.

Dr. Edward Ruzyllo

The Library as a Base for Postgraduate Teaching, Learning and Self-Education

General Goals

Lifelong learning has been a trademark of the medical profession and doctors are apt to be well read on any new developments in the medical sciences. That is why the most numerous means of scientific information exist in the field of medicine and in its many fields of specialities. Medical journals and books are the most numerous publications of all other fields of sciences in the world. A library should be used by a physician in his everyday work, and medical journals should be consulted in the course of his work. Postgraduate education requires utilisation of all possible means of scientific information. Modern libraries fulfil these requirements. An efficiently functioning library is considered a basic building stone in any training institution. Its validity is greatly considered as an infrastructure in Continuing Medical Education for the sake of efficiency and the development of health services. It is essential that provision be made for the library so that books, journals and A. V. materials that will reach the hospital can be properly accommodated. It is also essential that qualified personnel are engaged for the proper maintenance of these libraries. If no proper place is provided for the library and qualified staff are not there to maintain it, it will not serve the purpose even if the books are received.

Specific Services of a Postgraduate Medical Library are:

to collect, organise, and distribute medical information to meet the needs of those working in the field of medical services in hospitals, polyclinics, various departments or educational institutes;

to cooperate with the centres of information at the national level, such as: medical faculty, research centre and medical association, and at the international level with the National Medical Library in Washington, D.C., or the offices of the W.H.O.

to organise the network of information between itself and the above-mentioned information centre, for the benefit of Kuwait and the Gulf countries;

to prepare a training programme for those working in library services in hospitals or other ministry departments in order to raise the standard of technical performance. A good dynamic cooperative system should be initiated among all libraries for dissemination of information, feedback and interchange of knowledge and inter-library loan.

Principles of Organisation

According to the decision of the Joint Board and based on the opinion of the Council of the Undersecretary of the Ministry of Public Health, a Library for post-graduate medical teaching has been formed. The main body of the library will be in the location of the Joint Board (Training Division) but it will have its branches in all teaching hospitals in Kuwait.

All branches will have union catalogues of books and journals of the whole library. So any doctor will find a list of books he can get in each hospital, and the channel of intercommunication.

The library should serve doctors and should be of assistance in their learning and studies. To achieve these objectives the following arrangements are in the process of implementation:

1. General description of the accommodation given in each teaching hospital for its library and all necessary requirements needed for library activities.
2. To examine the manpower engaged in library services in each hospital.
3. Introducing thorough instructions for each branch of the Postgraduate Medical Library so that the same principles and rules for activities will exist in all branches.

These instructions of work, instructions for readers, for borrowing or lending books and journals, control the library's system. Statistical information about the utilisation of books and journals and all other instructions will ensure that each branch of the Postgraduate Medical Library in the teaching hospital is working on a modern level and utilises modern ways of functioning. Instructions are given that the records of *all books* of the Postgraduate Library should be in the catalogue to enable doctors of each hospital library to see where particular books are and in which branch (which hospital) of the Postgraduate Medical Library they may be found.

Library Services

The library offers its services to all doctors, nursing staff, paramedicals, social workers, and others. Membership is free for all staff members working in the Ministry of Public Health after having been issued proper membership cards which allow them to join the library. Library services include reading, borrowing, photocopying medical articles and preparing specialised bibliographies in scientific subjects that concern the community or that improve the performance in medical services. The library also participates effectively in representations in local conferences to collect documents as research and to specify and index them according to scientific principles. The library will inform the researchers step by step of all that is new in their fields of specialities (current awareness).

Forms of Activities and Detailed Forms of Organisation

1. Due to the fact that health care will develop progressively with increasing technical development, it is good to have the resources of information as quickly as possible. It is considered the basic function of the library to distribute the information in the proper time, to the proper person to take the appropriate decision. This is considered as the vital function of the librarian and he must work to increase the groups and the bibliographies in order to put the library services in proper perspective.
2. The postgraduate Medical Library is responsible for collecting all resources of information internally or with hospitals or departments and to produce a system to keep all these resources.
3. All the applications for books and periodicals are to be sent to the Library for review and for presentation to the specialised committee for its approval and to be forwarded to the concerned authorities.

4. To organise a library committee in each hospital.
5. To have a proper place in each hospital or scientific organisation that belongs to the Ministry of Public Health and to have it as a branch of the above-mentioned library.
6. The branch libraries are to be under the supervision of the Training Division and the Chief Librarian shall be responsible for them.
7. The budgets of the branch libraries are to be prepared by the library committees in each hospital or each department, and all are to go to the Training Division in order to prepare a unified budget to meet all the needs.
8. Each hospital director will assign a person to collect the medical books and journals in order to secure their safe handling.
9. To have a future plan for a mobile library for patients, especially for those who have chronic diseases. Such libraries ought to be mobile to reach the patient in his bed for light reading, local newspapers and weekly magazines.
10. To issue monthly or quarterly bulletins of the contents of branch libraries and the Postgraduate Medical Library in order to facilitate the exchange of information between them.
11. No library in the world can have all the important information in all fields of specialities unless it will cooperate with other libraries on the national and the international levels.

Dr. Edward Ruzyllo

General Outline of Postgraduate Medical Education in Oncology as an Example of Forming a Teaching Program

Many causes have been foreseen which may destroy mankind, but two of them have proved to be the most important:

— inside and outside intoxications of human beings and
— degeneration in which cancer may play the most important role.

The biological and social importance of cancer degeneration gives a strong motivation to develop a proper training for under- and postgraduate medical students and also for the health education of the general population. The first approach is to fight diseases, the second to try to prevent them and to cooperate with doctors during the process of treatment.

Curriculum for medical students in undergraduate schools includes a fair amount of oncology. But a general understanding of the disease, its pathologic and clinical specificity, as well as a proper treatment of patients can only be done by doctors who are specialists in the field of oncology. So the forming of specialists during a postgraduate medical education is very important.

Those doctors who do not specialise in oncology should keep in mind basic knowledge of the pathological and clinical facts of oncology. During their continuing postgraduate medical education doctors should be aware of the advances in that field of medicine and develop an alertness towards these diseases.

Mentioning the problem of postgraduate education as a whole, we have always to realise how difficult and how complex a problem is. It requires not only a sound knowledge of the given subject of medicine, but it requires first of all a proper methodical approach to it from the teacher's side and his full emotional engagement.

So far as methodology is concerned it could be compared with methods used in scientific investigations. The same method is to be applied in fulfilling teaching requirements in postgraduate medical education (Dr. J. R. McArthur).

Scientific or clinical investigations	Educational project or programme
What is to be proved? (Define hypothesis)	What is to be learned? (Develop educational objectives)
How is it to be proved? (Design experiment)	How is it to be learned? (Design learning process)
Has it been proved? (Evaluate results)	Has it been learned? (Evaluation)

Oncology is first of all a very large and complex science, comprising many different fields of science. It is this science that specialists should first of all master to be able to deal properly with the management of patients.

The components of general science in oncology come from different branches of such sciences as biology, pathology, histopathology, cellular metabolism, cytogenetics, cell kinetics, clinical pharmacology, immunology, haematology, endocrinology, metabolism, microbiology and biochemistry which introduce us to chemotherapy. Very important parts in oncology as a science come from physics, such as nuclear medicine, radiology and radiation medicine.

One is to mention again such sciences as biostatistics, and epidemiology which are important branches in searching out and judging the evolution of diseases in the population.

Oncology includes also such sciences as psychology and sociology which are necessary for proper management of an unhappy and depressed patient, his family members and social environment.

Oncology as a science is constantly developing, giving possibilities for better understanding or for better skill in the management of cancer diseases. Mankind is fully indebted to these numerous researchers and workers in basic sciences for their stubborn efforts and achievements which allow doctors to get better results in the treatment of patients.

From the educational point of view, of course, a science such as oncology requires time for learning and effort to master it. The teaching process requires the arrangement of proper timing and constant correlation between these different parts of oncology sciences.

Oncology as a clinical speciality has to serve the patients by this complex science. But the clinical management of the patient is divided into two basic clinical specialities:

— Medical oncology and
— Surgical oncology.

Oncology as a Clinical Speciality

Medical Oncology	*Surgical Oncology*
Internal Medicine	Surgery
Radiotherapy	E.N.T.
Chemotherapy	Ophthalmology
Clinical Pharmacology	Gynaecology
Hormone Therapy	Diagnostic Radiology
Nuclear Medicine	Natural History of Cancer
Diagnostic Radiology	Medical Treatment (indications for,
National History of Cancer	results of)
Paediatrics	Rehabilitation
Dermatology	
Gynaecology	
Surgical Treatment (indications for, results of)	
Rehabilitation	

The specialist in medical oncology has to first of all be fully trained in internal medicine and radiotherapy, then specialise in surgical oncology in surgery. Any specialists in clinical oncology should also fully be aware of the possibilities of the other oncologic specialities, namely surgical oncology and medical oncology.

Medical oncology as a speciality requires proper management from a non-surgical point of view and should cover also the requirements given to such clinical oncology as pediatrics, dermatology, gynaecology and others. On these bases of clinical oncology the doctor specialising in medical oncology should master also such problems as chemotherapy, hormone therapy, oncological pharmacology, and all forms of nuclear medicine and diagnostic radiology. Medical specialists in oncology should also consider the indications for surgical treatment and the results of such treatment. Psychological and social aspects should be included in the training programme as well as physical, psychological, sociological and professional rehabilitation.

Surgical oncology requires first of all good skill in general surgery and a specific programme for specialisation in surgical oncology. It should be based on general pathology and gross pathology of tumours and their behaviour in the patient's body. Of course, surgical oncology specialisation includes teaching surgery in E.N.T., ophthalmology, and gynaecology. Radiology and other diagnostic procedures are to be in the curriculum for specialisation of medical oncology. Specialists in surgical oncology should be well prepared to understand the indications for medical treatment and should be acquainted with the results of such treatment. Based on that, a specialist in surgical oncology may refer a patient to continue treatment in the care of the specialist in medical oncology.

Rehabilitation training for specialists of surgical oncology is as important as in medical oncology.

Rehabilitation of Oncologic Patients
Physical
Psychological
Sociological

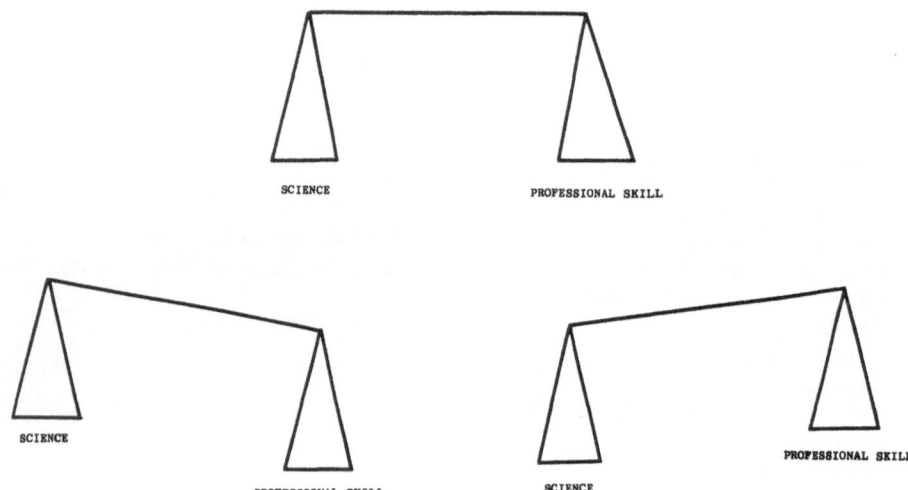

The programme on specialisation in clinical oncology should keep a very sound balance between the curriculum of the basic sciences and the curriculum of professional skills. Of course, if this teaching is properly balanced it is an ideal situation.

In case the specialist is skilled enough professionally, but is not fully aware of the achievements of science, he may make mistakes in the same way as the doctor whose professional skill is not as good as his knowledge of the oncological sciences.

Well-trained specialists in clinical oncology help to diminish the pain and suffering of the patient, the mortality rate and in many cases prolong the life of the patient.

But taking into consideration the specificity of the development of the tumour malignancy the most important factor in saving the patient from death is the role fulfilled by all practising doctors and in particular by the doctors who have the first contact with the patient.

That is why continuing medical education plays so important a role for diagnosis and treatment of the cancer.

These practising doctors should be involved continuously in postgraduate medical education with constant information about all the oncological sciences and clinical achievements. There are special facts which those who programme the teaching and administration should take into consideration. These important facts are:

early diagnosis of cancer
clinical skill in clinical oncology
psycho-social factors, and
rehabilitation of oncological patients.

The treatment of cancer is still not always effective. But we learnt by experience that early detection of the cancer is a most important factor for the management of this disease. This fact has been proved by clinical observation and by epidemiological and biostatistical studies. Early detection of cancer and immediate treatment of the diagnosed disease show that 95% of such patients overlive 5 years after the treatment, which is the accepted norm for curability of the malignant disease.

Early diagnosis of cancer requires:

— Alertness for cancer pathology both from the patient and the doctor's side,
— implementation of categoric diagnostic procedures by a specialist,
— repetition of diagnostic procedures, with full cooperation of a specialist and practitioner, and understanding of this necessity by the patient.

Clinical skill in clinical oncology is another factor in improving the rate of curability of this disease. It should be achieved during a proper postgraduate medical education during which

understanding of histopathological findings,
knowledge of the dynamism of different types of tumours,
knowledge of the medical possibilities of treatment, and
knowledge of the surgical possibilities of treatment

should be taught.

The danger of cancer is known by the whole population. Many people are afraid of it and some of them are developing some kind of defense. These kinds of patients require special attention from the practising doctor.

Some of the patients have a fatalistic approach to such a situation. They do not want to speak about the symptoms; they do not even want to begin treatment. They produce a state of apathy and resignation. Every doctor should be aware of the possibility of such a psychological state in the patient and deal accordingly with the proper approach to help the patient gaining confidence in himself. The social and economical conditions of the patient may have an influence on his cooperation with the doctor. Much depends again on the attitude of every doctor.

Psycho-social factors then should be important facts learnt during the continuing postgraduate medical education of doctors. The topics of training should recognise

the psychological approach of the doctor,
the psychologic and sociologic needs of the patient,
and personal attributes.

During the long time of treatment for cancer the patient may see not only specialists, but also the practitioners, and his family doctors. In such circumstances, the wise attitude of all doctors concerned based on understanding and knowledge of the oncological pathology may play a very important role in helping to manage the disease.

There is also a rehabilitation period after the oncological treatment which consists of

physical,
psychological,
sociological, and sometimes
professional rehabilitation.

That is why in postgraduate continuing medical education every doctor should be prepared to manage the rehabilitation of the patient in the above-mentioned fields.

To sum up, during postgraduate medical education we should see two important tasks:
— first, to properly train specialists in clinical oncology
— second, to train continuously all practising doctors in the early detection of the disease and in the ability to advise the patient during his prolonged period of treatment.

References

Guidelines for training in medical oncology from the American Board of Internal Medicine.
Cancer, November 1977, 2395—2399

Dr. Edward Ruzyllo

Community Medicine—Personal (Individual) Medicine

Kuwait State has a well organised National Health Care system. Such an existing system may give a lot of satisfaction to the managers, doctors and above all to society. At the same time we observe that each organised national health care system produces a lot of difficulties and misunderstandings. As every very complicated system, it requires constant study, improvements and further developments.

I am attracted by the report of the following two Committees:
1. Strategic Planning of Health Services in Kuwait prepared in April 1978 by: Dr. Abdulla M. Al-Rifai, Dr. Nouri Al-Kazemi and Mr. Leslie Fletcher.
2. Report of the Committee on the Programme for Community Medicine, submitted on 15th December, 1977 by: Dr. Richard Kurtz, Chairman; Dr. Ahmed Bayomi; Dr. Gafar Ezzat; Dr. Fahim Naser, Rapporteur; and Dr. Pritam Singh Sani.

Both these reports show a very sound knowledge of the modern requirements of medical care and also a very nice humanistic approach to this complex problem. Most of these ideas have been utilised and introduced in a thoroughly prepared report on National Health Care in the year 2000.

The crucial point of every system of national health care is always the doctor's first contact with the patient. This important, professional, social and national position of the doctor is the most traditional form of diagnostic and curative procedures, and is still the official continuation of old time activities and moral responsibilities. This professional work and the moral atmosphere of the practising doctor is dependent on many factors, some of which come from the doctor's attitudes and some from the patient's behaviour. But we observe nowadays that the practising doctor loses his complete independence in the field of these activities, and his moral and ethical obligations, for obvious reasons, are becoming more and more difficult.

The doctor's work is changing because of advances in technical possibilities both in diagnosis and treatment and also because of the development of many specialities in medical practice. This involves him in a system of technical and personal cooperation, and in this way he is limited in his complete independence in professional activities.

The patients' attitudes are also changing because they observe that their doctors are not completely free in their opinions and decisions depending on the above-mentioned conditions. On the other hand, the patient may notice that the condition of his life is also changing.

With the constantly growing population, the developing material and technical standard of living, modern human beings have adjusted to conditions in general, losing the personal aspects of the problem because of being closely linked with the above-mentioned changes. In effect, the economical pressures, society's regulations, environmental conditions and other factors may have priority over his personal requirements as an individual human being.

But having in mind these changing conditions both for doctors and patients, nobody should lose sight of the biological and moral purposes of life, and particularly the function and activity of medical care. In all situations doctors should look primarily for the requirement of an individual human being, and find him out from all modern structures and conditions covering him. In practise it means that the patient should be seen as living individual member of the community. The doctor should be seen as a traditional personal doctor, but as a member of the national health care system.

Nobody can deny that the process of medical treatment arises between the patient and the doctor. This is still understood too literally. Too little attention is given to the fact that the patient—doctor arrangement is not a single unit. For in the national system of health care the doctor only represents a complex medical system, and the patient, in the modern understanding of pathological phenomena, represents the environment in which he lives and works. The doctor in these conditions must know how to act within the prophylactic medical system and see and evaluate the patient on the background of his environment. The patient in his turn should gain confidence in the medical system and see in the doctor a qualified representative of this system. On the other hand, the patient should realise the conditioning of natural pathological phenomena, the existence of the confines of the biological, and at the same time subordinate his personal requirements to the potential possibilities of the country. The complexity of these problems calls for their constant discussion. For health care workers it means professional improvement. The lay society on the other hand must be taught to think in biological and socio-economic categories. It is an important task for primary schools, in the teaching of which an equilibrium must be maintained between thinking in technical, biological and social categories.

Hygiene, the most traditional public health science, was not sufficient to explain the medical science requirements of public health. Slowly it was developing a new term for this complex public health problem called "community medicine". As health services evolve, organisational structures and management practices change, and it is likely that new roles will open up for community medicine specialists with well-developed skills in epidemiology, and the planning and management of health services.

The confusion among public health, community medicine, industrial medicine, occupational medicine, family medicine, agricultural medicine, tropical medicine, ocean medicine and cosmos medicine is widely discussed, and gives rise to many differences of opinion. Therefore, everybody is free to express his own interpretation of these terms.

With the growing knowledge connected with the problem of public health or community medicine, is a greater demand of people who are concerned with its administration and general management. In some of the countries there is a new medical speciality called "Management of the Medical Services".

Community medicine is developed because of the rising standard of living modern human beings, because of the cultural, economical and organisational conditions of work, because of the climatic changes and so on. There is a constant study and development of the sciences looking after communities from the point of view of the general health situation. Anybody having the responsibility of the management of national health care should be well trained in public health and all aspects of these sciences. But also he should be additionally trained in the technique of management and administration of health care.

Community medicine doctors should be specialists in their professional activities, but doctors aiming at management of public health should be additionally trained in the organisation and management of public health care. It is also important because in many cases the administrator of national health care may come up with individual medicine, so-called clinical medicine, and he may have the same conditions and same values as for being the manager of national health care.

The definition of community medicine is not only a semantic problem, it is a problem not completely settled scientifically and it is still developing.

In Kuwait the following definition has been formulated (by Dr. R. Kurtz and others):

Community Medicine is the medical discipline which views the total community as its 'patient'. In taking this perspective, the Community Medicine physician is concerned with those community experiences (social, psychological, biological) which affect the occurrence of disease. In addition to this concern with antecedents, the Community Medicine physician also examines the community in terms of the consequences of health experiences. To obtain objective information about such phenomena, Community Medicine is concerned with the collection of accurate data and with data analyses which lead to a determination of disease rates and trends. Data collection and analysis is designed to understand community health experiences in both their general context and in differentials among various social, ecological, and demographic groupings. Directly related to this analysis is the focus on the prediction of future disease experiences for the total community and for different social groups within the community.

Community medical diagnosis is a description of the state of health of the community in terms of the important factors that determine this state. To express ourselves more clearly, one may say a "community-of-human-beings" medical diagnosis takes into consideration factors which may have an influence on the whole community; and again, it means an influence on all the people.

Naturally, community diagnosis deals with general factors of the state of health, overlooking individual problems or conditions if they have no obvious influence on the general state of health of the community. The "Community of people" medical diagnosis begins as an analytical process taking into consideration many fields of medical, biological and social sciences. The synthesis of this analytical process giving a proper diagnosis of the state of health of the community, aims at improving the conditions of life of the whole community of people. This improvement or change may usually be achieved after some time of proper management, arrangements or education and may not concern the state of health of every individual of the community.

Personal or individual medical diagnosis passes through the same process of analysis but takes into consideration the "community of organs" of the living body. A synthesis in the form of a clinical diagnosis has to consider different factors existing in the organs of the individual human being. This scholastic divagation serves the purpose of showing that in every example of diagnosis we are dealing always with complex problems.

In Kuwait the following definition of a General Practitioner or Primary Health Doctor has been formulated (by Dr. R. Kurtz and others):

Primary Health Care could be defined as an integrated comprehensive service (both curative and preventive) provided by a Primary Care physician to the individual, family and local population at the health centre peripheral level incorporating the functions of the lower tier of the health care delivery system.

If we still take the liberty of using scholastic divagations we could say that community medicine takes into consideration a group of people but deals with a collection of sciences, while a general practitioner (personal medicine) is concerned with one human being but dealing with collection of his organs.

One thing is common in both these examples. First, that we have to deal with complex problems which always include physical surrounding factors and the psychological insight of one or many human beings.

Community medicine is a general definition. Since we want to satisfy ourselves as to what kind of community we have in mind, we should explicitly define it. From the medical point of view there may be many kinds of communities: the municipal community, the factory community and so on. These communities usually have some physical, economical, social and other factors coming from outside the members of the community. They form the physical conditions of common life, but have different biological backgrounds and different biological factors from members of the community.

But there does exist one human collectivity which has a peculiar feature because it contains the attributes of all features of community medicine but at the same time consists of common biological elements characterising personal medicine. That human collectivity is the smallest social cell which is *the family*.

The family itself fully represents human beings collectively living in defined physical, economical, and social conditions. At the same time through its homely atmosphere and having common genetic factors, it also has the characteristic features of personal medicine.

In these conditions it is well understood that the family in the national health care system is an important subject of peculiar interest.

The practicing doctor engaged with personal medicine cannot step aside from the obligations of examining and controlling the state of health of the human collectivities to which a single patient belongs. In his everyday practice it is imperative to imagine or to see the patient as an individual in his closed environment which is formed by the family. During the treatment of the patient and the study of his conditions of life, even with his limited possibilities, a practising doctor enters automatically into the problems of community medicine. By this fact he again automatically engages himself in the basic problems of the national health care system.

That is why we notice the general trend of developing family medicine problems and we see it as an important branch of medical science. It is more and more obvious and will be more clear in the end, that the modern general practitioner should not lose anything from his traditional activities while practicing medicine. At the same time he should set the course for new directions of activity for the national health care system. By doing that he may discover important facts which have an influence on the general health state of the community.

The modern family doctor possesses all the best traditional characteristics of the personal doctor but at the same time is interested in the conditions of the family life of the patient. The doctor automatically begins to be an important element of exploration of the phenomena of the human collectivities, having a big influence on the state of general health of the collectivity.

The following table shows similarities and dissimilarities between community and personal medicine (thanks to Dr. Mustapha Khojali for submitting this table, which I modified slightly):

Practice of Medicine at the Personal (Individual) and Community Levels

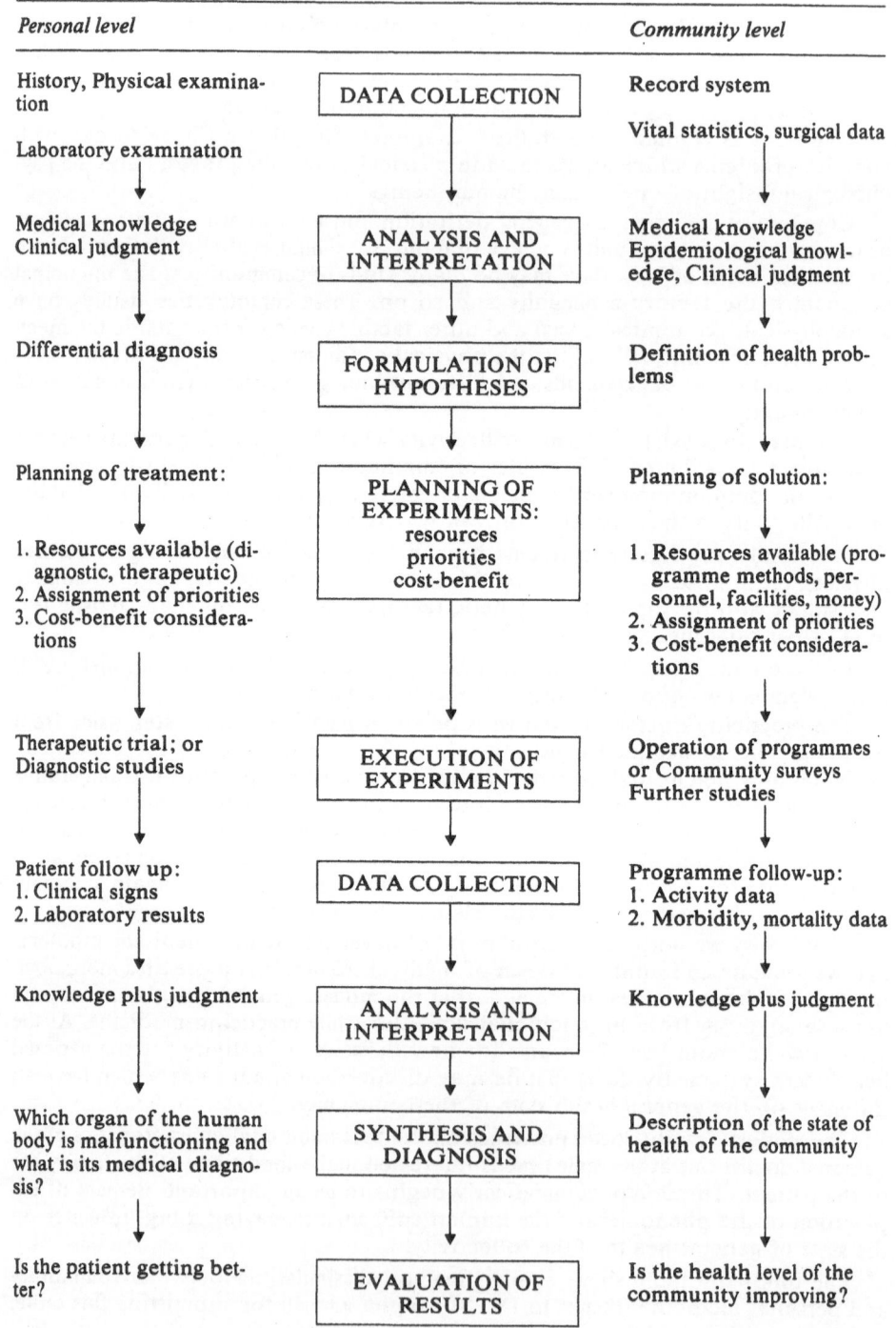

Personal level		Community level
History, Physical examination	**DATA COLLECTION**	Record system
Laboratory examination		Vital statistics, surgical data
Medical knowledge Clinical judgment	**ANALYSIS AND INTERPRETATION**	Medical knowledge Epidemiological knowledge, Clinical judgment
Differential diagnosis	**FORMULATION OF HYPOTHESES**	Definition of health problems
Planning of treatment: 1. Resources available (diagnostic, therapeutic) 2. Assignment of priorities 3. Cost-benefit considerations	**PLANNING OF EXPERIMENTS:** resources priorities cost-benefit	Planning of solution: 1. Resources available (programme methods, personnel, facilities, money) 2. Assignment of priorities 3. Cost-benefit considerations
Therapeutic trial; or Diagnostic studies	**EXECUTION OF EXPERIMENTS**	Operation of programmes or Community surveys Further studies
Patient follow up: 1. Clinical signs 2. Laboratory results	**DATA COLLECTION**	Programme follow-up: 1. Activity data 2. Morbidity, mortality data
Knowledge plus judgment	**ANALYSIS AND INTERPRETATION**	Knowledge plus judgment
Which organ of the human body is malfunctioning and what is its medical diagnosis?	**SYNTHESIS AND DIAGNOSIS**	Description of the state of health of the community
Is the patient getting better?	**EVALUATION OF RESULTS**	Is the health level of the community improving?

In Kuwait the Joint Board paid special attention to family medicine. Family medicine is formed not because of the organisational requirements but because of the biological, psychological, economical and cultural requirements of the different families. Families differ among themselves like individuals differ among themselves. Because we are seeing now that medicine as a whole demands prevention, cure and rehabilitation, features of family life have an important influence on the diagnosis and proper activities of the doctors.

The educational process in both of these medical science branches was well solved by the Joint Board on Postgraduate Medical Education in Kuwait by forming a Discipline Committee for Public Health and a Discipline Committee for Family Medicine. Family health, which includes all sciences may have an influence on the general state of health of the population. There are many fields which are developing and there are many fields which we do not expect to develop or arise in the future.

These prerequisites were the basic reasons why the authority of Kuwait has begun a serious activity for reorganisation of the work of the doctor of the first contact, calling him a family practise doctor. By this decision the medical authorities of Kuwait will restore the traditional authority of the personal doctor but at the same time give him the possibilities for realisation and also the objectives of community medicine.

Dr. Edward Ruzyllo

Preparatory Steps for Introducing Family Medicine Practice

Report
on
a Visit by the President and Chairman of Council
of the Royal College of General Practitioners of
the United Kingdom—February 1981

Summary

The Government of Kuwait is assessing the effectiveness and efficiency of the primary care services and their relation to hospital services. We were particularly asked to examine the role of the general practitioner within these health services and to make recommendations.

Recommendations

To improve the standard and status of primary medical care in Kuwait, the following measures, in our opinion, are needed:

1. A description of the role and responsibilities of the doctor as FAMILY DOCTOR.
2. The creation of at least one model practice
   a) as a demonstration
   b) for training both undergraduates and postgraduates.
3. The appointment of a Director for this practice, who will be responsible for training those doctors who work in it, to ensure that they are capable of providing cur-

ative and preventive services of a high standard to families in the population registered with the centre.

> TO ASSIST THIS DEVELOPMENT, OUR COLLEGE IS PREPARED TO ARRANGE A TRAINING PRO-GRAMME IN THE UNITED KINGDOM FOR THE DIRECTOR—OF THREE MONTH DURATION.

4. a) The development of a specific initial postgraduate training programme for family practice and its recognition by an educational authority of international standing.

b) The recognition at the end of the training period of successful completion of the programme by individual trainess—in the first place by the doctors from the model practice.

> WE ARE EXAMINING THE POSSIBILITY OF INVIT-ING SELECTED GENERAL PRACTITIONERS FROM THE UNITED KINGDOM TO VISIT KUWAIT FOR PERIODS OF A FEW WEEKS AT A TIME TO COOP-ERATE WITH THE DIRECTOR IN THE DEVELOP-MENT OF THE TRAINING PROGRAMME. WE ARE PREPARED TO SEND EXAMINERS FROM OUR COLLEGE TO VISIT KUWAIT AND TO UNDER-TAKE A MOCK EXAMINATION, TO ASSESS THE STANDARD OF LOCAL PRACTITIONERS IN RELA-TION TO THE EXISTING MRCGP EXAMINATION. COUNCIL OF THE COLLEGE HAS AGREED THAT, IF THE KUWAIT HEALTH AUTHORITIES WISH, A FORM OF EXAMINATION COULD BE PREPARED WHICH IS SUITABLE TO CANDIDATES WORKING IN THE MIDDLE EAST. ALTHOUGH PARTLY DIF-FERENT IN CONTENT, IT WOULD BE OF THE SAME STANDARD AS THE EXAMINATION IN THE UNITED KINGDOM. THIS COULD BE CONDUCT-ED IN KUWAIT.

5. A career structure for trained doctors.
6. A system of continuing education, aimed at sustaining the enthusiasm and self-criticism of trained doctors, and at helping them keep up-to-date with changing needs and changing knowledge.
7. Further development of family practice within the undergraduate programme of Kuwait University Medical School.

> WE BELIEVE THAT IT IS IMPORTANT TO APPOINT AN ACADEMIC GENERAL PRACTITIONER TO THE CHAIR OF FAMILY PRACTICE IN THE KUWAIT MEDICAL SCHOOL. WE WOULD TRY TO IDENTIFY SUCH A PERSON IN THE UNITED KINGDOM, IF ASKED TO DO SO.

Primary Medical Care in Kuwait

The Problems

Kuwait has had a primary care medical service since the expansion of the state began. But shortly afterwards—and until recently—priority was given to the building of hospitals and to developing medical and surgical specialities within them.

Few doctors—less than 10%—make primary care their first choice of career; the majority leave to study a speciality as soon as they can. Primary care has been used as a last resort for those who fail to reach an adequate standard when training for a speciality. A career in primary care is seen as lacking a structure, intellectual stimulation, and prestige, whether with patients or specialist colleagues or students.

There is unhappiness not only about the status of primary care doctors, but also about whether patients are getting proper treatment. There is no integration of care for the whole family—and very little continuity. Some patients are reaching hospital too late, whilst others are going there direct, when they do not need hospital care. There is inadequate follow-up of patients with chronic conditions. There are complaints. How is primary care to be revived and reorganised so that patients get preventive and curative care of high standard, and so that doctors of high quality value this career and are valued for the work which they do in it? There have been attempts to solve this problem already, but they have not been successful.

Strengths and Weaknesses of the Health Care System in Kuwait

Our opinions are based on the statements of senior doctors and administrators, from Dr. Abdel Rahman Al-Awadi, the Minister of Public Health, downwards. We see very strong determination in the government to improve the primary care service. There is a clear recognition of the contribution which it makes to the total health care of the community. Without an effective primary health care service the secondary and tertiary services in the hospital cannot be satisfactory.

The system of government is effective and can work on a salaried medical service to achieve what is planned. Kuwait is a country of action, backed by exceptional financial resources; the amount of building in progress makes this obvious to any visitor.

There are particular strengths where the population defined geographically is registered at an identifiable health centre, with an outlet to the same district hospital. This helps both planning and the evaluation of the outcome of care. An experiment in improving radically the work of one or two health centres as a teaching model might demonstrate, against the 'control' of the other centres, an impact both on the health of the population and on the use of the hospital—provided careful records are kept.

The weaknesses of primary care lie in the predominance of ex-patriate doctors whose undergraduate training has not been influenced by modern concepts of primary care. Their postgraduate training has seldom been planned with this work in view. Once in practice in Kuwait, they are under pressure from patients who have not known how best to use (or to refrain from using) the service. They are hurt by the desire of patients to be referred to hospital, or to bypass them altogether. There is a limitation on their ordering of x-ray or laboratory tests and on the prescription of important medicines. They can never look after their own patients within the local hospital. They come to realise that their hospital colleagues look down on them and attribute little worthwhile to the role of primary care, because of these limitations.

The shift system tends to diminish continuity of care for particular patients and the satisfaction which arises from a familiar and trusting relationship. The separation of obstetric and paediatric care removes any sense of being a family doctor and limits integration of care for the family unit. The absence of shared clinical records within the health centre and the almost complete absence of referral correspondence and replies from hospital intensifies the professional isolation of the general practitioner.

Good salaries, nearly equal to that of hospital colleagues, do not sufficiently compensate for the lack of prestige and intellectual satisfaction. We noticed a striking contrast between hospitals and primary care clinics in the standards of design, decoration, furnishing, and comfort (not to mention equipment), which is bound to remind doctors working in clinics that they are valued less than their colleagues.

Proposals

1. *Job Description*

It is important to define the aims to be achieved by the primary care clinics and to describe in outline the role and responsibility of the doctors working within it.

For example, is the clinic to undertake health education and disease prevention? Is the family doctor to cover paediatrics or is this a job for a separate doctor in the clinic?

The answer to the last question influences the name given to the primary care doctor. Can he be called family doctor? This is desirable for other reasons, chiefly its appeal to patients. Definitions are needed so that the doctor himself may know his responsibilities, the people in his district know what they can expect from him, and specialist colleagues understand better a role with which their own will increasingly interact.

It is impossible to plan the training programme unless the job is first defined to which the training is directed.

We have been given to understand that the Ministry of Health intends to reorganise primary care so that the same doctor deals with children and adults. He will also share in ante-natal care and undertake a number of preventive tasks with the help of other workers in the clinic.

2. *Training*

a) *Undergraduate*

Training for primary care begins at the beginning of the undergraduate course. If the subject does not appear until the end (or not at all), the doctor will be confirmed in the beliefs that medicine is hospital medicine, that all the interest of the subject is confined to the hospital setting and that anything beyond the hospital walls can only be the real thing diluted. Such attitudes take years to change, even in those who later make their career in general practice. The clinical problems facing primary care need to be demonstrated in as dramatic a way as possible at the start of the course, along with those facing some hospital specialists. They should preferably be demonstrated in patients' homes. This is a very real experience which the young student does not forget.

Primary care can contribute to the teaching of behavioural sciences—sociology, psychology and epidemiology—by providing living examples to theoretical subjects in which medical students are not easily interested. It can play an important part in the introduction to clinical medicine, particularly in the study of the consultation. When the patient presents one or more problems for the first time, the doctor's behaviour—what he says and does, and the way in which he responds—usually determines what happens afterwards. This first encounter is a rich source for essential learning.

There are opportunities to follow patients at home who have been seen already by the student in the hospital wards or in outpatients, so as to get a long-term view which includes the impact of social, personal and economic problems on physical ones.

The final year is generally regarded as the best time for the main teaching programme—accompanying the doctor, seeing patients before he does, visiting them in their homes by himself, doing projects (perhaps in cooperation with the Department of Community Health) and attending seminar discussions conducted by family doctors and by specialists working in the family practice setting.

Specialists in other branches of medicine, during their ward and outpatient teaching, must be encouraged in every possible way to remind students of the environment from which patients come and to which they return. For most people admission to hospital is only a rare and transient experience.

b) Initial Postgraduate Training

Hospital posts already used in Kuwait for the general professional training period for all doctors are well chosen, in our opinion, for primary care. These are: medicine, surgery, gynaecology, psychiatry, paediatrics. In the United Kingdom we would regard the period in surgery as unnecessarily long and might increase the paediatrics or psychiatry.

For those making a career in family practice a much longer period of training in the clinic setting is needed—not less than one year; probably two years will be needed until training is well established. This must be a supervised practice for the trainee, combined with a theoretical course and secondments to hospital departments. Each doctor should have an appointed trainer to supervise him. The trainers must be carefully selected for their enthusiasm, and then trained to teach. They should have the MRCGP diploma.

Community health should be taught during this period, but we believe that there is a special need to relate theory to practice by insistence on physical examination and by providing trainees with sufficient time to undertake this thoroughly and to discuss their findings. There is also a particular need for training in pharmacology. We enclose samples of educational objectives and curricula from Europe. These require study and will certainly require modification to fit the local circumstances and culture of Kuwait.

3. Clinical Work in Practice

It is possible to establish centres of excellence in primary care. In principle, family doctors should assume greater responsibility. To do this they require help in certain ways.

It seems likely that the range of subjects will be increased in the training programme to include paediatrics and ante-natal care and some activities. Family doctors will be encouraged to take greater responsibility in all areas, but particularly in psychiatry, which is inseparable from family practice. The amount of responsibility given to the present generation of primary doctors is limited. They are allowed to use only very restricted lists of drugs. We were told that only three out of 50 clinics have any x-ray equipment and only one out of five have simple laboratory tests on the premises. We are not certain how far direct access is available to these departments in hospitals, but would recommend that this is the most efficient system and that there should be daily delivery and daily reporting. There are no electro-cardiograms available nor lung function tests. All these are serious indications of the standard and status of family medicine.

Primary care doctors are sometimes seeing 70—100 patients in seven hours, i.e. an average of five minutes per patient or less (allowing for short breaks). Forty patients in seven hours would be a reasonable figure. Hurry is a major bar to good practice. To correct this may mean more doctors, but education in the use of the service by patients and delegation of tasks to nurses are also relevant measures. If time is available for more investigation at the level of primary care, hospital referrals will be more appropriate.

Case discussion of everday cases in small groups and case presentations by the family doctors themselves at least once a week are a valuable stimulus to interest and self-criticism. These discussions, once established, can be joined by other health workers in the clinic, and not least by consultants visiting from the hospital. We saw them already organised in one clinic. Continuity of care by one doctor is essential in certain types of case. It is an important feature of family practice and is helped by a limited appointment system. But it requires a certain discipline to maintain this in a clinic with two shifts and a number of doctors. The patients rightly complain that they see different doctors on different occasions, and receive contradictory advice; this is one of the most important reasons why they ask to be referred to specialists or go to specialists direct. However, they do not find continuity there, any more than in primary cases. Health education within the clinics is very much needed, not least education in the use of the service. But this purpose can also be served through radio and television. It would be particularly helpful if primary care doctors can be heard and seen to take part in such programmes. This is a rapid route to raising their prestige.

4. Interaction between Clinic and Hospital

In the United Kingdom general practitioners are usually able to deal themselves with nine out of ten new problems, referring only one out of ten or less. We are puzzled by the fact that less than this proportion is referred to hospitals in Kuwait, and yet hospital doctors (who vastly outnumber primary care doctors) complain that they get too many referrals. Are these not in fact patients who bypass the clinic and go direct (about 20% are said to do this)? Or is it that the patients referred by general practitioners are seen as inappropriate for hospital or specialist care? Continuity and trust in one family doctor is known to be a way of ensuring more appropriate referral and reducing the problem of direct access. Another important influence is in the quality of communication:

a) Letters

Do family doctors' referral letters describe the problem clearly and briefly? Ask a clear question of the specialist? Report what has already been done and what has already been said by the clinic doctor to the patient?

Do specialists routinely report back to the clinic doctor giving sufficient detail of their assessment, their recommendations and what they have said to the patient? Is there an adequate postal system between clinic and hospital? Do specialists normally return the patient to the clinic doctor, because they and the patient trust him to continue the care?

b) Telephone

This permits discussion of a difficult problem.

c) Meeting

The distance between clinic and hospital is small in Kuwait. The patients greatly appreciate seeing their own doctor visiting them in hospital, even if the visit is social. It is more difficult to arrange a clinical discussion with the specialist over the patient, but it can be done sometimes. An alternative which we recommend strongly is visits to the clinic by certain specialists—see below.

THE RELATIONSHIP BETWEEN SPECIALIST AND GENERALIST IS GREATLY HELPED BY MEETING FACE TO FACE.

5. *Continuing Education*

It is usual to think that the purpose of continuing education is to keep the general doctor up-to-date by informing him about recent advances in various specialities.

But this is only *one* purpose. It is just as important to maintain the generalist's enthusiasm for his own job and his critical attitude to what he is doing. It is easy for clinical skills to deteriorate through isolation and lack of contact with doctors doing the *same* work. If generalists are always taught by specialists, they see everyone as an expert except themselves, and everyone as a teacher except themselves. This is no way to raise their self-confidence or their status. It eventually helps to erode their standards of care. We believe that the central form of continuing education should be small group work in which each family doctor contributes from his experience and in which regular meetings create a group feeling which allows free discussion. Interesting or difficult cases are the main content, but there are many possible developments from that. By hearing what other doctors do, one questions what one is doing oneself. This offers greater hope of keeping the doctor's intellect and capacity for criticism alive than does listening to lectures. Moreover, the discussion is of his own problems and not those of a doctor who is seeing different ones.

There is a particular need for continuing education in therapeutics and pharmacology. This must be a condition for release of a full range of drugs for use in primary care clinics.

If there is a general movement to have one doctor looking after the whole family, those doctors who have been paediatricians hitherto will need further training in relation to older age groups, and adult doctors in relation to small children.

Different individuals have different needs for continuing education. Methods are available to identify them.

6. *A New Model*

The problems outlined at the start of this report have first to be attacked by setting up a model clinic—a *new* model.

This will be a centre for training and the demonstration of good practice. But it will also be an experiment in the revised pattern of family practice in which one doctor has responsibility for children under five, in addition to the parents. He will have limited responsibility in ante-natal and post-natal care and for personal preventive medicine.

The clinic at Hawalli lends itself to this experiment. But before any doctors can be trained, their trainers have to be trained. That in turn can be started only when a director has been selected and trained.

Training must include the main areas of clinical work, practice organisation, techniques of learning and teaching, and the evaluation of both education and performance.

We understand that the future trainers at Hawalli have already been selected and are in post. They are to have a 'crash course' later this year. If this is to increase their responsibility as clinicians and teachers, it must contain a high proportion of small group work in which discussion is initiated by the doctors themselves. The same purpose is not served by lectures from a variety of specialists, although their contribution will also be needed, preferably working as resource persons within groups.

The director will need to travel abroad for a period of perhaps three months before taking up his post. Much of this time should be spent in the United Kingdom, but he might also visit the Netherlands, Denmark and Norway. He should if possible *work* in a practice in the United Kingdom (i.e. see patients) and prepare to take the MRCGP examination. This is urgent and we recommend that it might be organised with a view to the examination in November 1981. In preparing his trainers for the same examination, it would be helpful if a United Kingdom doctor with teaching experience could come to Kuwait for a period of several months. Other teachers might come for shorter periods. If a relationship with a particular university department could be established, this would be the best basis.

Doctors in the model clinic should work in relatively ideal conditions. The premises should not differ in standard from those provided in Kuwait's new hospitals. The doctors should work at a reasonable speed, seeing not more than 40 patients daily (half this number when teaching). They should have full access to all relevant diagnostic tests and all relevant therapeutic agents.

It is of great importance that some doctors who are *Kuwaiti citizens* should work in primary care. If the model clinic is planned, resourced and promoted as an important experiment—relevant not only to Kuwait but to other Arab countries also—this may start to attract them.

Possible Assistance from the United Kingdom

Practical proposals are made in the summary at the beginning of this report. We believe it to be crucially important that any help provided should be seen as temporary and directed at introducing only what is appropriate to the culture, traditions and local needs of Kuwait. Kuwait needs better primary medical care, but the ultimate aim is for Kuwaiti doctors to provide this themselves to standards as high as can be found in any other country.

The Role of the Family Doctor and His Place in the National Health System

General Statement

1. The report takes into consideration the development of health services in Kuwait, the organisation of the health system and the social and cultural factors working within Kuwait Society.
2. It is generally accepted that the family doctor fulfils a crucial role in each national system of health care. Despite this fact, there are still many different opinions on the exact role family doctors should play in this systems. There are two basic reasons for this misunderstanding of the position:
   a) Because of constant change in the level of the community which are gaining more general knowledge, developing social requirements and economic conditions. On the basis of this fact, demands on the medical care system is growing.
   b) The second reason is that medical science is developing so quickly and specialising more and more both in knowledge and in professional skill, and using more sophisticated instruments for diagnostic purposes. This makes it impossible for one doctor to master everything intelligently and physically.

These above-mentioned reasons or aspects have possibly been foreseen and functionally solved. To fulfil this, there are many different obstacles that each of the countries face. One of the smaller problems which meet with obstacles is of a semantic nature—what exactly does "general practitioner" mean? "Family doctors" and other names are also used for this function. For this report we agreed that semantically it would be logical to use the name of *Family Doctor*.

Job Specification of Family Doctor

1. The Family Doctor is a licensed medical graduate who has completed two years of general professional training and one year in family practice training. He gives personal primary and continuing care to individuals, families and the general population, irrespective of age, sex, and illness.
2. He accepts responsibility for the patient's total health care, within the context of this environment, including the community and the family or comparable social unit.
3. He serves as the physician of first contact with the patient and provides a means of entry into the health care system. He will attend his patients in his consulting room in the clinic and sometimes in their homes or a hospital.
4. He evaluates the patient's total health needs and takes into consideration the physical, psychological and social factors.
5. He provides personal medical care and refers the patient when indicated to appropriate sources of care while preserving the continuity of his care.
6. He assumes responsibility for the patient's comprehensive and continuous health care and, when needed, acts as leader or coordinator of the team that provides health services.
7. He will intervene educationally, preventively and therapeutically to promote his patient's health.

Family Doctors Should Be Well Prepared for Their Duties

To introduce a physician to the role of Family Doctor he has not only to be properly trained but also educated in all aspects of his activities and responsibilities. If doctors are not prepared for these duties the whole system of national health care will suffer from it.

To fulfil this requirement we have to *find proper teachers* who will be able to teach new family doctors in this country.

Criteria for Selection of Trainers (Teachers)

1. Willingness to teach—by attending a trainer's course (before appointment, a commitment to attend trainer's course).
   i) Select 10 well recognised general doctors;
   ii) Release from work for the period of the course.
2. Ability to teach.
3. A readiness to make time to teach.
4. Clinical competence.
5. Experience — At least 3—5 years experience in family practice.

A Course for Teachers

A teacher's course should be organised on the following principles: 6 days week (one week) full day training, as an introductory beginning of the course, followed by a 3 months course twice a day weekly.

It is considered that the best place would be Farwania Hospital and the doctor responsible for this course would be Dr. Ashmawi Abdul Wahab.

A Clinic Suitable for Teaching Should Have the Following Criteria

1. Individual clinical records—well kept (so trainee learns good record keeping).
2. Sufficient consultation rooms.
3. A common room suitable for small group teaching.
4. Competent nurses and social workers.
5. Adequate secretarial and reception staff.
6. An effective appointment system.
7. Adequate access to laboratory, radiological and other diagnostic services.
8. Ready access to other medical services and close cooperation with the regional hospital—(Kuwait has five regional hospitals!).
9. Ready access to relevant literature.

Suggested Career

MEDICAL GRADUATE

	Professional Training	2 years
↓	Family Practice	1 year

FAMILY PRACTITIONER*

	Training (Courses)	3 years
	Certified after the	
	course approved by	
	the Joint Board.	
	Desirable examination e.g.	
↓	M.R.C.G.P.	

*FAMILY DOCTOR***

	Minimum	3 years
↓		

*SENIOR FAMILY DOCTOR****

	Minimum	5 years
	or more depending on	
	jobs but his increments	
↓	Continue.	

*CONSULTANT FAMILY DOCTOR*****

Payment:

   * Family Practitioner should have salary equivalent to **Registrar**
  ** Family Doctor should have salary equivalent to **Senior Registrar**
 *** Senior Family Doctor should have salary equivalent to **Specialist**
**** Consultant Family Doctor should have salary equivalent to **Consultant**.

Report on a Visit by the President and Chairman of Council of the Royal College of General Practitioners of the U.K.
(February 1981)

This report has been studied in Kuwait by two bodies:
— *First* from the Ministry of Public Health (Prof. E. Ruzyllo, Dr. Sami Matar, Dr. Ali Al Seif and Dr. Mustafa Khojali).
— *Second* from the Faculty of Medicine (Prof. F. Fenech, Prof. P. Vassalo Agius, Dr. Sami Matar and Dr. Mustafa Khojali).

The *First Body* discussed the report several times and on the basis of these discussions a report on "Role of the Family Doctor and its place in Kuwait National Health System" has been produced and presented to the Ministry of Public Health on 12th of July, 1981.

The *Second Body* also discussed the report of the representatives of R.C.G.P., London, and produced a report on 5th July, 1981 which was attached to the report of the First Body (see above).

Acknowledgement of the Report of Representatives of the Royal College of General Practitioners of the United Kingdom

All of us accepted the report as sound and appropriate for Kuwait's requirements. In the chapter on Primary Medical Care in Kuwait, the visiting doctors have a good picture of the situation except for some details with which they are not well oriented. This has no influence on the general assessment of Primary Medical Care in Kuwait.

Their discussion and proposition concerning Primary Health Care doctor's education are also appropriate ones and good, and easily adjustable to modern requirements as soon as the role of the Family Doctor in Kuwait's Medical Care System is settled. Based on the general assessment, they are proposing 7 recommendations:

The *job description* of the Family Doctor should be defined and his professional responsibility should be clearly stated. They properly stressed that it is impossible to plan the training programme unless the job is first defined to which the training is directed. Developing the problem of job descriptions and the visitor's advice that the Family Doctor should deal with children and others, that he should also share in antenatal care and undertake a number of preventive tasks with the help of other workers in the clinic, defining the jobs of doctors, etc., they came to the conclusion that the best title for such a doctor should be "Family Doctor".

Training: The visitors rightly expressed their view that proper training of the Family Doctor should be introduced in undergraduate training. That is why they proposed to form a *Chair in the Medical Faculty for "Family Medicine"*. They also advised us to form a model practice institution which has been carried out for some time in the Hawalli District (see report of Second Body).

This *model unit* which requires only a proper arrangement for teaching, has been discussed in the report of the First Body. To develop this problem the First Body decided to have a special *course for teachers*. The programme of it and the general management of the teaching programme is produced in the above-mentioned report of the First Body.

According to the suggestions of the visiting representatives of the Royal College of General Practitioners the name of *Director of the Practice* has been suggested by the First Body. It is advisable that this Director should attend the training programme in the United Kingdom for 3 months duration, arranged by the representatives of the Royal College of General Practitioners.

The representatives of the Royal College of General Practitioners also suggest that some of the *English general practitioners may visit Kuwait* for periods of a few weeks at a time to cooperate with the Director of the development of the training programme. This suggestion we consider as a sound one and we would like to see one or two English General Practitioners visit Kuwait.

Another suggestion by the visitors from the Royal College of General Practitioners was to send examiners from their College and to undertake a *MOCK* examination here to assess the standard of local practitioners in relation to existing *MRCGP examination*—we consider that this form of cooperation could be useful and in proper time we can take the initiative to invite such examiners to Kuwait.

The suggestion of the visiting doctors to elaborate *a career structure for the Family Doctor* has been proposed in a letter sent by the First Body.

A *system of continuing education* will be developed in due time and all Kuwait experience and advice given by the representatives of the Royal College of General Practitioners will be taken into consideration.

Program of Training in Community Medicine and Primary Health Care

According to our postgraduate medical training programme Community Medicine and Primary Health Care will be slowly adjusted to a new programme arranged for the Family Doctor, as being more suitable for the given tasks of these doctors. Of course community medicine will be an important subject of the programme as a part of public health science and its teaching will be continued with others, like preventive medicine and primary health care.

The actual programme of postgraduate medical education and primary health care is valid up to the end of the fiscal year 1981—1982.

In the same period of time we shall introduce the first course for the doctors chosen for the future teachers in Family Medicine. This proposition in detail is given in the report of the First Body.

The postgraduate medical education programme in the fiscal year 1982—83 should include a complete new programme laid down with the above accepted principles.

Dr. E. Ruzyllo
Dr. Mohd Sami Matar
Dr. Mustafa Khogali
Dr. Ali Al Sief

Kuwait,
26th July 1981

Role of the Family Doctor and His Place in the Kuwait National Health System

An Implementation Report

I. General Statement

The report takes into consideration the development of health services in Kuwait, the organisation of the health system and the social and cultural factors working within Kuwait Society.

It is our belief that the *Family Doctor* fulfils a crucial role in the national system of health care in Kuwait. Despite the fact, there are still many different opinions on the exact role family doctors should play in this system. There are two basic reasons for this misunderstanding of the position.

a) Because of constant change in the level of the Community which are gaining more general knowledge, developing social requirements and economic conditions. On the basis of this fact demands from the medical care system are increasing.

b) The second reason is that medical science is developing so quickly, specialising more and more both in knowledge and in professional skill and using more sophisticated instruments for diagnostic purposes. This makes it impossible for one doctor to master everything intelligently and physically.

These above-mentioned reasons or aspects have possibly been foreseen and functionally solved. To fulfil this, there are many different obstacles to overcome. One of the smaller problems which meet with obstacles is of a semantic nature— what exactly do general practitioner, family doctor and other names used for this function mean? For this report we agreed that semantically it would be logical to use the name "family doctor".

II. Job Specification of Family Doctor

1. The family doctor is a licensed medical graduate who has completed two years of general professional training and *one year in family practice training*. He gives personal primary and continuing care to individuals, families and the general population, irrespective of age, sex, or illness.
2. He accepts responsibility for the patient's total health care within the context of this environment, including the community and the family or a comparable social unit.
3. He serves as the physician of first contact with the patient and provides a means of entry into the health care system. He will attend his patients in his consulting room in the clinic and sometimes in their homes or a hospital.
4. He evaluates the patients total health needs and takes into consideration the physical, psychological and social factors.
5. He provides personal medical care and refers the patient when indicated to appropriate sources of care while preserving the continuity of his care.
6. He assumes responsibility for the patient's comprehensive and continuous health care and when needed, acts as leader or coordinator of the team that provides health services.
7. He will intervene educationally, preventively and therapeutically to promote his patient's health.

III. Training

a) *Undergraduate:*

The Faculty of Medicine have already included the teaching of Family Medicine in its curriculum. The curriculum extends over seven years but teaching of Family Medicine starts at the 6th year and continues through the 7th year when the students will have separate attachments to Family Doctors.

The Faculty had already advertised for a senior post in Family Medicine—aiming to establish a Department of Family Medicine. The person appointed will take part in both under- and postgraduate teaching.

b) *Postgraduate training:*

(i) *General professional training* in Kuwait provides during the first two years, 3 months of training in Family Medicine and Community Medicine. This course should be strongly coordinated and properly supervised by the Joint Board of Postgraduate Medical Education.

(ii) For those making Family Medicine their career—they should spend at least one year training in Family Practice under supervision. This *MUST BE A SUPERVISED PRACTICE FOR THE TRAINEE, combined with a theoretical COURSE and limited secondments to Hospital Departments.* (Such a detailed programme is being planned with aims derived from the job specification outlined above).

Each trainee should have an appointed trainer to supervise him. These trainers are very important during coming few years and we suggest that finding proper teachers and training them to become trainers is the *first* priority.

c) *Continuing Education:*

The purpose of continuing education is to:

i) Keep the Family Doctor up-to-date—by informing him about recent advances in various specialities.

ii) Maintain his enthusiasm for his own job and help him to develop a critical attitude toward what he is practicing. We recommend that continuing education can take different forms—one important form is through regular small group meetings in which each doctor participates under supervision.

IV. Trainers

a) *Criteria for Selection of Trainers:*

1. Willingness to teach—by responding to a specified questionnaire and by attending a trainers assessment interview—before appointment, commitment to attend a trainers course.

Ten doctors to be selected and released for the period of the course.

2. Ability to teach.
3. A readiness to make time to teach.
4. Clinical competence.
5. Experience at least 3—5 years in Family Medicine.

b) *Course for Trainers:*

The Trainers Course is very important—and should be organised in collaboration with the Royal College of General Practitioners who are willing to help and send staff for short periods to run this course.

The Course should be approximately 3 months—nearly full time with hospital attachment and duties. The *Farwania Hospital* is suggested as the centre for training in Family Medicine with Dr. Ashmawi Abd-El-Wahab as coordinator.

Also as agreed with RCGP—Dr. Ashmawi will go to the U.K. for a period of six weeks to be oriented in different aspects of Family Medicine.

We recommend that the process of selection should start in early January, 1982 and that the trainers course start in February, 1982.

c) *Health Centres Selected for Teaching and Training:*

To perform proper medical practice in Family Medicine and to teach it at the same time—a minimum requirement in each such Health Centre should be fulfilled.

1. Individual clinical records—Well kept (So trainee learns good record keeping).
2. Sufficient consultation room—with adequate necessary equipment.
3. A common room suitable for small group teaching.
4. Competent nurses and social workers.
5. Adequate secretarial and reception staff—with audiotyping, duplicating and photocopying machines.
6. An effective appointment system and an efficient communication system.
7. Adequate access to laboratory, radiological and other diagnostic services.
8. Ready access to other medical services and close cooperation with the regional hospital—(Kuwait has five regional hospitals).
9. Ready access to relevant literature.
10. Availability of transport to bring patients to clinic and to take them to hospital.
11. An epidemiological and vital health statistics unit.

Team Work in the Health Centre

Work in a health centre is team work—with the doctor as the leader of the team. It is very important that each member of the team should have a sound knowledge of the professional roles and responsibilities of every other member.

It is imperative that there *should be role definition* of *the Nurse, orderly, reception-ist,* and the administrative staff *of the Health Centre.* (This is under preparation.)

It is important to emphasise that the Family Doctor should be the head of the Health Centre as he is the one who plans the policy. We suggest that a board in the centres are formed with one Senior Family Doctor selected as *Director* of the Health Centre. Doctors frequently do not pay attention to the educational needs of their staff. In-service training should always be the going thing.

Career of the Family Doctor

The family doctor's role is a difficult one. If it is to be sustained and developed, he must become comprehensively well-educated and well paid at the same time.

We recommend the career structure as a career for Family Doctors in Kuwait. The consultant Family doctor at the top of the scale should have a salary equivalent to any other consultant in the Ministry of Health. The figure is self-explanatory but to promote a family practitioner to a Family Doctor requires that he attend recognised training courses with credits and certificates. If he performs satisfactorily—he will be a family doctor in three years. After two years as a FAMILY PRACTITIONER—a doctor can sit for the MRCGP and further qualifications. If he gets his MRCGP successfully he will be promoted to FAMILY DOCTOR immediately. An MRCGP or equivalent will be a requisite for family doctors to be appointed as trainers in accredited centres.

As a *FAMILY DOCTOR* he will also attend certain refresher courses and undergo continuous evaluation to be promoted to Senior Family Doctor after a minimum period of 3 years.

A Senior Family Doctor could become a Consultant Family Doctor after a minimum period of five years in his job and depending on the availability of posts at the consultant level.

Conclusion

The young doctor graduating from medical school and looking for his future career role in Kuwait should find Family Medicine an attractive option to choose. The aim of this report is to make Family Medicine a strong competitor to other specialities.

It is our strong conviction that a sound Family Medicine speciality is more rewarding and challenging than many other specialities, if properly practiced.

We strongly hope that the Ministry of Health will adopt the main points mentioned in this report which will result in raising the standard and status of Family Medicine and hence the standard and status of the Kuwait National Health Service.

Signed

Dr. Mustafa Khogali — Convenor
Prof. E. Ruzyllo   — Member
Dr. Sami Matar   — Member
Dr. Ali Al Sief   — Member

27 December, 1981

Dr. Nouri Al Kazemi
Chairman, Joint Board

Process of implementation of the system of Family Medicine

According to the decision of the Joint Board at the last meeting, I have met with Dr. Sami Matar, Dr. Khojali and Dr. Ali Al Seif to discuss the situation in the implementation of the decision of the Ministry of Public Health to introduce into the country the concept of Family Doctor and its organisation.

During the constructive discussion all confirmed the profound belief in a new approach to this complex problem and their willingness to cooperate in its full development.

General criteria for health centres and their organisation has been briefly reviewed. Also the career of Family Doctor has been confirmed as it was previously understood. The Medical Faculty of Kuwait University has chosen Dr. J. S. Berkeley from Aberdeen as the Acting Chairman of the Department of Family Medicine in the Faculty, to train undergraduates in this new field of teaching. So the implementation of Family Medicine in Kuwait is progressing along the foreseen directions.

Dr. Sami Matar, Director of the Department of External Health Services explained that he is developing the Al Adan region of National Health Service as a model region in which new principles of family medicine will be introduced and developed.

The Faculty is in the final stage of organising an outpatient clinic in East Hawalli as a base of training in Family Medicine for undergraduates.

Finally, all agreed that the Joint Board should take over the problem of postgraduate education in Family Medicine.

Discussing this point everybody realised that a proper Discipline Committee in the Joint Board should be formed and should begin to study the project of postgraduate medical education for such doctors.

To enable that, a special didactic area should be formed. Everybody agreed that such a training centre for postgraduate medical education should be formed at Farwania hospital, and therefore the Discipline Committee of Family Medicine should be composed of a bigger number of doctors from this hospital.

Dr. Edward Ruzyllo
Secretary, Joint Board

Trend of the Evolution of Medical Postgraduate Education

Postgraduate medical education is an overwhelming necessity to satisfy the growing, different modern requirements such as the biological, social, educational, and professional ones. In most of countries the requirements for developing this form of education is well understood but the complexity of the process of programming and organising postgraduate medical education raises difficulties in its understanding. This means that decisions taken in this matter are taken slowly and are not always of standard value. In many countries resourcefulness in forming a logical system of postgraduate medical education is often observed. This originated in most situations by a rigid traditional outlook on the problem. A proper proportion between the values of traditionalism and the necessity of vital evolution in education in general is very difficult to achieve when the collective decision is taken.

Postgraduate education is a relatively new phenomenon in the world. Constant development of the natural sciences and therefore also medical science means that knowledge acquired in universities is insufficient, and its supplementation by individual doctors difficult, particularly if they live far from medical centres. Modern development of technology ensuring ever better and fuller application of technical methods in the work of investigating natural phenomena creates, moreover, the need of not only supplementing basic knowledge, but acquiring the ability to use modern apparatus and modern methodology in professional work.

The results obtained in the application of technical methods of examination require the ability of their correct estimation and on that basis correct evaluation of disorders of systemic functions in humans.

At the moment we are witnessing great changes which are happening in biological conditions in the modern life of mankind. In these now conditions the doctors have to be actually prepared to fully meet the requirements.

It is foreseen that science will take a decidedly leading role in the development of humanity, and prominent scientists will play an increasingly important part in public life. Other conjectures see the 21st century as an age of rapid development of biology, which will leave far behind the magnificent development of the technical sciences of today, particularly physics.

Without judging how accurate these conjectures are, we all feel the approach of an era in which man will overstep many now acknowledged limits of possibilities.

We are already living in the period of a scientific, technical revolution when the dynamics of change is greatly precipitated, and the situation of man in the world of rapidly developing technology faces medicine with ever changing and new tasks. Medicine and science must keep pace with the development of other disciplines, but their particular social importance requires them to be sensitive to the problems of moral responsibility and matters of interhuman relations. For medicine is faced more and more often with questions of a socio-ethical nature, and a doctor in his practical activity is never free from making a choice of a moral character.

The progress of science and increasing requirements of society make it imperative for a doctor to follow intensive studies over many years in spite of the fact that medical studies were always among the longest, it has been and still is felt that they should yet be prolonged.

The development of the medical sciences has created the necessity of specialisation in the medical profession. The rise of medical specialities has aroused the admiration of laymen, but at the same time is a matter of deep concern to those responsible for medical care, especially if this specialisation is narrowly conceived. Discussions on specialisation and on the need of the integration of medicine are becoming increasingly frequent. Specialisation is often accused of introducing a narrow technological approach to medicine, and integration of medical specialisations is looked upon as the only means of restoring to medicine its human characteristics.

A doctor's subject of interest is *man* in all his complexity with all matters conditioning his life. It follows that a doctor, being in the first place a naturalist, should also embrace, with his knowledge and experience, the more important conditions of man in the modern world.

We see the world above all through the concrete reality nearest to us, which determines our attitudes and the conditions of our work.

Man's physical surroundings are rapidly being changed by the pollution of water, air and land, a circumstance which could generate changes in the world's climate. Even if active environmental protection is now pursued all over the world, future developments in industry and the community will probably cause even greater environmental destruction unless really drastic countermeasures are adopted. In addition to the grave problems posed by environmental pollution, we are also faced with the special problems presented by food additives, for there is no doubt that we are ingesting increasing quantities of various artificial additives whose long-range effects are unknown.

Climate may be regarded as a kind of metastable condition. We are indeed living in a period between long-range climatic fluctuations. But Man's influence on global, regional and local climate is the subject of increasing interest. Some of the subjects discussed are the effects of increased carbon dioxide release, i.e. the "greenhouse" effect, and increased particulate pollution of the air, affecting the reflectivity of the air blanket (the albedo), etc. The refrigeration effect is also involved. Local patches of heat, e.g. from urban areas are of concern. Air pollution, especially the release of chlorinated hydrocarbons into the upper layers of the atmosphere, may alter photochemical processes in the ozone layer whose powers of filtration are of vital importance to life on earth.

In other words we may expect pollution of our physical environment, the effects of artificial food additives and the increasing stress caused by our way of life to shrink our clinical margins so that extra loading on the organism will be more readily manifested in the form of illness. All these circumstances will probably complicate therapy employing a large number of concomitant medicines because of undesirable interaction between the drugs and pollutants.

Postgraduate medical education has to fulfil two basic and general objectives; to supply doctors with information and professional skill, and to deal properly with the changing conditions of life and with the advances of science.

Postgraduate medical education is not limited as to the time of its duration or as to its subject matter. It should be incorporated into the professional practice and should deal with all the aspects of this practice, as long as the physician remains professionally active.

In recent decades medical science has advanced at an increasingly rapid pace, thereby enhancing our knowledge and ability to provide aid. The society has kept apace of developments and made increasing resources available to public health. One might imagine that public confidence in doctors and hospitals would increase in step with general developments, but there is much evidence to suggest that this is definitely not the case. Quite the opposite. There appears to be a crisis of confidence between the people providing health services and the general public, a crisis whose magnitude appears to be growing. One of the most important tasks in the future will be to seek the causes of this crisis.

The diagnosis of disease is today a very complex task. For the modern doctor is not satisfied with only a global evaluation of the character of disorders of the function of an organ. He must grasp simultaneously the character of etiological factors, the mechanism of pathological phenomena and the dependence of these matters on the function of the organs whose efficacy is not directly disturbed by the pathological factor. This entire systemic view on organic disorders leads of necessity to the integration of pathological conceptions, and in consequence to the integration of the medical sciences. For this reason, the modern doctor must have an extensive supply of information from the sphere of human pathophysiology and from the border of various medical specialities. But the modern physician should not be just a medical technician. The character of diseases of which mankind is now suffering, the technical means facilitating the diagnosis and the increasing participation of the patient in the treatment process—all this calls for the modern physician being, first of all, well grounded in the basic medical sciences. The physician of the future will, by applying biochemical, biophysical and biological tests, and by making use of computers, obtain such extensive information about his patient, that he must be well prepared to handle and interpret such information. This too will be possible only if the physician has mastered the basic medical sciences.

The treatment of patients today is also a complex procedure. The versatility of methods of treatment, increasing number of drugs powerfully acting on the human system and the need of the application of various devices and apparatus in treatment creates the necessity of constant supplementation of knowledge in this respect.

The increasingly high standards of society and complicated conditions of life give rise to situations in which the physician must be prepared to solve many problems of contemporary life. To accomplish this, he must be knowledgeable in many fields, a number of which are not strictly medical. It is impossible today during the basic studies to teach mathematics, statistics, economics, psychology, and sociology, besides physics and chemistry, to the extent required by the physician. In practice, each branch of medicine makes use of these sciences, which however, cannot be adequately taught during the undergraduate studies. Their importance to the medical profession is increasing, however, especially to the physician when he comes into contact with the problems of life.

In these circumstances the possibility of independent supplementation of professional knowledge becomes very difficult, and in effect imperfect. Postgraduate education should be organised in view of this, and directed by an institution especially established for this purpose. It is not enough to be a good specialist in order to organise and conduct the postgraduate education of health service workers with higher education. It is necessary to be specially predisposed to this task, specially prepared for it and have a centre only for this purpose. The complete fulfilment of the task of conducting postgraduate education requires constant watching of the character and trends of development of medical sciences in the world, and the level of professional work of particular medical groups in the country, in order to be able promptly and widely to introduce new achievements of science into daily medical practice. Naturally, this task cannot be correctly performed spontaneously by doctors, but can only be carried out by an appropriately organised institution.

The diversity and extensive scope of the medical discipline renders the solution of this problem impossible without assuming the need of postgraduate studies. In his book "The Aims of Education", Whitehead has admirably stated that the study of medicine is a long one and consists of three stages: the stage of emotional and romantic approaches to a new field of learning, the stage of making sharp and precise acquaintanceship with new facts, and finally the stage of generalisation and synthesis.

Therefore not only progress of the sciences calls for organised postgraduate education, but also the need for prompt and efficient introduction of this progress to everyday life. National interest therefore requires that postgraduate education should he organised and coordinated.

How to deal with settling down properly and conducting the organisation of postgraduate medical education in a country is a complex and difficult problem.

This question has been and still is discussed in almost all countries of the world and up to now there are lot of differences of opinion in that respect. The reason the opinions are so differentiated are obvious, if one realises that much depends on the basic conditions in which different nations are living. To name a few of them I would enumerate the following important factors:

academic traditions

the traditions of the local doctor's societies

the economic state of the country

the kind of system of National Health Care

the number of medical schools and their territorial locations in the country

the number of doctors who whould be trained, load of work they have and their location inside the country.

Every organisation of education and its functional mechanism has to take into consideration all the above-mentioned factors.

In the above-mentioned circumstances and conditions the idea of forming a postgraduate medical education system should take into consideration some basic principles.

These basic principles of postgraduate medical education should acknowledge:

that such an education must be based on the local tradition of the country

that in the process of teaching, doctors who have didactic experience being teachers in academic schools, should primarily be engaged

that it should be conducted in the normal work condition of doctors in their professional environment. Only small parts of the training programme should be conducted in the lecture rooms

that is should be adjusted to the individual requirements of each doctor and should simultaneously satisfy the requirements of the national health care system.

These conditions are particularly important for the proper arrangement of the programme of postgraduate medical training. One could say that in strategic goals of training we should satisfy primarily the requirements of the national health care system, but on the tactical level of programming the training we should consider the requirements of particular doctors.

In conclusion we should observe the idea that postgraduate medical education should be primarily organised for the national health care system of the country where the individual requirements of each doctor should be satisfied as a result of his personal effort during the self-education process. Requirements for both of these aims of postgraduate medical education should be constantly examined, and training itself adequately suggested, organised, supported and aided.

In principles of postgraduate medical education the organisational process of self-education is quantitatively more important but methodologically more difficult. The programme of postgraduate medical education aiming at improving the level and efficiency of the national health care system should give better immediate results.

It is obvious that both the basic objectives of postgraduate medical education have to be very closely correlated and conditioned.

So far as organisation of the institution conducting the postgraduate medical education is concerned, one has to stress that it should be a logical consequence of the above-mentioned factors.

Broadly speaking, one may expect that smaller countries or smaller communities do not require big institutional forms for that purpose, but bigger countries having a number of medical faculties, a large number of doctors and other health workers require a more firm institutional organisation. Such an institution which leads the postgraduate medical education in the country should, of course, closely cooperate with all medical faculties and medical societies of that country.

The institution of a postgraduate education *should have an academic character*. Once it gets an administrative character only it loses its position and stops being of any value for the development of postgraduate medical education.

A national academy of postgraduate medical education has been proposed as far back as the years 1958 (2) and 1961 (1).

Passing to more concrete formulations, it may be assumed that to achieve high standards in medicine it is necessary to go through the following three stages:

— assimilation of the basic knowledge and experiments,
— specialisation,
— reflection and summing up of experience, and mastering the skills or related specialities. It is at this stage that every physician feels the need of integration of the medical disciplines.

These stages characterise the steps which lead to the full development of the physician, and illustrate the true character of the study of medicine. They are also significant for the effectiveness of the social health service. Obviously, the study of medicine consists of the continuous acquisition of professional experience, which alone imparts to medicine its true sense and leads to the expected benefits.

From this point of view, it must be concluded that full medical development can be achieved only after passing through all three stages that is, after many years of practising the profession.

To summarise it has to be stated that the need of increased training is superimposed by:

— intensive development of biology, chemistry and physics,
— introduction to medical practice of complex apparatus and technical methods,
— complexity and interdependence of the living conditions of modern society and increasingly higher intellectual levels which face the doctor with ever higher requirements,
— the cost of modern medicine and its socialisation place on the doctor the daily responsibility of handling large sums of money.

All these matters cannot be wholly included in the programme of undergraduate education, both on account of the necessary time limit and the fact that a young man, before he has obtained his diploma, is not able to grasp many problems accurately and realise them correctly. For in this sphere a certain amount of experience is absolutely necessary.

There arose therefore the necessity for the continuation of studies after a doctor has taken up his professional duties, and the concept of postgraduate education became a reality.

It appears from the above that medical studies are an entity which only for didactic and scientific purposes must be divided into pre- and postgraduate studies.

In these circumstances it is apparent that between these two stages of studies there is no clear essential division but there is a complete organisational, methodical and didactic difference.

Providing and consolidating suitable organisational and formal conditions for postgraduate medical education will make possible moving definite sections or problems from one stage of medical studies to another, which in effect may improve these studies and perhaps also shorten them. The present stiff requirements of undergraduate studies and their bursting programmes are consequences of the fact that postgraduate studies have not yet been essentially acknowledged and are not organisationally stabilised to the degree in which ages long tradition and experience established the role and importance of undergraduate studies.

Despite the ages long tradition and experience of higher education, the problems of the organisation of this education as well as the methods applied in it, is the subject of constant discussion and gradual change.

The development of sciences, increased requirements of the society and the complexity of modern life mean that everyone today is obliged to learn more and more over longer periods of time. As a result of this the programme of education can no longer be confined in formerly accepted periods of time. There arose a conception of continuous (permanent) learning, lasting in some spheres through the whole period of professional activity. Medical sciences belong to those spheres in which the need of constant learning is very clearly marked.

Continuous (constant, permanent) teaching cannot naturally be conducted according to classic school organisation and school methods, since this would make professional work impossible. In view of this continuous learning must be divided into two quite different forms:

1. In-service continuing education or departmental (hospital) education.
2. Nation-wide (widespread) continuing education or institutional continuing education.

The first form includes principally everyday professional work, the second, nation-wide organised postgraduate studies.

Continuing medical education should take place on all levels of the medical hierarchy, therefore of:

— family doctors (health centres),
— doctors of specialised outpatient clinics,
— doctors and paramedical personnel of preventive medicine units (public health),
— hospital doctors,
— consultants.

The goal of continuing medical education is to maintain and improve the competence of physicians. Feasible and acceptable methods to determine competence in practice do not exist. The distinction between *competence* and *performance* is also not easily made. Some define competence as the possession of the potential (knowledge, skills and attitudes) to perform adequately over time. Such a potential can be examined in its several components, at any given point in a career. Performance is the sustained expression of that competence (3). Traditionally, lifelong learning has been a trademark of the medical profession and physicians are apt to be well read on any new development in their field, even though they may not immediately incorporate the new developments in their practice. The concept of continuing medical education is itself complex. The words "continuing" and "medical" each carry very definite implications, if not always clear operational definitions. Continuing Medical Education in fact, is not a program, it is an idea, a synonym for a physician's lifelong learning. There is consensus, however, that motivation, workload, supportive personnel and facilities, integrity, mental and emotional health, clinical judgement, data gathering and assessment skills and communication skills are more apt to figure in quality of care deficits than knowledge.

It would be less than realistic to believe that a general practitioner or a specialist could competently practice for a lifetime with the knowledge and skills acquired during formal undergraduate and graduate education. The continuing expansion of medical knowledge and technology makes continuing medical education essential if the physician is to maintain or improve the quality of care delivered to his patients.

Because of its "continuing" aspect and its intensely personal attributes, continuing medical education requires a highly heuristic form of education as contrasted with the more didactic mode characterstic of the classroom. Therein lies a major problem, since the dominant organisation of undergraduate and graduate education has a predominantly didactic orientation. The didactic deals primarily with the acquisition of cognitive and motor skills, which are capable of relatively simple objective expression and measurement. The heuristic implies a strong attitudinal component with an evolving adjustment of the "curriculum" by the learner based upon his own perception of his needs. It is a serious error to transfer the values of the didactic mode to an educational sphere which is heuristic by its very nature.

In the absence of national goal definitions, it is very difficult to discuss continuing medical education holistically, since there are no reference points of common previous agreement. There is constant confusion about both the physician-learners and the educational principles involved (3).

The programme of continuing medical education should meet the requirements of each individual doctor. From the perspective of the competent physician, certification programs are insignificant. From the point of view of the public interest in quality of care or control of the incompetent physician, certification programs are inadequate.

In terms of the physician-learners, or audience, one may be talking about either the medical profession at large, or the profession as part of a greater health profession, of subsets of the medical profession arranges along disciplinary or geographic boundaries, or of the individual practitioner himself. The discussion is entirely different depending upon this variant.

In terms of education goals, there is confusion between ultimate and more immediate goals, the former having to do with issues of performance, and the latter being more directly related to the programmatic educational process itself. The issues of quality control are different from those of continuing education. Confusion of these issues, which eventually places a recredentialing value on continuing medical education credits, can only frustrate the larger educational purposes of continuing medical education (3).

Because a postgraduate teaching institution is not in a position to get such information, careful study of the general development of medical science and evidence of doctor's practical activities should be the guiding lights for forming a programme of continuing medical education.

So the programme of continuing medical education requires high skill and knowledge both of the possibilities of academic activities and of the level and efficiency of the national health care system.

Methods of postgraduate education are varied and open to discussion. There is a lack in the whole world of uniform opinions in this respect. The general tendency is to withdraw from school forms and teaching methods.

Postgraduate training must have traits of individual education, and therefore cannot resemble school teaching. The realisation of such education requires methodical aid, up-to-date cooperation of specialist pedagogues and financial means. Training of a doctor in his place of work may be both individual and collective. Individual training must be a basic form of eduction. Collective teaching, on the other hand, is an economic necessity, when the problems dealt with in individual training must be presented to a large group of doctors in conditions or places as required by the subject concerned.

The doctor's training in his place of work (in-service training) should be based on the following estimations:

— assessment of organisation and methods of his work and on this basis giving him organisational-methodical indications,
— assessing the professional qualifications of the doctor and accordingly working out for him a programme of education,
— assessing the results of the doctor's work, determining accordingly the need of, and the frequency and type of professional consultations needed for the individual doctor of for a group of them.

On the basis of these evaluations, individual talks and discussions prepared and supplemented with educational aids should systematically take place.

For it must be accepted that the basic form of medical postgraduate education should be *self-education*.

Depending on the professional position of the doctor and the concrete purpose of his training, this self-education should be confronted either with the progress of science, or with the efficacy of his daily activity. In practice both of these aspects must always be considered in postgraduate education. Well prepared seminars and practical work with patients are considered the best forms and methods. Equal partnership in the didactic process of the teacher and the learner is accepted today as compulsory in postgraduate education. It requires on the part of teachers a thorough essential and organisational preparation. Therefore postgraduate training is for them a very time-consuming occupation.

Institutional (nation-wide) postgraduate medical education may be organised in different ways. In this activity universities, colleges and societies could be and should be involved. But having such different institutions involved there is usually a lack of continuity of policies and responsibility for continuing teaching activity. There is also a lack of teachers who require special training to teach the programme of postgraduate medical education. To overcome these difficulties the best solution would be to have a separate institution specialising in postgraduate medical education and responsible for its performance.

Teaching courses in nation-wide programmes of postgraduate education should be short as a rule, since their aim should only be to provide a possibility for exchange of experiences and confrontation of acquired knowledge. The process itself of acquiring information should take place before the course. Courses should be organised when the constant presence of the learners is absolutely necessary or when they come for training from distant localities.

The enforcing of obligatory postgraduate education provides the possibility of realising the best forms and methods of training without interfering with the doctors' professional work. Such a situation reduces greatly the number of courses increasing at the same time as the number of learning doctors. This circumstance should be fully taken advantage of. It necessitates the working out of an appropriate system of education. It seems that the best would be a system, in which it would be possible constantly to up-date and to discuss with the doctors the observed shortcomings and achievements respectively. The importance of performed tasks and the responsibility for the manner of conducting postgraduate education is very great. Both the doctors teaching and those learning must be active participants of transformations which occur in the manner of fulfilling the tasks of national health care, as well as adapting the teaching forms and methods to the developing new technical possibilities and changing social conditions.

Some of these problems depend wholly on health care workers and some to a large extent on society's attitude, on its understanding of the natural and socio-economic possibilities of medical activity.

The complexity of educational tasks, its universality, the fact that doctors should not be disturbed in their professional occupations, and the fact that doctors as people with high social positions have no predisposition to take a passive part in collective lectures, results in the tendency of postgraduate education to establish *directed and aided self-education*. The realisation of such education is a complex task and the difficulties concern both the teachers and the learners.

For the teacher must work out his subject in such a way as to make it sufficiently attractive and adequate to the needs of the learning doctors. In transmitting his knowledge the teacher must apply such methods as would meet the requirements—intellectual, psychic and professional—of the learner.

In view of the various possibilities of the learner, the teacher should work out his lecture (subject) in as many variants as there are types of personality in the learners, depending on their individual intellectual, psychic and professional level. It may probably be assumed that there are similar personalities and as a result it may be theoretically assumed that a particular lecture may be presented in three of five various ways suitable for the particular personalities, that in effect will meet the requirements of the whole community of learners. This is a theory of probability of qualitative classification which could practically be realised only by way of empiric procedures, constantly controlled. There arises therefore a reversible activity which means that the teacher must simultaneously evaluate the result of training, analyse the influence of educational methods on this result, and in consequence change the manner of conducting his teaching.

The learner, on the other hand, must have the possibility of choosing a method of education (manner of instruction), which will suit his socio-professional conditions. No one can determine in advance which method of instruction will meet the requirements of a particular learner in view of non-cognisance of the personality of the learner as to his intellectual and professional level. Also the learner will not be able to determine the optimum for his system of instruction, not knowing the methods of the teacher. So there remains on this part also the need of empirical determination of appropriate teaching methods.

In effect it means that at present we have no definitely worked out theories of didactic methods suitable for medical postgraduate education and that in this respect we must use empirical methods. This manner of teaching and learning may be realised with the aid of the oldest organisation, that is the team—one learner—one teacher—or else with the aid of technical means (radio, television) presenting the same lecture in different ways. Then the recipients of the lecture will absorb the information which will best suit their purpose.

Each lecture, seminar and conference should form an important pillar in the whole process of postgraduate education. That is why each form of postgraduate medical study should be fully studied and carefully prepared by the academicians and professional representatives and doctors attending the studies should participate actively in it.

Postgraduate medical education is being developed in all countries of the world. Almost all countries develop their own system of postgraduate education, because this section of education is closely connected with the culture, customs and traditions of every country and must be adapted to its economic level and its system of health care.

Postgraduate medical education is an important academic activity aiming to satisfy the needs of growing sciences and the growing demands of society. The variety of courses and topics presented during the year may give an impression of lack of unity and continuity of the whole process of postgraduate medical education. But if one looks at doctors' life-long work and their responsibility to keep abreast of the constant development of science and professional skill then one may better understand the complexity of the development of these studies. Postgraduate medical studies should be judged by the efficiency and level of existing national health care.

These briefly formulated opinions point to the fact that we feel the trend of the evolution of postgraduate medical education, but at the present stage cannot yet put it fully into practice.

References

1. Darley W., Cain, As.: A proposal for a national academy of continuing medical education. J. Med. Educ. *33*, 33—37 (1961).
2. Ruzyllo, E.: Necessity of Modern Approach to Postgraduate Medical Education (in Polish). Med. Studia Podyplom. *2*, 6—11 (1958).
3. Gonnella, J. S., Storey, P. B.: Continuing Medical Education and Clinical Conference: A Matrix Approach to a Complex Problem. Jefferson Medical College (Original paper not available).

Dr. Edward Ruzyllo